Clinical Dilemmas in

Viral Liver Disease

EDITED BY

Graham R. Foster, PhD, FRCP

Professor of Hepatology
Queen Mary's University of London
Blizard Institute of Cell and Molecular Science
The Liver Unit
London, UK

K. Rajender Reddy, MD, FACP, FACG, FRCP

Professor of Medicine
Professor of Medicine in Surgery
Director of Hepatology
Medical Director of Liver Transplantation
University of Pennsylvania
Philadelphia, PA, USA

 **WILEY-BLACKWELL**

A John Wiley & Sons, Ltd., Publication

Blackwell Publishing was acquired by John Wiley & Sons in February 2007. Blackwell's publishing program has been merged with Wiley's global Scientific, Technical and Medical business to form Wiley-Blackwell.

Registered office: John Wiley & Sons Ltd, The Atrium, Southern Gate, Chichester, West Sussex, PO19 8SQ, UK

Editorial offices: 9600 Garsington Road, Oxford, OX4 2DQ, UK

The Atrium, Southern Gate, Chichester, West Sussex, PO19 8SQ, UK

111 River Street, Hoboken, NJ 07030-5774, USA

For details of our global editorial offices, for customer services and for information about how to apply for permission to reuse the copyright material in this book please see our website at www.wiley.com/wiley-blackwell

Library of Congress Cataloging-in-Publication Data
Clinical dilemmas in viral liver disease / edited by Graham R. Foster, K. Rajender Reddy.
p. ; cm.
Includes bibliographical references and index.
ISBN 978-1-4051-7905-8
1. Hepatitis, Viral.   I. Foster, Graham   II. Reddy, K. Rajender.
[DNLM: 1. Hepatitis, Viral, Human–diagnosis.   2. Hepatitis, Viral, Human–therapy.   3. Diagnostic Techniques, Digestive System.   4. Hepatitis, Chronic–diagnosis.   5. Hepatitis, Chronic–therapy.   6. Liver Cirrhosis–diagnosis. 7. Liver Cirrhosis–therapy. WC 536 C641 2010]
RC848.H43C65 2010
616.3′623–dc22

2009046373

ISBN: 9781405179058

A catalogue record for this book is available from the British Library.

Set in 8.75/12pt Minion by Graphicraft Limited, Hong Kong
Printed and bound in Singapore by Fabulous Printers Pte Ltd

1   2010

Contents

Contributors

Nezam H. Afdhal, MD
Associate Professor of Medicine
Harvard Medical School
Beth Israel Deaconess Medical Center
Boston, MA, USA

William Alazawi, MA, PhD, MRCP
Barts and The London School of Medicine
London, UK

Alfredo Alberti, MD
Venetian Institute of Molecular
    Medicine (VIMM);
Department of Histology, Microbiology and
    Medical Biotechnologies
University of Padova
Padova, Italy

Mohsin Ali, MD
Thomas Jefferson University
Philadelphia, PA, USA

Angelo Andriulli
Head
Division of Gastroenterology
Hospital Casa Sollievo della Sofferenza
IRCCS
San Giovanni Rotondo, Italy

**Quentin M. Anstee, BSc,
MB BS, PhD, MRCP**
Clinical Lecturer in Medicine & Hepatology
Department of Hepatology &
    Gastroenterology
St Mary's Hospital Campus
Imperial College London
London, UK

Brenda Appolo, MS, PA-C
Division of Gastroenterology
Hospital of the University of Pennsylvania
Philadelphia, PA, USA

Tarik Asselah, MD, PhD
Service d'Hépatologie
Hôpital Beaujon
University of Paris
Clichy, France

Ranjeeta Bahirwani, MD
Fellow Gastroenterology
Research/Gastroenterology Sections
Philadelphia Veterans Administration
    Medical Center;
Division of Gastroenterology
Department of Medicine
University of Pennsylvania School of Medicine
Philadelphia, PA, USA

Pierre Bedossa, MD, PhD
Professor and Head
Department of Pathology
Hôpital Beaujon
Université Paris Diderot
Paris, France

**A. Mithat Bozdayı,
MD, PhD**
Professor of Molecular Biology and
    Biochemistry
Deputy Director
Hepatology Institute
University of Ankara
Ankara, Turkey

Hakan Bozkaya, MD
Professor of Gastroenterology
Department of Gastroenterology
University of Ankara Medical School
Ankara, Turkey

**William F. Carman, MBBCh,
MMed, PhD, FRCPath**
Director, West of Scotland Specialist
    Virology Centre

Gartnavel General Hospital
Glasgow, UK

Grace M. Chee, PhamD
Hepatology Department
Cedars-Sinai Medical Center
Los Angeles, CA, USA

Antonio Craxì, MD
Professor of Internal Medicine
    and Gastroenterology
University of Palermo
Palermo, Italy

Olav Dalgard, MD, PhD
Medical Department
Oslo University Hospital
Rikshospitalet
Oslo, Norway

Janet Dearden, MRCP
Hepatology Fellow
Department of Hepatology
The Royal London Hospital
London, UK

Guohong Deng, PhD
Associate Professor
Department of Infectious Diseases
Southwest Hospital
Third Military Medical University
Chonqqing, China

Paul Desmond, MB, BS, FRACP
Gastroenterology Department
St Vincent's Hospital
Fitzroy, Victoria, Australia

Douglas T. Dieterich, MD
Professor of Medicine
Division of Liver Diseases
Mount Sinai School of Medicine
New York, NY, USA

Rosa Di Stefano, BSc
Department of Hygiene and Microbiology
University of Palermo
Palermo, Italy

Geoff M. Dusheiko,
MB BCh, FCP(SA), FRCP,
FRCP (Edin)
UCL Centre for Hepatology and Royal Free
Hospital
London, UK

Yasser El sherif,
MBBch, MSc, MRCP
National Liver Institute
Menoufia University
Menoufia, Egypt

Alexander Evans, MB, BS
Institute of Hepatology
University College London
London, UK

Gregory T. Everson, MD
Professor of Medicine
Director of Hepatology
University of Colorado Denver
Aurora, CO, USA

Fabrizio Fabrizi, MD
Staff Physician
Division of Nephrology
Maggiore Hospital
IRCCS Foundation
Milano, Italy, and
Division of Hepatology
School of Medicine
University of Miami
Miami, FL, USA

Harald Farnik, MD
Department of Medicine
Division of Gastroenterology, Hepatology
and Endocrinology
Frankfurt University Hospital
Frankfurt am Main, Germany

Peter Ferenci, MD
Professor of Medicine
Department of Internal Medicine III
Division of Gastroenterology and Hepatology
Medical University of Vienna
Vienna, Austria

Steven L. Flamm, MD
Professor of Medicine and Surgery
Medical Director, Liver Transplantation

Department of Internal Medicine
Northwestern Feinberg School of Medicine
Chicago, IL, USA

Chris Helen Ford, MB ChB,
MRCP, FRCGP
Clinical Lead SMMGP and GP
Lonsdale Medical Centre
London, UK

Kimberly A. Forde, MD, MHS
Instructor of Medicine
Division of Gastroenterology
University of Pennsylvania
Philadelphia, PA, USA

Lisa M. Forman, MD, MSCE
Assistant Professor of Medicine
Gastroenterology and Hepatology Division
University of Colorado Denver
Aurora, CO, USA

Daniel M. Forton, PhD, FRCP
Consultant Hepatologist and Senior Lecturer
St Georges' University of London
London, UK

Brett E. Fortune, MD
Fellow, Gastroenterology and Hepatology
University of Colorado Denver
Aurora, CO, USA

Graham R. Foster, FRCP, PhD
Professor of Hepatology
Queen Mary's University of London
Blizard Institute of Cell and Molecular Science
The Liver Unit
London, UK

Alyson N. Fox, MD
Fellow, Gastroenterology
Hospital of the University of Pennsylvania
Division of Gastroenterology
Philadelphia, PA, USA

Dennis A. Freshwater,
MB BS, MD, MRCP(UK)
Consultant Hepatologist
The Liver and Hepatobiliary Unit
Queen Elizabeth Hospital
Birmingham, UK

Michael W. Fried, MD
Professor of Medicine
Director of Hepatology
Division of Gastroenterology and
Hepatology
University of North Carolina at Chapel Hill
Chapel Hill, NC, USA

Markus Gess, MRCP
Specialist Registrar in Gastroenterology and
Hepatology
Department of Gastroenterology and
Hepatology
St George's Hospital and Medical School
London, UK

Jenny Heathcote, MD, FRCPC
Professor of Medicine
Division of Gastroenterology
Toronto Western Hospital
University Health Network
University of Toronto
Toronto, Ontario, Canada

Ramazan Idilman, MD
Professor of Medicine
Ankara University Faculty of Medicine
Department of Gastroenterology
Ankara, Turkey

Ira M. Jacobson, MD
Professor of Medicine
New York Presbyterian Hospital – Weill
Cornell Medical Center
Division of Gastroenterology and Hepatology
New York, NY, USA

Maureen M. Jonas, MD
Senior Associate in Medicine
Children's Hospital Boston;
Associate Professor of Pediatrics
Harvard Medical School
Boston, MA, USA

David E. Kaplan, MD, MSc
Gastroenterology Staff Physician
Research/Gastroenterology Sections
Philadelphia Veterans Affairs Medical Center;
Assistant Professor of Medicine
Gastroenterology Division
Department of Medicine
University of Pennsylvania School of Medicine
Philadelphia, PA, USA

Banu W. Kaya,
BM, BS, BSc, MRCP, MRCPath
Consultant Haematologist
Barts and The London NHS Trust
London, UK

Ronald L. Koretz, MD
Emeritus Professor of Clinical Medicine
David Geffen-UCLA School of Medicine
Los Angeles, CA, USA;
Division of Gastroenterology
Olive View-UCLA Medical Center
Sylmar, CA USA

Kris V. Kowdley, MD, FACP
Director, Center for Liver Disease
Digestive Disease Institute
Virginia Mason Medical Center
Seattle, WA, USA

Olivier Lada, PhD
Service d'Hépatologie
Hôpital Beaujon
University of Paris
Clichy, France

Michelle Lai, MD, MPH
Beth Israel Deaconess Medical
    Center
Boston, MA, USA

Stephen Locarnini,
MBBS, BSc (Hon), PhD, FRC (Path)
Head, Research and Molecular
    Development
Victorian Infectious Diseases Reference
    Laboratory
North Melbourne, Victoria, Australia;
Director, WHO Collaborating Centre for
    Virus Reference and Research
Melbourne, Australia

Bryan D. Maliken, BA
Benaroya Research Institute and Center for
    Liver Disease
Digestive Disease Institute
Virginia Mason Medical Center
Seattle, WA, USA

Alessandra Mangia
Liver Unit
Division of Gastroenterology
Hospital Casa Sollievo della Sofferenza
IRCCS
San Giovanni Rotondo, Italy

Patrick Marcellin, MD
Professor of Medicine
Service d'Hépatologie
Hôpital Beaujon
University of Paris
Clichy, France

Richard Marley, PhD, FRCP
Consultant Hepatologist
Department of Hepatology
The Royal London Hospital
London, UK

Jorge A. Marrero, MD
Professor of Medicine
Division of Gastroenterology

University of Michigan
Ann Arbor, MI, USA

Paul Martin, MD
Professor of Medicine
Director, Division of Hepatology
School of Medicine
University of Miami
Miami, FL, USA

Steven Masson,
MB ChB, MRCP
Specialist Registrar in Hepatology
Department of Hepatology
The Royal London Hospital
London, UK

Rami Moucari, MD
Service d'Hépatologie
Hôpital Beaujon
University of Paris
Clichy, France

David J. Mutimer, MB BS, MD,
FRACP, FRCP
Reader in Hepatology and Honorary
    Consultant Hepatologist
The Liver and Hepatobiliary Unit
Queen Elizabeth Hospital
Birmingham, UK

Tin Nguyen, MBBS(Hons)
Gastroenterology Department
St Vincent's Hospital
Fitzroy, Victoria, Australia;
Victorian Infectious Diseases
    Reference Laboratory
North Melbourne, Victoria, Australia

Venessa Pattullo, MB BS,
FRACP
Division of Gastroenterology
University Health Network
Toronto Western Hospital
University of Toronto
Toronto, Ontario, Canada;
Faculty of Medicine
University of Sydney at Westmead
    Hospital
Sydney, Australia

Valeria Piazzolla
Liver Unit
Division of Gastroenterology
Hospital Casa Sollievo della
    Sofferenza
IRCCS
San Giovanni Rotondo, Italy

Fred Poordad, MD
Associate Professor of Medicine
David Geffen School of Medicine at
    UCLA
Chief, Hepatology and Liver
    Transplantation
Cedars-Sinai Medical Center
Los Angeles, CA, USA

Kaiser Raja, MD
Division of Liver Diseases
Mount Sinai School of Medicine
New York, NY, USA

K. Rajender Reddy, MD, FACP,
FACG, FRCP
Professor of Medicine
Professor of Medicine in Surgery
Director of Hepatology
Medical Director of Liver Transplantation
University of Pennsylvania
Philadelphia, PA, USA

William Rosenberg,
MA, MBBS, DPhil, FRCP
Professor of Hepatology
The Centre for Hepatology
University College London
London, UK

Vinod K. Rustgi, MD
Clinical Professor of Medicine and Surgery
Georgetown University Medical Center
Fairfax, Virginia, VA, USA

Christoph Sarrazin, MD
Professor of Medicine
Division of Gastroenterology, Hepatology,
    and Endocrinology
J.W. Goethe-University Hospital
Frankfurt am Main, Germany

Giada Sebastiani, MD
Department of Digestive Diseases,
    Hepatology and Clinical Nutrition
Dell'Angelo Hospital
Venice, Italy;
Venetian Institute of Molecular Medicine
    (VIMM)
Padova, Italy

Pari Shah, MD
Fellow Gastroenterology
Division of Gastroenterology
Department of Medicine
University of Pennsylvania
Philadelphia, PA, USA

M. Shadab Siddiqui, MD
Division of Hepatology
Department of Medicine
Northwestern Feinberg School of
 Medicine
Chicago, IL, USA

Amit G. Singal, MD
Division of Gastroenterology
Department of Internal Medicine
University of Michigan
Ann Arbor, MI, USA

Belinda C. Smith,
MBBS, MD, FRACP
Consultant Hepatologist
St Mary's Hospital Campus
Imperial College
London, UK

Mark Sulkowski, MD
Associate Professor of Medicine
Department of Medicine
Divisions of Infectious Diseases and
 Gastroenterology/Hepatology;
Medical Director, Viral Hepatitis
 Center
Johns Hopkins University School
 of Medicine
Baltimore, MD, USA

Simon D. Taylor-Robinson,
MD, FRCP
Professor of Translational
 Medicine
Liver and Antiviral Unit
Department of Medicine
Faculty of Medicine
Imperial College London

St Mary's Hospital Campus
London, UK

Paul Telfer, MA, DM, FRCP,
FRCPath
Senior Lecturer in Haematology
Barts and The London School of
 Medicine and Dentistry;
Honorary Consultant Haematologist
Barts and The London NHS
 Trust
London, UK

Howard C. Thomas, PhD, FRCP,
FRCPath, FMedSci
Professor of Medicine
Head of Department of Hepatology and
 Gastroenterology
Division of Medicine
Imperial College London
St Mary's Hospital Campus
London, UK

Mark R. Thursz, MD, FRCP
Professor of Hepatology
Imperial College
St Mary's Hospital
London, UK

Tram T. Tran, MD
Associate Professor of Medicine
Geffen UCLA School of Medicine;
Medical Director, Liver Transplant
Cedars Sinai Medical Center
Los Angeles, CA, USA

Kelly C. Vranas, MD
Resident Physician
Department of Internal Medicine

Hospital of the University of
 Pennsylvania
Philadelphia, PA, USA

Hank S. Wang, MD
Fellow, Gastroenterology
Geffen UCLA School of Medicine
Los Angeles, CA, USA

Ilan S. Weisberg, MD, MS
Fellow, Gastroenterology
New York Presbyterian Hospital – Weill
 Cornell Medical Center
Division of Gastroenterology and
 Hepatology
New York, NY, USA

Eleri S.W. Wilson-Davies,
MB BS, MSc
Specialty Registrar
West of Scotland Specialist Virology
 Centre
Gartnavel General Hospital
Glasgow UK

Cihan Yurdaydın, MD
Professor
Department of Gastroenterology
University of Ankara Medical School
Ankara, Turkey

Stefan Zeuzem, MD
Professor of Medicine
Director of the Department of
 Medicine
Division of Gastroenterology, Hepatology
 and Endocrinology
Frankfurt University Hospital
Frankfurt am Main, Germany

Preface

Viral hepatitis is a global problem of enormous magnitude and the consequences of chronic liver disease due to hepatitis B virus (HBV) and hepatitis C virus (HCV) have significant economic implications. Globally, approximately 170 million people are estimated to be infected with HCV and another 350–400 million with HBV. Chronic hepatitis and cirrhosis evolve to a varying degree and the propensity to devolop cirrhosis and its consequences is variable and depends on several factors. Suffice to say that with HBV infection, approximately 15–40% develop cirrhosis, liver failure or hepatocellular carcinoma, whereas HCV infection generally requires two to three decades to evolve into cirrhosis and its consequences, albeit in 20–30% of patients over this time period. The leading predisposing cause for hepatocellular carcinoma in the Western world is HCV cirrhosis, with an annual incidence of approximately 1–1.5%, while HBV regardless of the presence of cirrhosis is the leading cause in areas where this infection is endemic.

Although hepatitis, perhaps manifesting as jaundice, has been recognized for over 2000 years, dating back to several centuries BC, the advances made over the past few decades have been fundamental to the proper classification of viral hepatitis. Ingenious molecular biology techniques have led to the identification of HCV. Diagnostic assays, including viral molecular assays, are reliable in the diagnosis of these hepatitis virus infections and, further, help in monitoring therapeutic response. Screening, diagnosis and therapeutic algorithms and recommendations have been made by experts from various parts of the world but these are inevitably based on the highly selected populations that participate in seminal clinical studies. Many patients present with complications or characteristics that have not been adequately researched and evidence-based medicine cannot be applied. In these controversial areas there is considerable debate about the most appropriate management. This book, *Clinical Dilemmas in Viral Liver Diseases*, has been compiled to address these controversial understudied questions that arise in our day-to-day practice while dealing with patients with viral hepatitis. This is not intended to be an exhaustive review of a specific topic but to be a focused approach, supported by literature and expert opinion, looking at the controversial questions and topics where there is divergence of opinion. We have assembled a number of globally recognized investigators and clinicians to address these issues in viral hepatitis B and C. Readers will find the issues tackled to be unique and not readily accessed in standard textbooks. The style is simple and has key learning points. This book was assembled in a few months, making the material up to date in this rapidly moving area that frequently has new developments. We believe the reader will have a rewarding experience while going through the various sections.

Graham R. Foster, FRCP, PhD
K. Rajender Reddy, MD, FACP, FACG, FRCP

PART I
Investigating the Liver

1 Non-invasive markers of liver fibrosis: useful or useless?

Pierre Bedossa

Department of Pathology, Hôpital Beaujon, Université Paris-Diderot, Paris, France

---

LEARNING POINTS

- Liver biopsy enables accurate evaluation of stage of fibrosis using semi-quantitative scoring systems, including both architectural disturbance and evaluation of fibrous deposition.

- Non-invasive markers of fibrosis are useful for screening for cirrhosis but not sufficiently accurate for staging fibrosis.

- Liver fibrosis is only one facet of chronic viral hepatitis, which needs to be interpreted in its full histological context.

Introduction

Liver fibrosis is a non-specific tissue response to chronic inflammation related to an unresolved tissue injury. In the liver, cirrhosis, the end-point of fibrosis, is the major cause of morbidity and mortality in chronic liver diseases [1]. Therefore, assessment of the degree of fibrosis (stage) is often a prerequisite for the management and follow-up of patients with chronic liver disease. Because fibrosis is tissue damage, biopsy is, by definition, the only direct, albeit invasive, tool that assesses fibrosis whereas non-invasive methods (either serum markers or physical and/or imaging techniques) are surrogate indirect approaches. In this chapter, the strengths and weaknesses of non-invasive markers and liver biopsy are reviewed and their respective roles in management of patients with chronic viral hepatitis discussed.

Clinical Dilemmas in Viral Liver Disease, 1st edition. Edited by Graham R. Foster and K. Rajender Reddy. © 2010 Blackwell Publishing.

Non-invasive markers

The main alternative to liver biopsy is based on two very different methods, serum markers and liver stiffness. These have substantially different underlying principles, but both have an obvious advantage: they are non-invasive. Although they generate a significant cost and are not universally available, non-invasive markers are easy to use and well adapted to mass screening and, with some adequate precautions, can be considered highly reproducible procedures.

Stiffness, as assessed by ultrasound (Fibroscan) and more recently by magnetic resonance imaging (MRI), evaluates the velocity of propagation of a shock wave within the liver tissue. This method measures a physical parameter of liver tissue that is related to its elasticity. The rationale is that normal liver is viscous and not favourable to wave propagation, whereas fibrosis increases the hardness of the tissue and favours more rapid wave propagation. The main drawback is that additional space-occupying lesions within the liver, such as steatosis, oedema and inflammation, develop within an organ wrapped in a distensible but non-elastic envelope (Glisson's capsule). This contributes to modification of liver texture and acts as a confounding factor where stiffness is concerned (see ref. 2 for review). Nevertheless, the results of large studies evaluating several thousands of patients confirm that elasticity parallels the state of fibrosis at pre-cirrhotic or cirrhotic stages. A recent meta-analysis of Fibroscan has shown that the area under the receiver operating curve (AUROC) is very highly correlated with the presence of cirrhosis [3]. However, it is noteworthy that this approach is essentially valid for the diagnosis of cirrhosis but is not adequate for assessing milder fibrosis or transition from one stage to a higher one. Finally, a potential additional advantage of Fibroscan is that it provides a wide range of stiffness values within the broad group of cirrhotic livers, which would overcome one of the major limitations of biopsy (i.e. one histological stage for all types of cirrhosis) and thus could provide additional prognostic value within this group.

Serum markers represent combinations of blood constituents that are optimized to mirror the histological stage of liver fibrosis. Several markers are available, with some only obtainable commercially (for review see ref. 4). Despite the wide number of proposed combinations, they are all designed in the same way: a predefined choice of blood parameters is combined and optimized in order to match as closely as possible the histological stages of fibrosis in a group of patients undergoing both liver biopsy and serum marker measurement. This is fundamentally different from Fibroscan. While Fibroscan assesses a genuine characteristic of liver tissue (i.e. stiffness), the serum marker algorithm is designed to mimic biopsy results irrespective of biopsy accuracy. Therefore, any limitation of the biopsy procedure (e.g. sampling variation) will decrease the functionality of serum marker measurement. Nevertheless, the most widely tested serum marker has demonstrated acceptable accuracy in the differential diagnosis of significant and non-significant fibrosis [5].

Surrogate markers have been set up and tested to dicholomize between significant vs. non-significant fibrosis. This is imposed by the use of AUROC, which tests a binary hypothesis. Using this approach there is significant loss of information. In most studies these limitations have been artificially bypassed by considering the different histological stages as linear variables and extrapolating intermediate values for each of the stages. However, this is an erroneous supposition since scores are categories not continuous variables. Such an approximation explains why, when considering only adjacent stages (F1 vs. F2, or F2 vs. F3), AUROC values are unacceptably low, leading to the supposition that these surrogates are inadequate tools for individual staging [6].

Liver biopsy

Liver biopsy has been considered the gold standard for the evaluation of tissue damage including fibrosis. However, the well-recognized limitations involved in this procedure have fuelled discussion on the position of liver biopsy in the management of patients with chronic viral hepatitis.

The main drawbacks of liver biopsy are sampling and observation errors. These errors are specific to biopsy and theoretically should be eliminated when using serum marker measurements. Because liver biopsy involves only a very tiny part of the whole organ, there is a risk that the area biopsied might be irrelevant for evaluation of any lesion in the whole liver due to heterogeneity in its distribution. Extensive literature has shown that increasing the length of liver biopsy decreases the risk of sampling error [7,8]. Except for cirrhosis, for which microfragments may be sufficient, a 25-mm biopsy is considered an optimal specimen for accurate evaluation, although 15 mm is considered sufficient in most studies.

Observer variation is another potential limitation of biopsy, related to the discordance between pathologists in biopsy interpretation. The use of histopathological scoring systems for evaluation of fibrosis and necroinflammation has limited this drawback and several studies have shown that concordance between pathologists is considered satisfactory, especially when staging of fibrosis is performed by specialized liver pathologists [9]. Thus, although liver biopsy has its limitations, appropriate precautions may reduce the flaws inherent to this method.

Because liver biopsy is invasive, the only serious limitations to its use are potential adverse effects and complications, which have been comprehensively reviewed in several studies [10]. Transient and moderate pain, along with anxiety and discomfort, are common. Severe complications such as haemoperitoneum, biliary peritonitis and pneumothorax are rare (0.3–0.5%). Death is exceedingly rare, but has been occasionally reported for biopsies in advanced liver disease and haemorrhagic tumours and in patients with major comorbidities. A biopsy via the transjugular route greatly reduces the risk of bleeding in patients with advanced liver disease and coagulation disorders. Performance of biopsy by a trained physician, use of only a limited number of passes and ultrasound guidance can significantly decrease the risk of complications, thereby enhancing the safety of biopsy. Nevertheless, liver biopsy should be performed only after carefully balancing the risks of the procedure with the potential benefits in terms of patient management. Overlooking these limitations, liver biopsy provides invaluable information that none of the non-invasive markers provide. Because of their accuracy, standardized scoring systems for evaluation of fibrosis (staging) have proven to be relevant for describing the natural history of chronic liver diseases by assessing the rate of progression of disease.

Although strongly favoured as a major decision criterion for hepatologists, fibrosis is only one of many elementary histopathological features present simultaneously on liver biopsy. Indeed, fibrosis is not an autonomous feature but rather scar tissue resulting from other pathobiological mechanisms such as inflammatory, degenerative or dystrophic processes. Simultaneous evaluation of necroinflammation (portal tract inflammation, interface hepatitis, lobular inflammation) enables an assessment about whether fibrosis is the result of a past event that has stabilized or even regressed, or is an ongoing process that may continue to worsen. Biopsy also frequently detects associated lesions such as steatosis, steatohepatitis and iron overload, providing useful information for patient management and prognosis.

Finally, it is noteworthy that in diseases with a high burden like hepatitis C, liver biopsy may also reveal that abnormal liver function tests are related to another unexpected and additional liver disease. Clearly, all this information may influence patient management. Therefore, equating chronic liver disease only with the extent of fibrosis is an oversimplification that may be misleading.

Markers of non-invasive fibrosis: useful or useless?

Based on the evaluation of non-invasive markers in several thousands of patients, it appears that surrogate markers are useful methods for assessing significant fibrosis or cirrhosis but are useless for individual follow-up or in the case of associated comorbidities (often discovered when reading the biopsy). This suggests that surrogate markers alone should be used when there is no disagreement about the indications for treatment, for example patients with relatively recent onset hepatitis C virus (genotype 2 or 3) who will always be treated or patients where treatment is mandatory for other reasons such as severe extrahepatic manifestations. In addition, patients with contraindications to antiviral drugs should not undergo liver biopsy on first evaluation. In these situations, a simple evaluation of significant versus non-significant fibrosis with one or several non-invasive markers seems sufficient, although biopsy should be performed if any abnormal symptom or atypical evolution occurs. Similarly, biopsy is not mandatory in patients with obvious cirrhosis, where the excellent performance of non-invasive markers allows confirmation of the diagnosis.

When there is disagreement about whether or not to treat a patient, then biopsy comes first. This encompasses all patients with hepatitis B virus and hepatitis C virus (genotype 1). Because antiviral drugs are far from completely efficacious and have significant adverse effects, an accurate evaluation of liver lesions with biopsy is needed. The level of accuracy provided by liver biopsy is particularly important in this context, where staging is often used to endorse the decision to treat a patient with antiviral therapy or to screen and prevent complications such as portal hypertension and hepatocellular carcinoma. Such evaluation will rely on biopsy since non-invasive markers can confidently diagnose only cirrhosis, a stage where antiviral treatments are less effective and the chances of cure are lower.

There is an urgent need to pursue the development of surrogate markers for staging fibrosis. Because of the conditional relationship with biopsy, the development of serum markers will always have limitations. Hopefully, physical imaging will eventually be refined to an acceptable level of accuracy, especially for evaluation of early stages of fibrosis. In the future these considerations might become invalid as antiviral treatment evolves towards much efficient drugs with fewer side effects.

References

1. Khan MH, Farrell GC, Byth K et al. Which patients with hepatitis C develop liver complications? *Hepatology* 2000;31: 513–520.
2. Rockey D. Noninvasive assessment of liver fibrosis and portal hypertension with transient elastography. *Gastroenterology* 2008;134:8–14. **Review of elastography in advanced fibrosis.** ⚷
3. Friedrich-Rust M, Ong MF, Martens S et al. Performance of transient elastography for the staging of liver fibrosis: a meta-analysis. *Gastroenterology* 2008;134:960–974.
4. Manning DS, Afdhal NH. Diagnosis and quantitation of fibrosis. *Gastroenterology* 2008;134:1670–1681.
5. Poynard T, Morra R, Halfon P et al. Meta-analyses of FibroTest diagnostic value in chronic liver disease. *BMC Gastroenterology* 2007;7:40. **Review of one of the leading serological markers of liver fibrosis.** ⚷
6. Lambert J, Halfon P, Penaranda G et al. How to measure the diagnostic accuracy of noninvasive liver fibrosis indices: the area under the ROC curve revisited. *Clinical Chemistry* 2008;54:1372–1378.
7. Regev A, Berho M, Jeffers LJ et al. Sampling error and intraobserver variation in liver biopsy in patients with chronic HCV infection. *American Journal of Gastroenterology* 2002;97:2614–2618.
8. Bedossa P, Dargère D, Paradis V. Sampling variability of liver fibrosis in chronic hepatitis C. *Hepatology* 2003;38:1449–1457.
9. Rousselet MC, Michalak S, Dupre F et al. Sources of variability in histological scoring of chronic viral hepatitis. *Hepatology* 2005;41:257–264.
10. Cadranel JF, Rufat P, Degos F. Practices of liver biopsy in France: results of a prospective nationwide survey. For the Group of Epidemiology of the French Association for the Study of the Liver (AFEF). *Hepatology* 2000;32:477–481.

2 Liver biopsy in hepatitis C patients with easy-to-treat characteristics: should we bother or just do biomarkers?

Michelle Lai, Nezam Afdhal

Beth Israel Deaconess Medical Center, Boston, Massachusetts, USA

LEARNING POINTS

- The utility of routine liver biopsy in chronic HCV is debated.

- Biomarkers are excellent alternatives to liver biopsy in HCV patients with easy-to-treat characteristics.

- HCV patients with easy-to-treat characteristics are defined as those with genotype 2 or 3 or with three or more of the following characteristics: Caucasian or Asian race, pretreatment viral load < 250 000 IU/mL, fibrosis stage 0–3, BMI < 30, no insulin resistance, age < 40 years, and female.

- The two indications for liver biopsy in chronic HCV patients with easy-to-treat characteristics are (i) determination of the stage of fibrosis in cases where the treatment course is undecided and biomarker values are indeterminate and (ii) determination of the presence of concomitant diseases and the degree to which these conditions contribute to the liver disease.

Liver biopsy and hepatitis C: role, indications and limitations

Hepatitis C virus (HCV) infection is the most common chronic blood-borne infection in the USA, with approximately 3.2 million persons chronically infected [1]. Of chronically infected persons, 60–70% develop chronic liver disease. While most patients undergo liver biopsy prior to treatment of chronic HCV infection, the utility of routine biopsy continues to be debated. A survey conducted in

Clinical Dilemmas in Viral Liver Disease, 1st edition. Edited by Graham R. Foster and K. Rajender Reddy. © 2010 Blackwell Publishing.

2004 asked 61 expert hepatologists whether they would recommend a liver biopsy in 12 clinical scenarios of chronic HCV [2]. The survey found great divergence of management opinion, with most of the experts recommending liver biopsy in four to eight of the 12 clinical scenarios.

Liver histology is useful for determining the stage and prediction prognosis of the disease. Patients with cirrhosis, for example, should undergo screening for hepatocellular carcinoma according to the American Association for the Study of Liver Diseases (AASLD) guidelines and upper endoscopy every 2 years to evaluate for varices. When considering a difficult treatment with toxic side effects, the stage of disease and the chance of success of treatment are both very important factors to consider. Advanced fibrosis and a high chance of success both provide impetus to treat, whereas minimal fibrosis and a low chance of success tip the decision scales the other way.

Once treatment has started, the threshold for discontinuing therapy may be relatively high in patients who have advanced histological features. In addition to staging, a liver biopsy is also useful in establishing the presence of concomitant diseases, such as iron overload or fatty liver disease, and the degree to which these conditions contribute to the liver disease.

The limitations of liver biopsy include cost, its invasive nature with the accompanying risk of complications, and sampling error. Minor biopsy complications such as pain occur in up to 30% of patients, with more severe complications like bleeding or perforated viscus occurring in 0.3% and mortality rates approaching 0.01% [3]. The third and perhaps most important limitation of liver biopsy is its significant sampling error. Bedossa *et al.* [4] examined the sampling variability of liver biopsy in chronic HCV. Image analysis of liver biopsies showed a coefficient of variation of 55% for 15-mm biopsies and 45% for 25-mm biopsies. Using the Metavir scoring system, the variation improved to 35% and 25% for the respective biopsy sizes. Poynard *et al.* [5] found that only 13.8% of 537 liver biopsies performed at an experienced medical centre were greater than 25 mm. In addition to the issues with biopsy size, there is also variablity in sampling that can lead to incorrect staging of disease. A study compared percutaneous biopsy with laparoscopic biopsy and demonstrated that cirrhosis was missed in almost 30% of cases by percutaneous biopsy [6]. The potential for error in staging disease can be as high as 35% and even cirrhosis can be missed in 30% of patients. These findings reflect the heterogeneity of liver disease in HCV, the small sampling size of biopsy (1 in 25 000 to 1 in 50 000 of the liver) and interobserver variability in interpreting biopsy results. Because of the many limitations of liver biopsy, there has been ongoing research to seek better alternatives.

Biomarkers in hepatitis C

Commercially available serological biomarkers in the USA include FibroSure, FibroSpect and Hepascore. These biomarkers and others are available to varying degrees in other parts of the world as well. They consist of combinations of several blood and clinical parameters that are optimized to reflect the stage of liver fibrosis. While all these tests have demonstrated acceptable accuracy in differentiating early from advanced disease [7–9], they lack sensitivity for quantifying the amount of fibrosis and monitoring fibrosis progression and regression. For this reason, biomarkers are excellent alternatives to liver biopsy for patients in whom we need to determine whether or not cirrhosis is present. Therefore, they are valid approaches for assessing for significant fibrosis or cirrhosis in the following HCV patient groups: (i) patients who will always be treated (e.g. those with easy-to-treat characteristics), (ii) those with obvious cirrhosis, and (iii) those with absolute contraindications to treatment. The role of these biomarkers is more limited for patients in whom more detailed information on exact stage of fibrosis is necessary for management of disease. Besides the commercially available serological markers mentioned above, a large number of other serological markers and elastography have been evaluated for the assessment of liver fibrosis. The strengths and limitations of these non-invasive markers are all similar in that they are excellent for evaluating the presence or absence of significant fibrosis, but lack sensitivity for quantifying the amount of fibrosis [10].

Patients with easy-to-treat characteristics in hepatitis C

What are easy-to-treat characteristics?

For each patient it is important to weigh the chance of a sustained virological response (i.e. cure) and the risk of disease progression against the risks of treatment. The major predictors of a sustained virological response (SVR) are HCV genotype, race or ethnic group, viral load, and degree of liver fibrosis. Multivariate analyses have identified two major predictors of SVR among all populations studied: the viral genotype and pretreatment viral load [11–13]. SVR rates were higher in patients infected with genotype non-1 (mostly genotype 2 and 3) and in those with a viral load of less than 250 000 IU/mL [13]. In the VIRAHEP-C (Viral Resistance to Antiviral Therapy of Chronic Hepatitis C) study of patients infected with HCV genotype 1, sponsored by the National Institutes of Health, black race was associated with lower rates of SVR (28%) compared with Caucasian race (52%) [14]. Other less consistently reported baseline characteristics associated with a favourable response include female gender, age less than 40 years, lower body weight (< 75 kg), the absence of insulin resistance, and the absence of bridging fibrosis or cirrhosis on liver biopsy (Table 2.1) [11,12,15].

Recommended management approach (Figure 2.1)

For the purposes of management, we define HCV patients with easy-to-treat characteristics as those with genotype 2 or 3 or with three or more of the following characteristics: Caucasian or Asian race, pretreatment viral load less than 250 000 IU/mL, fibrosis stage 0–3, body mass index (BMI) less than 30, no insulin resistance, age under 40 years, and female. In patients meeting these criteria, we recommend biomarkers to assess for advanced fibrosis prior to initiating treatment.

TABLE 2.1 Characteristics that predict response to treatment.

Characteristics	Easy to treat	Hard to treat
Genotype	2 or 3	1 or 4
Race/ethnicity	Caucasian, Asian	Black, Hispanic
Pretreatment viral load	< 250 000 IU/mL	≥ 250 000 IU/mL
Fibrosis stage	0–3	4
BMI	< 30	≥ 30
Insulin resistance	Absent	Present
Age (years)	< 40	≥ 40
Gender	Female	Male

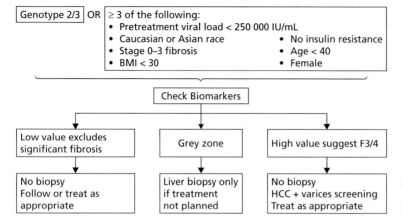

FIG. 2.1 Algorithm for HCV patients with easy-to-treat characteristics. HCC, hepatocellular carcinoma.

If the biomarkers indicate advanced disease, regular screening for hepatocellular carcinoma and varices should be initiated.

There are two indications for liver biopsy in this subgroup of HCV patients. One is to determine the stage of fibrosis in cases where the treatment course is undecided and biomarker values are indeterminate. Another indication is to establish the presence of concomitant diseases (such as haemochromatosis, alcoholic hepatitis and hepatic sarcoidosis) and the degree to which these conditions contribute to the liver disease.

References

1. Centers for Disease Control. Hepatitis C. Available at http://www.cdc.gov/hepatitis/HCV.htm.

2. Almasio PL, Niero M, Angioli D et al. Experts' opinions on the role of liver biopsy in HCV infection: a Delphi survey by the Italian Association of Hospital Gastroenterologists (AIGO). Journal of Hepatology 2005;43:381–387.

3. Cadranel JF, Rufat P, Degos F. Practices of liver biopsy in France: results of a prospective nationwide survey. For the Group of Epidemiology of the French Association for the Study of the Liver (AFEF). Hepatology 2000;32:477–481.

4. Bedossa P, Dargere D, Paradis V. Sampling variability of liver fibrosis in chronic hepatitis C. Hepatology 2003;38:1449–1457. **This key paper was important in highlighting the limitations of liver biopsy in staging liver disease.**

5. Poynard T, Munteanu M, Imbert-Bismut F et al. Prospective analysis of discordant results between biochemical markers and biopsy in patients with chronic hepatitis C. Clinical Chemistry 2004;50:1344–1355.

6. Regev A, Berho M, Jeffers LJ et al. Sampling error and intraobserver variation in liver biopsy in patients with chronic HCV infection. American Journal of Gastroenterology 2002;97:2614–2618.

7. Becker L, Salameh W, Sferruzza A et al. Validation of hepascore, compared with simple indices of fibrosis, in patients with chronic hepatitis C virus infection in United States. Clinical Gastroenterology and Hepatology 2009;7:696–701.

8. Poynard T, Morra R, Halfon P et al. Meta-analyses of Fibro Test diagnostic value in chronic liver disease. BMC Gastroenterology 2007;7:40.

9. Zaman A, Rosen HR, Ingram K, Corless CL, Oh E, Smith K. Assessment of FIBROSpect II to detect hepatic fibrosis in chronic hepatitis C patients. American Journal of Medicine 2007;120:280.e9–e14.

10. Manning DS, Afdhal NH. Diagnosis and quantitation of fibrosis. Gastroenterology 2008;134:1670–1681. **This comprehensive review of fibrosis biomarkers is important for understanding the strengths and limitations of biomarkers and their role in the evaluation of patients with chronic hepatitis C.**

11. Fried MW, Shiffman ML, Reddy KR et al. Peginterferon alfa-2a plus ribavirin for chronic hepatitis C virus infection. New England Journal of Medicine 2002;347:975–982.

12. Manns MP, McHutchison JG, Gordon SC et al. Peginterferon alfa-2b plus ribavirin compared with interferon alfa-2b plus ribavirin for initial treatment of chronic hepatitis C: a randomised trial. Lancet 2001;358:958–965.

13. Zeuzem S, Buti M, Ferenci P et al. Efficacy of 24 weeks treatment with peginterferon alfa-2b plus ribavirin in patients with chronic hepatitis C infected with genotype 1 and low pretreatment viremia. Journal of Hepatology 2006;44:97–103.

14. Conjeevaram HS, Fried MW, Jeffers LJ et al. Peginterferon and ribavirin treatment in African American and Caucasian American patients with hepatitis C genotype 1. Gastroenterology 2006;131:470–477.

15. Romero-Gomez M, Del Mar Viloria M, Andrade RJ et al. Insulin resistance impairs sustained response rate to peginterferon plus ribavirin in chronic hepatitis C patients. Gastroenterology 2005;128:636–641.

3 Screening for hepatocellular carcinoma in viral liver disease: is ultrasound enough?

Amit G. Singal, Jorge A. Marrero

Division of Gastroenterology, University of Michigan, Ann Arbor, Michigan, USA

LEARNING POINTS

- The best currently available surveillance strategy for HCC is ultrasound and AFP, although it only has a sensitivity of 70% for early-stage tumours.

- Radiological tests, such as CT or MRI, have not been adequately studied as surveillance tests or with regard to early-stage HCC.

- Serological tests, such as AFP-L3 and DCP, increase the number of false positives and do not significantly improve the sensitivity for early-stage HCC.

Cirrhosis is the most important risk factor for the development of hepatocellular carcinoma (HCC), with an annual risk of 2–7% [1]. Two large prospective studies have shown that underlying hepatitis C virus (HCV) or hepatitis B virus (HBV) are independent risk factors for HCC in these patients. HCV-associated cirrhosis is largely responsible for the increase in HCC in the USA and Europe, while HBV is the leading cause of HCC worldwide, with a particularly high prevalence in Asia and Africa [2].

Surveillance in these patients strives to detect HCC at an early stage, when it is amenable to curative therapy, in order to reduce mortality. Current American, European and Asian-Pacific guidelines recommend surveillance in high-risk individuals (i.e. patients with cirrhosis) using ultrasound with or without alpha-fetoprotein (AFP) every 6–12 months [3].

There are two types of surveillance test: serological and radiological. Ultrasound is the most widely used radiological test for HCC surveillance, although some physicians also use computed tomography (CT) or magnetic resonance imaging (MRI). The sensitivity of ultrasound for early-stage HCC (i.e. Barcelona Clinic Liver Cancer stage A) is only 63% (95% CI 49–76%), which can be improved to 70% by performing ultrasound every 6 months compared with less frequent intervals [4]. Moreover, a systematic review has shown that the level of evidence for ultrasound as a surveillance test is weak (grade C), and currently available data are limited by small sample size, variable surveillance intervals, unspecified liver disease severity, and verification bias [5]. Furthermore, ultrasonography is operator dependent and its reproducibility has never been tested so its sensitivity for HCC in less experienced centres may be even lower, further limiting its widespread utility.

Some studies have proposed that CT or MRI may be more sensitive as alternative imaging studies for the detection of HCC. A systematic review found that the sensitivity of CT for HCC at any stage was 68% (95% CI 55–80%) and the sensitivity of MRI was 81% (95% CI 70–91%) [6]. Although these numbers are encouraging, it is important to note that CT and MRI were only studied as diagnostic tests and not as surveillance tests with regard to early-stage HCC in patients with cirrhosis. Additionally, the increased cost and potential adverse effects, such as radiation exposure, limit their utility in surveillance. There is currently insufficient evidence for their use in routine clinical practice, and ultrasound should remain the radiological test of choice until further studies have been performed.

AFP is the best-studied serological test for HCC surveillance. A large randomized trial of surveillance with AFP alone versus no surveillance in China demonstrated a sensitivity and specificity for HCC of 80.0% and 80.9%, respectively [7]. Although surveillance with AFP led to a higher percentage of tumours being discovered at an early stage, there was no difference in 5-year mortality between the two

Clinical Dilemmas in Viral Liver Disease, 1st edition. Edited by Graham R. Foster and K. Rajender Reddy. © 2010 Blackwell Publishing.

arms due to ineffective treatment options at the time. This study was able to establish that AFP alone has good performance characteristics in HBV carriers. Recent systematic reviews of the literature show that the quality of other evidence supporting the use of AFP as a diagnostic and screening test for HCV-related HCC remains limited [6,8]. The included studies had significant limitations such as small sample size, lack of blinding, verification bias, and heterogeneous patient populations with varying risks of HCC [5]. Given these concerns about the validity of the underlying data, the authors could not calculate conclusive summary estimates of the sensitivity and specificity of AFP as a diagnostic test for HCC. A level of 20 ng/mL has become the most commonly used cut-off in clinical practice to trigger further evaluation,

although it is important to note that this value was determined in a study where only one-third of patients had early-stage HCC [9]. A systematic review of five studies evaluating AFP at this cut-off in patients with cirrhosis showed sensitivities ranging from 41 to 65% and specificities ranging from 80 to 94% for HCC at any stage [8]. A more recent multicentre phase 2 biomarker study showed that AFP, using a new cut-off of 10.9 ng/mL, had a sensitivity of 66% for early-stage HCC [10]. Better-quality studies, using the guidelines from the National Cancer Institute [11], are still needed to further evaluate the role of AFP in surveillance.

Other tumour biomarkers, including des-γ-carboxyprothrombin (DCP) and the *Lens culinaris*-agglutinin reactive fraction of AFP (APF-L3), have been used but there is

TABLE 3.1 Cohort studies evaluating ultrasound (US) and alpha-fetoprotein (AFP) for the detection of hepatocellular carcinoma (HCC) in patients with cirrhosis. Adapted from Singal *et al.* [16].

Study	No. of patients	Mean follow-up (months)	Surveillance method	HCC incidence (N)	Early-stage HCC (N)
Kobayashi (1985)	95	50	AFP, US, and CT	8 (8%)	6 (75%)
Sheu (1985)	223	17	AFP and US	7 (3%)	7 (100%)
Cottone (1988)	147	24	AFP and US	5 (3%)	4 (80%)
Oka (1990)	140	41	AFP and US	39 (28%)	27 (82%)
Oka (1990)	260	39	AFP and US	55 (21%)	50 (91%)
Colombo (1991)	417	33	AFP and US	26 (6%)	9 (35%)
Degos (1991)	416	68	AFP and US	60 (14%)	37 (62%)
Imberti (1993)	228	44	AFP and US	38 (17%)	14 (37%)
Cottone (1994)	147	65	AFP and US	30 (20%)	25 (83%)
Pateron (1994)	118	36	AFP, DCP, and US	14 (12%)	5 (36%)
Zoli (1996)	164	28	AFP and US	34 (21%)	32 (94%)
Bruno (1997)	163	68	AFP and US	22 (13%)	16 (73%)
Tradati (1998)	40	48	AFP and US	6 (15%)	2 (33%)
Henrion (2000)	94	34	AFP and US	6 (6%)	5 (83%)
Bolondi (2001)	313	56	AFP and US	57 (18%)	53 (87%)
Tong (2001)	173	35	AFP and US	31 (18%)	18 (58%)
Caturelli (2002)	1599	43	AFP and US	269 (17%)	253 (94%)
Iavarone (2003)	201	50	AFP and US	27 (13%)	17 (63%)
Santagostino (2003)	66	72	AFP and US	8 (12%)	2 (25%)
Velazquez (2003)	463	39	AFP and US	38 (8%)	18 (47%)
Sangiovanni (2004)	417	148	AFP and US	112 (27%)	27 (24%)
Van Thiel (2004)	100		AFP, US, and triple-phase CT	14 (14%)	13 (93%)

DCP, des-γ-carboxyprothrombin.

insufficient evidence for their use in clinical practice currently [12]. A large multicentre study recently demonstrated that AFP, at the cut-off of 10.9 ng/mL, is likely more sensitive for early-stage HCC than both of these new biomarkers. AFP-L3 had a sensitivity of 37% (95% CI 31–45%) for early-stage tumours and DCP had a sensitivity of 56% (95% CI 53–75%), whereas AFP had a sensitivity of 66% (95% CI 56–77) using the cut-off of 10.9 ng/mL [10]. Further studies are necessary to better determine the role of AFP-L3 and DCP in clinical practice, but the use of these markers for HCC surveillance is not supported with currently available evidence.

There has been considerable debate regarding the additional benefit of AFP to ultrasound during surveillance. The prospective cohort studies evaluating surveillance for HCC have shown significant variability in sample size, follow-up time, and number developing early HCC (Table 3.1). A recent meta-analysis demonstrated that the addition of AFP to ultrasound only minimally improves the sensitivity of surveillance for early-stage HCC, independent of the cut-off level used (Figure 3.1a) [4]. Although the pooled sensitivity for early-stage HCC increased from 63% with ultrasound alone to 69% with both tests, this was not statistically significant ($P = 0.65$) [4]. Despite this minimal

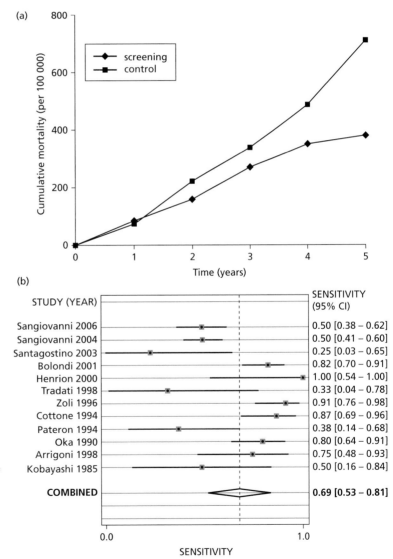

FIG. 3.1 Efficacy of surveillance ultrasound and alpha-fetoprotein (AFP) for the detection of early-stage hepatocellular carcinoma. (a) Survival curves in the large randomized trial of surveillance in chronic hepatitis B carriers. (From Zhang *et al.* [15] with kind permission of Springer Science and Business Media.) (b) Forest plot of prospective cohort studies determining sensitivity of ultrasound and AFP in the detection of early-stage hepatocellular carcinoma (From Singal *et al.* [4] with permission of Wiley-Blackwell.)

additional benefit, the combination of ultrasound and AFP at 6-month intervals remains the most cost-effective strategy [13]. In this cost-effective analysis, AFP detected some early-stage tumours missed by ultrasound and vice versa so this strategy led to the highest percentage of tumours discovered at a stage amenable to curative therapy. Furthermore, there is evidence to suggest that persistent elevations in AFP are correlated with an increased risk of HCC over time and can help identify high-risk patients [14].

The best evidence supporting the strategy of using a combination of AFP and ultrasound comes from a large randomized controlled trial in China, which demonstrated that routine surveillance is highly effective in reducing mortality in HBV carriers [15]. The surveillance arm had a 59.9% 2-year survival compared with 7.2% in patients not undergoing regular surveillance (Figure 3.1b). To date, there have not been any randomized controlled trials conducted in patients with cirrhosis. Although the benefit of surveillance with AFP and ultrasound has been demonstrated in several prospective cohort studies, it should be noted that these suffered from limitations such as verification bias, lack of adequate follow-up, lead-time bias and referral bias [4].

In theory, the best surveillance test should ideally be readily available, reproducible, accurate for early-stage disease, and cost-effective. So, is ultrasound enough for surveillance of patients at risk for HCC? The answer is no. The combination of AFP and ultrasound is the most cost-effective strategy and furthermore is the only surveillance method that has been shown to reduce mortality in a large randomized trial. AFP and ultrasound both have suboptimal sensitivities when used alone, and using the tests in combination maximizes the likelihood of finding early-stage tumours. Other tests, such as CT, MRI, AFP-L3 and DCP, have not been adequately evaluated as surveillance tests and should not be used at this time. There is an urgent need for high-quality studies to better evaluate the performance of these surveillance tests, better understand their false-positive rates, and study their reproducibility. Until that time, ultrasound with AFP at 6-month intervals remains the best surveillance strategy for those at risk for HCC.

References

1. Collier J, Sherman M. Screening for hepatocellular carcinoma. *Hepatology* 1998;27:273–278.
2. El-Serag HB, Rudolph KL. Hepatocellular carcinoma: epidemiology and molecular carcinogenesis. *Gastroenterology* 2007;132:2557–2576.
3. Bruix J, Sherman M. Management of hepatocellular carcinoma. *Hepatology* 2005;42:1208–1236.
4. Singal A, Volk ML, Waljee A *et al.* Meta analysis: surveillance with ultrasound for early stage hepatocellular carcinoma in patients with cirrhosis. *Alimentary Pharmacology and Therapeutics* 2009;30:37–47. **This meta-analysis shows that surveillance with ultrasound and AFP has a 70% sensitivity for early-stage tumours, which can be optimized by performing these tests at 6-month intervals.** ⚷
5. Gebo KA, Chander G, Jenckes MW *et al.* Screening tests for hepatocellular carcinoma in patients with chronic hepatitis C: a systematic review. *Hepatology* 2002;36(5 Suppl 1):S84–S92.
6. Colli A, Fraquelli M, Casazza G *et al.* Accuracy of ultrasonography, spiral CT, magnetic resonance, and alpha-fetoprotein in diagnosing hepatocellular carcinoma: a systematic review. *American Journal of Gastroenterology* 2006;101:513–523.
7. Chen JG, Parkin DM, Chen QG *et al.* Screening for liver cancer: results of a randomised controlled trial in Qidong, China. *Journal of Medical Screening* 2003;10:204–209.
8. Gupta S, Bent S, Kohlwes J. Test characteristics of alpha-fetoprotein for detecting hepatocellular carcinoma in patients with hepatitis C. A systematic review and critical analysis. *Annals of Internal Medicine* 2003;139:46–50.
9. Trevisani F, D'Intino PE, Morselli-Labate AM *et al.* Serum alpha-fetoprotein for diagnosis of hepatocellular carcinoma in patients with chronic liver disease: influence of HBsAg and anti-HCV status. *Journal of Hepatology* 2001;34:570–575.
10. Marrero JA, Feng Z, Wang Y *et al.* Alpha-fetoprotein, des-gamma carboxyprothrombin, and lectin-bound alpha-fetoprotein in early hepatocellular carcinoma. *Gastroenterology* 2009;137:110–118.
11. Pepe MS, Etzioni R, Feng Z *et al.* Phases of biomarker development for early detection of cancer. *Journal of the National Cancer Institute* 2001;93:1054–1061.
12. Marrero JA. Screening tests for hepatocellular carcinoma. *Clinics in Liver Disease* 2005;9:235–251, vi.
13. Thompson Coon J, Rogers G, Hewson P *et al.* Surveillance of cirrhosis for hepatocellular carcinoma: systematic review and economic analysis. *Health Technology Assessment* 2007;11:1–206.
14. Gonzalez SA, Jacobson IM. Clinical course of chronic hepatitis C in patients with very high serum alpha-fetoprotein levels and normal hepatic imaging. *American Journal of Gastroenterology* 2005;100:977–978.
15. Zhang BH, Yang BH, Tang ZY. Randomized controlled trial of screening for hepatocellular carcinoma. *Journal of Cancer Research and Clinical Oncology* 2004;130:417–422. **This randomized controlled trial showed that surveillance with ultrasound and AFP detects a higher percentage of tumours at an early stage and improves survival in chronic hepatitis B patients.** ⚷
16. Singal A, Marrero JA. Screening for hepatocellular carcinoma. *Gastroenterology and Hepatology* 2008;4(3):201–208.

4 Genomic investigations in viral hepatitis: likely to help or hinder?

Guohong Deng[1], Yasser El sherif[2], Mark R. Thursz[3]

[1]Department of Infectious Diseases, Southwest Hospital, Third Military Medical University, Chonqqing, China
[2]National Liver Institute, Menoufia University, Menoufia, Egypt
[3]Department of Hepatology and Gastroenterology, Division of Medicine, Imperial College, St Mary's Hospital, London, UK

LEARNING POINTS

- Host genetic background plays an important role in determining the outcome of viral hepatitis infections.

- A number of genetic associations have been reported but only a few are reproducible.

- Identification of disease susceptibility genes tells us a lot about the biology of these infections but has not yet been translated into clinical practice.

Introduction

Infection with the hepatitis B virus (HBV) or hepatitis C virus (HCV) may result in a number of different outcomes, ranging from asymptomatic self-limited (*acute*) infection to persistent (*chronic*) infection with liver cirrhosis, liver failure or hepatocellular carcinoma (HCC). While it has been shown that viral factors such as genotype, sub-genotype, viral variation and viral load have an important influence on the outcome of HBV and HCV infection, it is also evident that host genetic background plays a major role in determining many aspects of viral liver disease including early viral clearance, disease progression, vaccine efficacy and response to interferon. None of the genetic associations reported to date are simple Mendelian traits and they should be considered as complex traits where viral (or

Clinical Dilemmas in Viral Liver Disease, 1st edition. Edited by Graham R. Foster and K. Rajender Reddy. © 2010 Blackwell Publishing.

vaccine), environmental and host genetic variables contribute to the outcome. Furthermore, unlike simple Mendelian traits, many polymorphic genes will exert effects on the outcome, rather than one major gene. Thus we may expect the influence of any particular gene to be small and, if odds ratios are used as the measure of increased susceptibility conferred by possession of an allele, then values in the range of 1.2–2 would be expected [1].

Genetic mapping by linkage and association studies

Viral clearance/chronicity

HBV infection

Self-limiting infection with either HBV or HCV is associated with a vigorous polyclonal and multispecific CD4+ T-helper cell responses, in contrast to the weak responses seen in persistent infection. Therefore, polymorphism in the major histocompatibility complex (MHC) class II region is a potential explanation for the variation in outcome. The alleles DRB1*1301/2 are consistently associated with resistance to persistent HBV infection in sub-Saharan African, Oriental and Caucasian populations. Other alleles such as DRB1*07 and DRB1*0301 have also been associated with persistent HBV infection. DRB1*0901, DQA1*0301, DQA1*0501 and DQB1*0301 are consistently associated with persistent HBV infection in different ethnic populations [2]. Several population studies have also revealed that some non-human leucocyte antigen loci, including interferon (IFN)-γ, tumour necrosis factor (TNF)-α, vitamin D receptor (VDR), interleukin (IL)-10, estrogen receptor α (ESR1),

MHC class II transactivator (C2TA) and T-bet (TBX21), are associated with persistent HBV infection or HBV clearance [3].

Recently, in a cohort of 200 sibling pairs with persistent HBV infection from Gambia, a genome-wide scan has been conducted for susceptibility genes. The initial scan revealed linkage of markers on chromosome 21. Fine-mapping with additional markers revealed a maximum linkage located within a cluster of cytokine receptor genes. Family association studies using pedigree disequilibrium analysis revealed an IL-10 receptor B (IL10-RB) haplotype that includes the minor allele at both the IL-10RB-K47E and IFN-α receptor 2 (IFNAR2)-F8S loci, which conferred resistance to persistent HBV infection [4].

HCV infection

Several consistent associations have been observed between MHC alleles and HCV outcomes. Perhaps the most interesting and consistent finding has been the association of the human leucocyte antigen (HLA) class II allele DQB1*0301 and self-limiting HCV. In a meta-analysis of the effects of DQB1*0301 and DRB1*11 employing molecularly genotyped studies conducted among Caucasians, DQB1*0301 had a relatively strong correlation with self-limiting HCV infection [summary estimates of 3.0 (95% CI 1.8–4.8) and 2.5 (95% CI 1.7–3.7) for DQB1*0301 and DRB1*11, respectively]. Other non-HLA loci, such as IL-10, TNF-α and IFN-stimulated genes (*MxA*, *PKR* and *OAS1*), are also reported to associate with HCV clearance or persistence [2].

Disease progression

The outcome of chronic HBV infection is variable, with 80% of cases reaching a stable and relatively safe disease state with low viral loads, normal liver biochemistry and no histological evidence of necroinflammatory disease. In contrast, 20% of cases will progress to cirrhosis and HCC [5]. In chronic HCV infection the rate of disease progression varies such that probably the majority of patients will die with, rather than from, their infection [6]. The rate of disease progression varies substantially between individuals; while it is influenced by a number of demographic and environmental factors, these account for only a small proportion of the variability. Numerous case–control, candidate gene, allele-association studies have examined the relationship between host single-nucleotide polymorphisms (SNPs) or other genetic mutations and disease progression in patients with HBV or HCV infection.

HBV infection

In East Asian populations, it is consistently demonstrated that IL-10 gene promoter polymorphisms influence disease progression (acute liver failure, liver cirrhosis and HCC), mode and sequelae of HBeAg seroconversion in patients with chronic HBV infection [7]. Recently, Chong *et al.* [8] demonstrated that low-expression promoter haplotypes of *MBL* were associated with the occurrence of cirrhosis and HCC in patients with HBsAg persistence and disease progression. Deng *et al.* [9] identified a regulatory SNP, G201A, in the promoter region of *CXCL10* that was associated with susceptibility to disease progression of chronic HBV infection, while Zhai *et al.* [10] reported that estrogen receptor α gene haplotypes were associated with HBV-related HCC.

Numerous studies have demonstrated strong familial clustering of cirrhosis and liver cancer. Formal segregation analysis of HCC, performed by several groups, consistently demonstrate a sibling risk of 3.9 or higher. However, the predicted mode of inheritance varies between datasets, with some studies finding evidence of a major gene with a recessive effect and others predicting an autosomal dominant gene with incomplete penetrance [11].

HCV infection

Studies of the MHC and the progression or severity of HCV have largely been inconsistent. However, there is a trend towards an association with DRB1*11 alleles and 'less severe' liver disease. Hellier *et al.* found a protective role for CCR5-Δ32 carriage against severe fibrosis and CCR5-Δ32 homozygotes had milder portal inflammation, while Knapp *et al.* observed an association between the low-IL-10-producing genotype and haplotype with fast fibrosis progression. TNF variants have also been studied with respect to the progression of HCV-related liver disease, and the results have been inconsistent. Wright *et al.* [6] found that median fibrosis rates were higher among patients who were heterozygotes for the factor V Leiden variant, while Promrat *et al.* [12] examined six chemokine system polymorphisms and demonstrated that HCV-seropositive Caucasians with the RANTES-403A allele were less likely to have severe hepatic inflammation compared with those without. Recently, it has been reported that IFN regulatory factor 7 (*IRF-7*) polymorphisms are associated with increased risk of cirrhosis in Japanese patients with chronic hepatitis C [13].

Huang *et al.* [14] tried to identify clinically significant SNPs in 433 patients with chronic HCV infection through a low-resolution genome-wide scan (consisting of 24 823 SNPs, 68.3% coding functional SNPs, 24.9% non-coding putative regulatory SNPs, and 6.8% other types of SNPs) covering 12 248 genes and tried to validate their findings in a separate cohort of 483 patients. A missense SNP in the DEAD box polypeptide 5 gene causing an amino acid replacement at position 480 (S480A) in exon XIII was associated with an increased risk of advanced fibrosis, while a missense SNP in the carnitine palmitoyltransferase 1A gene caused an amino acid change with a decreased risk for advanced fibrosis. Seven SNPs (one in the antizyme-inhibitor-1 gene, one in the Toll-like receptor-4 gene, and five in five other genes of unclear function) with the highest predictability for cirrhosis (odds ratio 1.86–3.23) were used to build a cirrhosis risk score (CRS) signature. CRS offered a better prediction of cirrhosis compared with clinical factors (age, gender and alcohol abuse): area under the receiver operating characteristic curves 0.73–0.75 for CRS, 0.53 for clinical factors and 0.76 for CRS and clinical factors together. Two cut-off CRS values (range 0–1) were eventually suggested as potentially identifying the majority of low-risk (< 0.50) and high-risk (> 0.70) patients for development of cirrhosis.

Response to interferon therapy

HBV infection
Currently, predictive factors for responsiveness to IFN-α-based treatment include viral genotypes, baseline alanine aminotransferase level, serum HBV DNA, female gender, fibrosis on liver biopsy and pre-existing T-cell immune responses. King et al. [15] examined genes in the IFN pathway involved in antiviral and signalling activities and demonstrated that SNPs of eIF-2α and MxA affected IFN response in patients from Taiwan. Chen et al. [16] developed a new approach for identifying whole-genome short tandem repeat (STR) markers that allowed the prediction of IFN response in HBV-infected patients. The study subjects could be divided into six groups based on 11 STR markers, which correlated with IFN response rate.

HCV infection
Studies of the MHC and responsiveness to anti-HCV therapy have yielded conflicting results. Conflicting observations have also been observed with respect to CCR5-Δ32 variant and HCV therapy. Several studies have demonstrated a lack of association between TNF variants and the response to anti-HCV therapy. Hijikata et al. observed the presence of MxA −88G/G homozygotes to be lower in sustained type I

IFN responders (31%) than in non-responders (62%). These effects appeared to be independent of HCV genotype. Knapp et al. reported that the MxA gene −88G/G genotype was also correlated with non-response to IFN. A similar association was found in an independent Japanese population. The −88MxA SNP lies in a region that is highly homologous to the IFN-stimulated response element consensus sequence, with T substitution increasing the homology [2]. Persico et al. reported that SNPs of SOCS3 (suppressor of cytokine signaling 3) were positively and negatively associated with response to antiviral therapy in HCV genotype 1-infected patients. The concept of SOCS3 being involved in modulating antiviral response mechanisms is appealing, because it acts as a negative regulator of the cytokine-induced JAK/STAT pathway. Asselah et al. reported that the expression of three genes (IFI-6-16, IFI27 and ISG15) coding for IFN-inducible proteins are upregulated in non-responders to anti-HCV therapy. They further showed that a two-gene signature including one of these three genes (IFI27) predicts treatment outcome reasonably well [17]. Wada et al. [18] demonstrated that genetic polymorphisms in IFN signalling pathway-related genes were associated with IFN-induced neutropenia (10848A→G and 4757G→T) and thrombocytopenia (789G→A) in chronic HCV-infected patients.

Chen et al. [19] conducted genome-wide linkage disequilibrium screening for loci associated with genetic differences between responder and non-responder HCV patients by using 382 autosomal STR markers. They identified 19 STR markers displaying different allele frequencies between the two patient groups. In addition, based on their genomic location and biological function, the authors selected the CD81 and IL-15 genes to perform SNP genotyping. Four SNPs of the CD81 gene region and three SNPs in the IL-15 gene region showed significant association, with P-values ranging from 0.0135 to 0.0013 and from 0.0168 to 0.0034, respectively.

Recently, three independent genome-wide association studies (GWAS) identified rs12979860 (located ~3 kb upstream of IL28B) [25] and rs8099917 (located ~8 kb upstream of IL28B) [26,27] in the IL28B region as the variant most strongly associated with sustained virological response to pegylated interferon-alpha/ribavirin treatment among HCV-infected individuals of European, African and Asian ancestry. The specific causal variant(s) accounting for this effect remains to be determined, however, this seems a biologically plausible candidate for a role in HCV infection. IL28B encodes a protein also known as interferon-λ3, which is found adjacent to *IL28A* (interferon-λ2) and *IL29* (interferon-λ1) [28]. The significantly different responses to interferon-alpha/ribavirin therapy between European, African and Asian patients with HCV now seems in partly due to population differences in the frequency of the advantageous *IL28B* genotype. This exciting discovery raises the possibility of personalized therapy for HCV, and encourages a combination treatment regimen including both interferon-alpha and interferon-λ.

Vaccine efficacy

The alleles DRB1*0701 and DRBI*0301 have been associated with failure to respond to HBsAg-based vaccine, although this finding needs to be replicated in other populations [2]. Hennig *et al.* [20] analysed 715 SNPs across 133 candidate genes in 662 infant vaccinees from the Gambia, assessing peak vaccine-induced anti-HBs level and core antibody (anti-HBc) status. A replication study comprised 43 SNPs in a further 393 individuals assessing genetic determinants of HBV vaccine-induced immunity. A coding change in *ITGAL*, which plays a central role in immune cell interaction, was shown to exert beneficial effects on induction of peak antibody level in response to HBV vaccination. Variation in this gene does not appear to have been studied in relation to immune responses to viral or vaccine challenges previously. The findings suggest that genetic variation in loci other than the HLA region affect immunity induced by HBV vaccination.

Hohler *et al.* [21] aimed to assess the heritability of the HBsAg (anti-HBs) and anti-hepatitis A virus (anti-HAV) immune response and to estimate the effect of the HLA-DRB1 locus and other genetic loci unlinked to HLA. They did an open prospective study and vaccinated 202 twin pairs with a combined recombinant HBsAg/inactivated HAV vaccine. Anti-HBs and anti-HAV showed heritabilities of 0.61 and 0.36, respectively. For the anti-HBs immune response, 60% of the phenotypic variance was explained by additive genetic and 40% by non-shared environmental effects. The heritability of the HBsAg vaccine response accounted for by the DRB1* locus was estimated to be 0.25, leaving the remaining heritability of 0.36 to other gene loci. Their results demonstrate that genetic factors have a strong effect on the immune response to HBsAg. Although genes encoded within the MHC are important for this immune response, more than half the heritability is determined outside this complex. Hohler *et al.* [22] further investigated the influence of IL-10 promoter polymorphisms on anti-HBs and anti-HAV responsiveness. In the multiple regression analysis account-

ing for smoking, gender, body mass index and age, the ACC haplotype (−1082, −819 and −592) had a strong influence on anti-HBs production. Individuals carrying the ACC haplotype had anti-HBs titres almost twice as high as individuals without this haplotype. In contrast, anti-HAV production was suppressed by the presence of the −1082A allele in comparison with individuals homozygous for the −1082G allele. The contribution of the shared IL-10 promoter haplotype accounted for 27% of the genetic influence on anti-HBs antibody response.

Dilemmas and lessons

Genetic association studies are fuelled in almost every disease by the unlimited availability of SNPs, the relative ease and low price of performing genotyping assays based on polymerase chain reaction technology, and the desire to identify major disease susceptibility genes. However, genetic association studies generate enthusiasm, suspicion and even confusion among readers and reviewers. Many results have generally been unrepeatable and disappointing because of small sample size, poor study design, and diverse viral or environmental confounding factors [23]. For viral hepatitis there are a number of confounding factors that need to be taken into account when assessing genetic mapping studies.

Diversity of viral genotypes and sub-genotypes

One major problem in genetic association studies in viral hepatitis is that different genotypes and subtypes of HBV and HCV are prevalent in different ethnic populations, and parallel evolution of virus–host interactions occurs in geographically distinct areas [24]. It is not feasible to replicate genetic association results in different major ethnic groups for the same genotype or sub-genotype of hepatitis viruses because there are only one or two genotypes prevalent in most geographical regions. On the other hand, we have to collect at least twice the number of samples to maintain statistical power, if there are two or more viral genotypes in the same ethnic population.

Effect sizes for common variants are typically modest

Studies so far indicate that for the vast majority of common variants, the estimated effects are small, mostly increases in risk by a factor of 1.2–1.5 per associated allele. Furthermore, the frequency of a genetic variant is not related to the magnitude of its effect nor to the potential clinical value that may be obtained [25].

Confounding factors are heterogeneous

The age at infection and the age of disease onset are important determinants for outcome, but are difficult to identify and match. Outcome is also significantly different between male and female viral carriers. Host DNA is stable throughout life and easy to measure. However, the viral sequence varies and evolves with age and with clinical stages of disease (e.g. HBeAg/eAb seroconversion and precore/core mutation in HBV).

Links between genetic association and disease biology

Although genetic association studies show that a particular gene might be important in the pathogenesis of viral hepatitis, many of them are unable to reveal anything about the links between these associations and disease mechanisms. Gene products are subject to several levels of regulation from transcription to elaboration of final protein, which might suppress, attenuate or amplify the functional consequences of a given polymorphism [17].

Translation into clinical practice

Many genetic associations are difficult to translate into clinical and therapeutic benefit, such as association with MHC class II alleles. At present, only few results are expected to be applied in clinical practice, such as the seven-gene-signature CRS established by Celera Diagnostics, and a clinical trial of warfarin anticoagulation in patients transplanted for HCV-related diseases (arising from the genetic association study which demonstrated that the thrombophilic factor V Leiden mutation conferred susceptibility to rapid fibrosis).

Prospects for the future

The outcome and course of HBV/HCV infection are determined by a complex interplay of genetic, immunological, virological and environmental factors. The successful determination of genetic signatures for outcomes of HBV/HCV infection will require multicentre collaborations using genome-wide association studies with large, phenotypically well-defined sample sets. Although these studies will require a significant financial commitment, a successful understanding of the genetic architecture is essential not only to gain better and new insight into the mechanisms of viral hepatitis, but also to offer the potential for personalized therapy and better patient management. Additionally, genetic mapping for previously unidentified phenotypes, such as HBV/HCV-exposed uninfected individuals, HAV and hepatitis E, may open new windows onto the mechanisms of viral hepatitis. Finally, translation of genetic risks into biological mechanisms is here with us today, but translation into clinical practice for patients with HBV/HCV infection remains an aspirational goal rather than a reality.

References

1. Thursz M. Pros and cons of genetic association studies in hepatitis B. *Hepatology* 2004;40:284–286. **Review of the associations reported to date.**
2. Yee LJ, Thursz M. Hepatitis B and hepatitis C infection. In: Kaslow RA, McNicholl JM, Hill AVS, eds. *Genetic Susceptibility to Infectious Diseases*. Oxford: Oxford University Press, 2008: 318–332.
3. Deng G, Zhou G, Zhai Y *et al*. Association of estrogen receptor alpha polymorphisms with susceptibility to chronic hepatitis B virus infection. *Hepatology* 2004;40:318–326.
4. Frodsham AJ, Zhang L, Dumpis U *et al*. Class II cytokine gene cluster is a major locus for hepatitis B persistence. *Proceedings of the National Academy of Sciences USA* 2006;103:9148–9153.
5. Thursz M, Thomas HC. Pathogenesis of chronic hepatitis B. In: Thomas HC, Lemon S, Zuckerman AJ, eds. *Viral Hepatitis*, 3rd edn. Oxford: Blackwell, 2005: 308–321.
6. Wright M, Goldin R, Fabre A *et al*. Measurement and determinants of the natural history of liver fibrosis in hepatitis C virus infection: a cross sectional and longitudinal study. *Gut* 2003;52:574–579.
7. Tseng LH, Lin MT, Shau WY *et al*. Correlation of interleukin-10 gene haplotype with hepatocellular carcinoma in Taiwan. *Tissue Antigens* 2006;67:127–133.
8. Chong WP, To YF, Ip WK *et al*. Mannose-binding lectin in chronic hepatitis B virus infection. *Hepatology* 2005;42:1037–1045.
9. Deng G, Zhou G, Zhang R *et al*. Regulatory polymorphisms in the promoter of *CXCL10* gene and disease progression in male hepatitis B virus carriers. *Gastroenterology* 2008;134:716–726.
10. Zhai Y, Zhou G, Deng G *et al*. Estrogen receptor α polymorphisms associated with susceptibility to hepatocellular carcinoma in hepatitis B virus carriers. *Gastroenterology* 2006;130:2001–2006.
11. Yu MW, Chang HC, Liaw YF *et al*. Familial risk of hepatocellular carcinoma among chronic hepatitis B carriers and their relatives. *Journal of the National Cancer Institute* 2000;92:1159–1164.
12. Hellier S, Frodsham AJ, Hennig BJ *et al*. Association of genetic b variants of the chemokine receptor *CCR5* and its

ligands, *RANTES* and *MCP-2*, with outcome of HCV infection. *Hepatology* 2003;38:1468–1476.

13. Knapp S, Hennig BJ, Frodsham AJ *et al.* Interleukin-10 promoter polymorphisms and the outcome of hepatitis C virus infection. *Immunogenetics* 2003;55:362–369.

14. Promrat K, McDermott DH, Gonzalez CM *et al.* Associations of chemokine system polymorphisms with clinical outcomes and treatment responses of chronic hepatitis C. *Gastroenterology* 2003;124:352–360.

15. Papatheodoridis GV, Paraskevis D. Role of genetic polymorphisms in the progression of liver fibrosis in chronic hepatitis C virus infection. *Liver International* 2008;28:764–766.

16. Huang H, Shiffman ML, Friedman S *et al.* A 7 gene signature identifies the risk of developing cirrhosis in patients with chronic hepatitis C. *Hepatology* 2007;46:297–306.

17. King JK, Yeh SH, Lin MW *et al.* Genetic polymorphisms in interferon pathway and response to interferon treatment in hepatitis B patients: a pilot study. *Hepatology* 2002;36:1416–1424.

18. Chen PJ, Lin CGJ, Lin FY *et al.* Genetic structural differences between responders and non-responders to interferon therapy for chronic hepatitis-B patients. *Journal of Human Genetics* 2006;51:984–991.

19. Hijikata M, Ohta Y, Mishiro S. Identification of a single nucleotide polymorphism in the *MxA* genene promoter (G/T at nt −88) correlated with the response of hepatitis C patients to interferon. *Intervirology* 2000;43:124–127.

20. Knapp S, Yee LJ, Frodsham AJ *et al.* Polymorphisms in interferon-induced genes and the outcome of heptatis C virus infection: roles of *MxA*, *OAS-1* and *PKR*. *Genes Immun* 2003;4:411–419.

21. Persico M, Capasso M, Russo R *et al.* Elevated expression and polymorphisms of *SOCS3* influence patient response to antiviral therapy in chronic hepatitis C. *Gut* 2008;57:507–515.

22. Asselah T, Bieche I, Narguet S *et al.* Liver gene expression signature to predict response to pegylated interferon plus ribavirin combination therapy in patients with chronic hepatitis C. *Gut* 2008;57:516–524.

23. Wada M, Marusawa H, Yamada R *et al.* Association of genetic polymorphisms with interferon-induced haematologic adverse effects in chronic hepatitis C patients. *Journal of Viral Hepatitis* 2009;16:388–396.

24. Chen PJ, Hwang Y, Lin CG *et al.* The genetic differences with whole genome linkage disequilibrium mapping between responder and non-responder in interferon-alpha and ribavirin combined therapy for chronic hepatitis C patients. *Inter-national Journal of Immunogenetics* 2008;35:153–157.

25. Ge DL, Fellay J, Thompson AJ *et al.* Genetic variation in *IL28B* predicts hepatitis C treatment C treatment-induced viral clearance. *Nature* 2009;461:399–401. **Pivotal study identifying a novel and important polymorphism that influences response to therapy and outcome of infection in patients with chronic hepatitis C.** 🔑

26. Suppiah V, Moldovan M, Ahlenstiel G *et al.* IL28B is associated with response to chronic hepatitis C interferon- and ribavirin therapy. *Nat Genet* 2009;41:1100–1104.

27. Tanaka Y, Nishida N, Sugiyama M *et al.* Genome-wide association of *IL28B* with response to pegylated interferon-α and ribavirin therapy for chronic hepatitis C. *Nat Genet* 2009;41:1105–1109.

28. O'Brien TR. Interferon-α, interferon-λ and hepatitis C. *Nat Gene* 2009;41;1048–1050.

29. Hennig BJ, Fielding K, Broxholme J *et al.* Host genetic factors and vaccine-induced immunity to hepatitis B virus infection. *PLoS ONE* 2008;3:e1898.

30. Hohler T, Reuss E, Evers N *et al.* Differential genetic determination of immune responsiveness to hepatitis B surface antigen and to hepatitis A virus: a vaccination study in twins. *Lancet* 2002;360:991–995.

31. Hohler T, Reuss E, Freitag CM *et al.* A functional polymorphism in the IL-10 promoter influences the response after vaccination with HbsAg and hepatitis A. *Hepatology* 2005;42:72–76.

32. Jonsson JR, Purdie DM, Clouston AD *et al.* Recognition of genetic factors influencing the progression of hepatitis C: potential for personalized therapy. *Molecular Diagnosis and Therapy* 2008;12:209–218.

33. Fung SK, Lok AS. Hepatitis B virus genotypes: do they play a role in the outcome of HBV infection? *Hepatology* 2004;40:790–792.

34. Altshuler D, Daly MJ, Lander ES. Genetic mapping in human disease. *Science* 2008;322:881–888. **Overview of the strengths and weaknesses of genetic mapping studies from one of the leading groups in the field.** 🔑

35. Starkel P. Genetic factors predicting response to interferon treatment for viral hepatitis C. *Gut* 2008;57:440–442.

5 Affective and cognitive disorders in hepatitis C infection: are they real and what are the mechanisms?

Markus Gess[1], Daniel M. Forton[1], Howard C. Thomas[2], Simon D. Taylor-Robinson[3]

[1]Department of Gastroenterology and Hepatology, St George's Hospital and Medical School, London, UK
[2]Department of Hepatology and Gastroenterology, Imperial College London, London, UK
[3]Division of Medicine, Faculty of Medicine, Imperial College London, London, UK

LEARNING POINTS

- Chronic HCV infection is associated with significant impairment in quality of life.

- Cognitive dysfunction and aberrant neuroimaging using a variety of different techniques have confirmed that patients with chronic HCV have altered higher cerebral function.

- The mechanisms underlying this impairment remain unclear, although intracerebral infection and/or virus-induced cytokine release remain the most attractive models.

Introduction

Most textbooks state that chronic hepatitis C virus (HCV) infection is an asymptomatic disease. However, both general *physical complaints*, such as fatigue and musculoskeletal and right upper abdominal discomfort, and *neuropsychological complaints*, including depression, mental clouding ('brain fog') and a perceived inability to function effectively, are common and have led to a number of published reports documenting the prevalence of such symptoms and their impact on quality-of-life scales in cohorts of patients with HCV infection. Hepatic encephalopathy is the most obvious neurological consequence of chronic HCV infection in the

context of advanced liver disease. Vasculitic neurological complications of HCV-associated mixed cryoglobulinaemia are uncommon and present as a peripheral sensory or motor neuropathy, although there are sporadic case reports of cryoglobulin-related central nervous system (CNS) vasculitis. The possibility of HCV infection *itself* leading to cerebral dysfunction in the absence of a vasculitic process or advanced liver disease has been the subject of intense debate.

The presence of neuropsychological symptoms in the context of HCV infection does not imply causality, since there are many associated factors that may independently affect patients' perceptions of well-being, such as anxiety regarding diagnosis, prognosis and treatment, previous or ongoing substance abuse and associated emotional problems or personality traits [1]. In addition to epidemiological evidence linking HCV infection with neuropsychological impairment, there is emerging evidence from imaging, neuro-physiological, neuropsychological and virological studies demonstrating a biological effect of HCV on cerebral function.

Health-related quality of life, fatigue and depression

The results from several large studies challenge the perception that HCV infection is an asymptomatic disease, with general agreement that physical and mental health-related quality of life (HRQL) is significantly reduced in HCV-infected patients compared with published normative data [2]. This reduction in HRQL appears independent of the severity of the liver disease and is seen in all domains of

HRQL, including mental health. In one study, SF-36 scores were lower in patients with HCV infection compared with both healthy controls and patients with chronic hepatitis B virus (HBV) infection. These findings, together with large studies, which have shown significant improvements in HRQL in combined cohorts of many thousands of patients after successful antiviral therapy, suggests that the viral infection itself is an important determinant of reduced HRQL [3]. However, whether a biological mechanism underlies this remains controversial. Other relevant determinants of HRQL, which have been described in the literature, include medical comorbidity, the effect of the diagnosis, depression and labelling [4]. Importantly, many studies did not blind their subjects to HCV polymerase chain reaction status and the impact of diagnosis or knowledge of antiviral response is likely to affect reported HRQL.

Fatigue is often said to be the commonest symptom in patients with chronic HCV infection, affecting up to 80% of patients referred for treatment. It is an important determinant of reduced HRQL. Although improvements in fatigue have been reported after treatment [5], it appears to persist in some individuals despite a virological response. Fatigue in chronic HCV infection is a multidimensional symptom and is influenced by multiple interrelating social, behavioural, psychological and personality factors [6]. Indeed, it has been argued that because most studies have been methodologically flawed in some way and fail to take account of all confounding factors, there is no evidence of a causal association between HCV infection *per se* and fatigue [7]. It is likely that the fatigue reported by HCV-infected patients is due to multiple coexistent causes and the relative contribution of a biological mechanism remains unclear.

Depression is a common and clinically important finding in HCV-infected patients [8]. Antiviral therapy with interferon alfa may precipitate or exacerbate depression [9] and hence this symptom may limit the tolerability of treatment and reduce compliance [10]. The relationship between HCV and depression is undoubtedly complex. The greatest reservoir of HCV infection is in intravenous drug users, many of whom have clinical depression [11]. Conversely, depression may exist as a secondary phenomenon to HCV infection. This may take the form of a reactive depression, related to the diagnosis and concerns over long-term health or may be associated with symptoms such as fatigue and cognitive impairment [12].

It has become clear that objective measures of cerebral function are needed in order to elicit more precisely the nature and extent of CNS dysfunction in HCV infection. In recent years, significant advances have been made and a number of published studies have focused on cognitive function, brain metabolism and neurophysiological parameters in HCV-infected patients. There is increasing evidence of measurable biological abnormalities, which are summarized below:

Evidence for impaired cognitive function in HCV-infected individuals

Impairments in the domains of psychomotor speed, visual perception and attention are common in otherwise asymptomatic patients with cirrhosis, constituting the syndrome of minimal hepatic encephalopathy [13]. Clinical studies of cognitive function in HCV infection therefore need to exclude or control for the effect of cirrhosis. Forton *et al.* [14] used a computer-based cognitive testing battery and reported selective impairments in attention, concentration and working memory in a cohort of patients with biopsy-proven minimal HCV hepatitis attending a tertiary treatment centre. These impairments were significantly less common in a comparable group of patients who had recovered from HCV infection. The findings were independent of depression and fatigue scores and were not related to the presence or absence of a history of substance abuse. In an expanded cohort of HCV patients with mild liver disease, the same investigators demonstrated impaired cognitive testing scores in 38% of HCV-infected individuals.

Hilsabeck *et al.* [15] found evidence of mild cognitive impairment in up to 49% of HCV-infected patients with varying stages of liver fibrosis. The same group of researchers used a similar testing battery in an independent cohort of HCV-infected individuals to test the relationship between neuropsychiatric symptoms (e.g. complaints of cognitive dysfunction) and objective neuropsychological test performance. Similar rates of impairment in complex attention, concentration and working memory were reported, but no significant differences on any of the cognitive measures were found between individuals reporting high or low levels of fatigue, depression or perceived cognitive function, raising questions about the clinical significance of the measured impairments. Weissenborn *et al.* [16] addressed this issue in a study designed to determine whether patients' subjective impression of fatigue was associated with objective evidence of cerebral dysfunction; 30 HCV-infected patients with normal liver function, 15 with mild and 15 with moderate to severe fatigue on the fatigue impact scale, underwent a battery of well-validated neuropsychological tests, which again revealed deficits in attention and higher executive function. These deficits were more pronounced in the more severely fatigued patients.

The clinical significance of cognitive impairment in HCV was questioned by McAndrews et al. [17], who studied a highly selected cohort of HCV-infected patients with minimal liver disease; patients with cirrhosis, depression and substance misuse were excluded. They reported less cognitive dysfunction than in the earlier studies, detecting impaired learning efficiency in only 13% of 37 patients. Likewise, Cordoba et al. [18] showed no cognitive impairment in HCV-infected patients without cirrhosis and in those who had compensated cirrhosis. Cognitive impairment was only detected in those patients who had had previous episodes of hepatic decompensation (almost certainly explained by hepatic encephalopathy). Patients in this study were enrolled after a diagnosis of HCV infection had been made at blood donation, which means this cohort may have been positively selected for good health and is therefore probably not comparable to groups of patients recruited from hospital-based treatment centres.

Neuroimaging in chronic HCV infection

Neuroimaging has been employed in an attempt to provide an objective measure of cerebral function in HCV infection. Proton magnetic resonance spectroscopy (^{1}H-MRS) is an established imaging technique that has been used in the investigation of hepatic encephalopathy and CNS infections such as HIV. This technique gives information on brain metabolism. Forton et al. [19]. showed that HCV-infected patients with mild liver disease had significantly elevated choline to creatine ratios in the basal ganglia and frontal white matter compared to patients with chronic HBV infection and also healthy controls. These findings were unrelated to previous substance use. In a later study [20] of a similar patient cohort, the same group of researchers demonstrated elevated myoinositol/creatine ratios in the frontal white matter, which were associated with impairments in working memory.

Similarly, Weissenborn et al. [16] used ^{1}H-MRS to study 30 HCV-infected patients with normal liver function who also had cognitive testing. They found decreased N-acetylaspartate (NAA)/creatine ratios in occipital grey matter compared

with healthy controls, but no abnormalities in any other brain regions or in choline-containing compounds. There were no significant associations between the MRS data and the neuropsychological or fatigue scores. McAndrews et al. [17] studied 37 HCV-positive patients with minimal hepatitis and found elevated cerebral levels of choline and reduced levels of NAA in the central white matter, in keeping with the previous studies by Forton and Weissenborn. There was also no statistical correlation between cognitive dysfunction and cerebral metabolite ratios in this study.

Elevated myoinositol/creatine and choline/creatine ratios have been demonstrated in HIV-related minor cognitive–motor disorder and are thought to represent CNS immune activation. In early HIV disease, elevations in white matter myoinositol/creatine are the most consistently found MRS abnormalities associated with abnormal cognitive processing. The MRS data from the studies in HCV infection suggest that cerebral immune activation may also occur in this setting and may underlie some of the mild neurocognitive impairment seen in a proportion of HCV-infected patients.

This has been studied further in a study combining cerebral positron emission tomography, using a selective ligand for microglial/brain macrophage activation, $[^{11}C](R)$-PK11195, and MRS [20]. Mean PK11195 binding potential was significantly increased in the caudate nucleus of 11 patients with histologically mild HCV infection compared with controls. This was more significant in the subgroup of six patients with genotype 1 HCV infection and correlated with viral load. Again, elevations were seen in cerebral myoinositol/creatine ratios. These data provide further in vivo evidence for immune activation within the CNS as a consequence of HCV infection.

Possible underlying mechanisms

The pattern of neurocognitive dysfunction in HCV patients is consistent with the involvement of subcortical brain systems. Similar impairments have been reported in the asymptomatic stages of HIV infection. The ^{1}H-MRS findings in HCV-infected subjects are similar to those that are well documented in HIV infection, where viral infection of microglia is well established. The recent demonstration of in vivo microglial activation in HCV infection raises the question of whether this virus, like HIV, also infects the CNS.

Although the hepatocyte is the major cell for HCV replication, there is evidence of low-level replication in extrahepatic sites. Different HCV quasi-species have been detected in liver and peripheral blood monocuclear cells [21], supporting the concept of independent viral replication in different compartments. This methodology has been applied to the CNS and distinct viral quasi-species have been identified in post-mortem brain samples, suggesting that brain-specific variants of HCV may replicate within brain [22]. Furthermore, Radkowski et al. [23] detected negative-strand HCV RNA, the replicative intermediate, in post-mortem brain tissue. Most recently, negative-strand HCV RNA has been detected in microglia/macrophages derived from post-mortem brain tissue of HCV-infected patients [24]. It is therefore possible that, in certain individuals, the immune response to viral proteins within the CNS may constitute the underlying mechanism leading to cognitive dysfunction.

An alternative hypothesis is that peripherally derived cytokines may result in CNS immune activation and/or changes in neurotransmission. The therapeutic use of cytokines such as interferon alfa is associated with the induction of depressive symptoms in patients with viral hepatitis. Interferon alfa increases serum kynurenine concentrations and reduces serum serotonin and tryptophan concentrations and these changes have been shown to correlate with depression ratings. Interactions between the immune system and serotonergic neurotransmission have been demonstrated at a number of levels, both peripherally and within the CNS [25]. However, there are few data on the role of endogenous cytokines and CNS effects in chronic HCV infection.

Alterations in monoaminergic neurotransmission in patients with HCV infection have been documented using single-photon emission computed tomography: reduced serotonin and dopamine receptor binding capacity was associated with impaired performance on cognitive testing [26]. These novel findings were interpreted as implicating a role for disturbed monoaminergic neurotransmission in the pathophysiology of HCV-associated cerebral dysfunction. It is therefore conceivable that some individuals, possibly predisposed as a result of HCV neuroinvasion, may develop neuropsychological symptoms and cognitive impairment as a consequence of both central and peripheral immune activation, mediated by disturbances in serotonergic neurotransmission.

In summary, there is increasing evidence for CNS dysfunction in HCV infection which is associated with abnormal metabolism within brain structures. It is hypothesized that, as in HIV, HCV neuroinvasion may lead to the observed CNS abnormalities, even though progressive disease, as in HIV dementia, is not seen. The mechanisms which may mediate these CNS abnormalities remain unclear and need to be investigated further.

Acknowledgements

H.C.T. and S.D.T.-R. are grateful to the NIHR Biomedical Facility for infrastructure funding support and to the British Medical Research Council, the British Engineering Physics and Science Research Council (EPSRC) and the Alan Morement Foundation for funding support. We are grateful to Dr Bob Grover, Sr Mary Crossey and the late Professor Andres Blei for useful discussions.

References

1. Forton DM, Taylor-Robinson SD, Thomas HC. Reduced quality of life in hepatitis C: is it all in the head? *Journal of Hepatology* 2002;36:435–438.

2. Bonkovsky HL, Woolley JM. Reduction of health-related quality of life in chronic hepatitis C and improvement with interferon therapy. The Consensus Interferon Study Group. *Hepatology* 1999;29:264–270. **An important study showing that effective antiviral therapy for patients with chronic HCV infection is associated with an improvement in quality of life.** 🔑

3. Ware JEJ, Bayliss MS, Mannocchia M, Davis GL. Health-related quality of life in chronic hepatitis C: impact of disease and treatment response. The Interventional Therapy Group. *Hepatology* 1999;30:550–555.

4. Fontana RJ, Hussain KB, Schwartz SM, Moyer CA, Su GL, Lok AS. Emotional distress in chronic hepatitis C patients not receiving antiviral therapy. *Journal of Hepatology* 2002;36:401–407.

5. Cacoub P, Ratziu V, Myers RP et al. Impact of treatment on extra hepatic manifestations in patients with chronic hepatitis C. *Journal of Hepatology* 2002;36:812–818.

6. Obhrai J, Hall Y, Anand BS. Assessment of fatigue and psychologic disturbances in patients with hepatitis C virus infection. *Journal of Clinical Gastroenterology* 2001;32:413–417.

7. Wessely S, Pariante C. Fatigue, depression and chronic hepatitis C infection. *Psychological Medicine* 2002;32:1–10.

8. Goulding C, O'Connell P, Murray FE. Prevalence of fibromyalgia, anxiety and depression in chronic hepatitis C virus infection: relationship to RT-PCR status and mode of acquisition. *European Journal of Gastroenterology and Hepatology* 2001;13:507–511.

9. Zdilar D, Franco-Bronson K, Buchler N, Locala JA, Younossi ZM. Hepatitis C, interferon alfa, and depression. *Hepatology* 2000;31:1207–1211.

10. Kraus MR, Schafer A, Csef H, Faller H, Mork H, Scheurlen M. Compliance with therapy in patients with chronic hepatitis C: associations with psychiatric symptoms, interpersonal problems, and mode of acquisition. *Digestive Diseases and Sciences* 2001;46:2060–2065.

11. Johnson ME, Fisher DG, Fenaughty A, Theno SA. Hepatitis C virus and depression in drug users. *American Journal of Gastroenterology* 1998;93:785–789.

12. McDonald J, Jayasuriya J, Bindley P, Gonsalvez C, Gluseska S. Fatigue and psychological disorders in chronic hepatitis C. *Journal of Gastroenterology and Hepatology* 2002;17:171–176.

13. Ferenci P, Lockwood A, Mullen K, Tarter R, Weissenborn K, Blei AT. Hepatic encephalopathy: definition, nomenclature, diagnosis, and quantification: final report of the working party at the 11th World Congresses of Gastroenterology, Vienna, 1998. *Hepatology* 2002;35:716–721.

14. Forton DM, Thomas HC, Murphy CA *et al.* Hepatitis C and cognitive impairment in a cohort of patients with mild liver disease. *Hepatology* 2002;35:433–439. **One of many studies showing that there is objective impairment in cerebral processing in patients with chronic HCV infection.** 🔑

15. Hilsabeck RC, Perry W, Hassanein TI. Neuropsychological impairment in patients with chronic hepatitis C. *Hepatology* 2002;35:440–446.

16. Weissenborn K, Krause J, Bokemeyer M *et al.* Hepatitis C virus infection affects the brain: evidence from psychometric studies and magnetic resonance spectroscopy. *Journal of Hepatology* 2004;41:845–851.

17. McAndrews MP, Farcnik K, Carlen P *et al.* Prevalence and significance of neurocognitive dysfunction in hepatitis C in the absence of correlated risk factors. *Hepatology* 2005;41:801–808.

18. Cordoba J, Flavia M, Jacas C *et al.* Quality of life and cognitive function in hepatitis C at different stages of liver disease. *Journal of Hepatology* 2003;39:231–238.

19. Forton DM, Allsop JM, Main J, Foster GR, Thomas HC, Taylor-Robinson SD. Evidence for a cerebral effect of the hepatitis C virus. *Lancet* 2001;358:38–39.

20. Forton DM, Hamilton G, Allsop JM *et al.* Cerebral immune activation in chronic hepatitis C infection: a magnetic resonance spectroscopy study. *Journal of Hepatology* 2008;49:316–322.

21. Grover VPB, Pavese N, Koh SB *et al.* Evidence of neuroinflammation in patients with chronic hepatitis C: a cerebral positron emission tomography (PET) study. Poster presentation at the British Association for the Study of the Liver Annual Meeting 2007.

22. Afonso AM, Jiang J, Penin F *et al.* Nonrandom distribution of hepatitis C virus quasispecies in plasma and peripheral blood mononuclear cell subsets. *Journal of Virology* 1999;73:9213–9221.

23. Forton DM, Karayiannis P, Mahmud N, Taylor-Robinson SD, Thomas HC. Identification of unique hepatitis C virus quasispecies in the central nervous system and comparative analysis of internal translational efficiency of brain, liver and serum variants. *Journal of Virology* 2004;78:5170–5183.

24. Radkowski M, Wilkinson J, Nowicki M *et al.* Search for hepatitis C virus negative-strand RNA sequences and analysis of viral sequences in the central nervous system: evidence of replication. *Journal of Virology* 2002;76:600–608.

25. Wilkinson J, Radkowski M, Laskus T. Hepatitis C virus neuroinvasion: identification of infected cells. *Journal of Virology* 2009;83:1312–1319.

26. Forton DM. Altered monoaminergic transporter binding in hepatitis C related cerebral dysfunction: a neuroimmunological condition? *Gut* 2006;55:1535–1537.

27. Weissenborn K, Ennen JC, Bokemeyer M *et al.* Monoaminergic neurotransmission is altered in hepatitis C virus infected patients with chronic fatigue and cognitive impairment. *Gut* 2006;55:1624–1630.

PART II
Today's Therapies

Section 1: HCV

6 Acute hepatitis: treat immediately or give a chance to spontaneously clear?

Ranjeeta Bahirwani[1,2], David E. Kaplan[1,2]

[1]Research/Gastroenterology Sections, Philadelphia Veterans Administration Medical Center, Philadelphia, Pennsylvania, USA

[2]Division of Gastroenterology, Department of Medicine, University of Pennsylvania School of Medicine, Philadelphia, Pennsylvania, USA

LEARNING POINTS

- Acute HCV infection is defined as new occurrence of viraemia with conversion from HCV antibody negative to positive status.

- Symptomatic acute HCV infection occurs in only 25–30% of patients; acute HCV infection is rarely fulminant.

- Symptomatic patients have a higher chance of spontaneous viral resolution by 12–24 weeks after exposure.

- Antiviral treatment with pegylated interferon monotherapy is extremely effective in treating acute HCV infection, with sustained virological response rates over 80% when initiated within 48 weeks of infection.

- Duration of therapy is controversial; however, most authorities recommend treatment for 12–24 weeks with longer duration of treatment advised for patients with genotypes 1 and 4 or those with HCV/HIV co-infection.

Introduction

The lack of universal diagnostic criteria, the asymptomatic nature of most acute cases of hepatitis C virus (HCV) infection, and a lack of screening programmes result in the vast majority of HCV diagnoses being made when the infection is in the chronic state [1,2]. However, detection of acute HCV, often defined as HCV viraemia of shorter than 6 months'

Clinical Dilemmas in Viral Liver Disease, 1st edition. Edited by Graham R. Foster and K. Rajender Reddy. © 2010 Blackwell Publishing.

duration, affords clinicians an opportunity to intervene and prevent long-term complications of HCV infection.

The majority of HCV infection in the acute phase remains subclinical, with only 25–30% of patients presenting with symptoms [1]. An estimated 15% of all symptomatic cases of acute liver injury in the USA result from acute HCV. Acute HCV infection should be suspected in patients with (i) new-onset elevation of serum aminotransferases, (ii) documented HCV viraemia, (iii) exclusion of other causes of acute hepatitis, (iv) optimally in the setting of documented seroconversion from hepatitis C antibody (HCVAb) seronegative to seropositive status, and (v) a risk factor for exposure. However, many patients have never been previously tested for HCVAb and up to 20% do not have clearly identifiable risk factors such as parenteral drug use or high-risk sexual behaviour. Ancillary findings that may be considered for the diagnosis include the receipt of graft tissue or blood products known to be contaminated with HCV, large fluctuations of HCV RNA titres (> 1 log), and documentation of persistently normal liver-associated enzymes prior to the acute episode.

After needlestick exposures, HCV RNA can generally be detected in the serum within 1–2 weeks but clinical hepatitis does not occur until 6–8 weeks after exposure. Antibody seroconversion usually also occurs after 6–8 weeks; however, seroconversion can be delayed in immunocompromised patients. Sensitive HCV RNA polymerase chain reaction (PCR) testing should be used to confirm the diagnosis of acute HCV infection in patients with clinical suspicion who remain HCVAb-negative on initial evaluation. During the acute phase, spontaneous clearance occurs in 16–46% of patients usually by 12–16 weeks after exposure [1,2].

While in established chronic infection interferon-based antiviral therapy only cures 46–54% of patients, therapy in the acute phase has a much greater chance of success, with greater than 80% sustained virological response (SVR) rates [3]. The timing of therapy (in light of fairly high spontaneous resolution rates) and the composition and duration of therapy (standard vs. pegylated interferon, the use of ribavirin, 24 vs. 48 weeks) remain debated.

Epidemiology

A precise estimation of the incidence of acute HCV infection is difficult to determine since most acute infections remain undiagnosed and the rates of spontaneous resolution are variable. The epidemiology of acute HCV has changed over the past decade, particularly in the western world. In the USA, the incidence of acute HCV decreased from 130 per 100 000 in the 1980s to 0.2 per 100 000 in 2005, with approximately 40 000 acute HCV cases reported per year [4]. The falling incidence of acute HCV is attributed to improvements in blood donor screening, needle exchange programmes, and education among injection drug users. As a result of these efforts, other modes of transmission such as needlestick injuries and sexual and perinatal transmission have gained relative importance.

Injection drug use accounts for about 25–54% of acute HCV cases in Europe and the USA. The risk of HCV transmission via contaminated needlestick injuries is 0.3%. Acquisition of HCV infection via perinatal transmission occurs in approximately 6.5% of infants born to HCV-infected mothers. The role of sexual transmission of HCV remains controversial. In approximately 15% of individuals diagnosed with acute HCV infection, sexual transmission is the only identifiable risk factor. This is of particular concern in HIV-positive men who have sex with men, associated with traumatic sexual practices and concomitant sexually transmitted diseases. Blood transfusions from unscreened donors and unsafe therapeutic procedures remain the major modes of transmission of HCV in the developing world [5].

Clinical presentation and diagnosis

Diagnosing acute HCV with certainty can be difficult given the high proportion of asymptomatic cases as well as the absence of a reliable IgM-based serological test. However, a series of clinical features can lead to the diagnosis of acute HCV infection, including known or likely exposure to HCV during the previous 2–12 weeks, development of symptoms (particularly jaundice) in a previously healthy individual, and an acute increase in alanine aminotransferase (ALT) levels to more than 10–20 times the upper limit of normal coupled with detectable HCV RNA by PCR-based techniques. HCV-specific antibodies are detected 6–8 weeks after infection, although seroconversion may often be delayed or absent in the immunocompromised host.

Acute HCV infection is rarely fulminant (<< 1%). Symptoms occur in about 25–30% of patients with acute HCV. Flu-like symptoms, fever, jaundice, dark urine, fatigue, nausea, vomiting, anorexia and abdominal pain are commonly reported by symptomatic patients. Symptoms when present usually develop 6–8 weeks after exposure and may last for 3–12 weeks in self-limited disease, subsiding as ALT and HCV RNA titres decline. Most patients with self-limiting infection experience HCV RNA clearance within 3 months of disease onset. Detectable HCV RNA titres beyond 6 months after infection is usually associated with chronic evolution.

Spontaneous clearance

Spontaneous clearance occurs in up to one-third of patients with acute HCV infection. Although no reliable predictors of spontaneous resolution of acute HCV have been identified, several clinical features have been associated with spontaneous viral clearance. The presence of jaundice, HCV genotype 3 infection, female gender, white ethnicity, low peak viral load and a rapid decline in viral load within the first 4 weeks of diagnosis are associated with spontaneous viral clearance. Factors associated with viral persistence include co-infection with HIV or *Schistosoma mansoni*, and infection at the time of receipt of an organ transplant [6].

Cellular immune responses seem to play a crucial role in the spontaneous resolution of acute HCV infection. Clearance of HCV is associated with the development of vigorous and multispecific CD4+ and CD8+ T-cell responses in the blood and the liver that can be maintained for years following recovery from acute disease. It has been suggested that viral clearance occurs more frequently in patients with acute HCV infection whose peripheral blood mononuclear cells proliferate well and display a Th1 phenotypic profile, associated with secretion of interleukin (IL)-2 and interferon-γ, compared with those who express a Th2 phenotype (associated with secretion of IL-4 or IL-10) [7].

Treatment of acute HCV infection (Figure 6.1 and Table 6.1)

There are several factors providing a rationale for treating patients with acute HCV infection, including the high rate of chronic evolution, the lack of reliable factors to predict the outcome of acute infection, and high treatment success rates.

Large randomized controlled trials in acute HCV infection do not exist to guide therapeutic decisions. Studies in this field show considerable heterogeneity in trial design, inclusion criteria, patient characteristics, duration between exposure and treatment onset, and treatment dosages and duration.

In a sentinel study by Jaeckel *et al.* [8] assessing the outcomes of 44 patients with acute HCV treated with standard

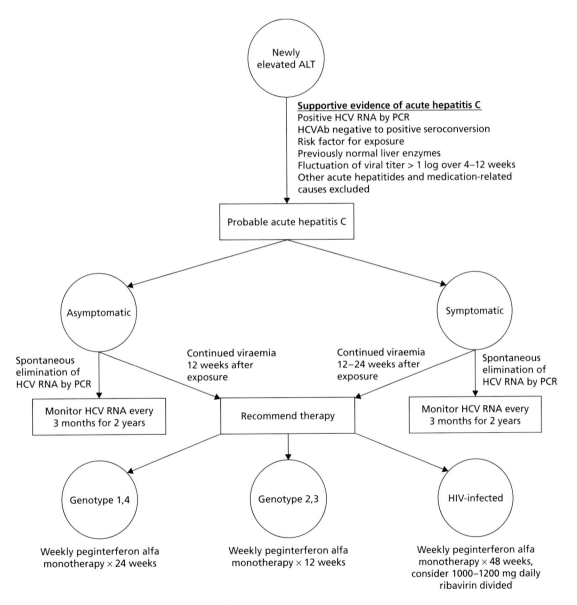

FIG. 6.1 Algorithm for treatment of acute HCV infection.

TABLE 6.1 Trials comparing therapies for acute HCV infection.

Study	Design	No. of patients	Regimen	Time to initiation of therapy	Treatment duration	SVR
Jaeckel et al. [8]	Non-randomized	44	Interferon alfa-2b 5 MU/day for 4 weeks followed by interferon alfa-2b 5 MU three times weekly	89 days from infection	24 weeks	98%
Wiegand et al. [9]	Non-randomized	89	Peginterferon alfa-2b 1.5 µg/kg	76 days after infection	24 weeks	71%
Kamal et al. [11]	Randomized controlled trial	173	Peginterferon alfa-2b 1.5 µg/kg per week	12 weeks	8 weeks 12 weeks 24 weeks	68% 82% 91%
Dominguez et al. [12]	Non-randomized	25 (HIV/HCV)	Peginterferon alfa-2a 180 µg/week and ribavirin 800 mg/day	3–24 weeks	24 weeks	71%

MU, million units.

interferon alfa monotherapy (5 million units daily for 4 weeks followed by 5 million units three times weekly for 20 weeks), 43 subjects (98%) attained SVR. In this study, the average time from infection to the start of therapy was 89 days. The effectiveness of standard interferon monotherapy has been confirmed in a number of other studies, with SVR rates between 75 and 100%. With the introduction of pegylated interferon alfa (peginterferon alfa), a preferred medication due to the once-weekly dosing schedule and lower side effects, several randomized and non-randomized studies were conducted to assess its efficacy in acute HCV. Monotherapy with peginterferon alfa-2b (1.5 µg/kg per week) for a duration of 24 weeks has been shown to result in SVR rates of 71–94%, with significant impact on outcomes related to patient adherence to therapy [9]. One randomized controlled trial reported by Kamal et al. [10] showed no benefit with the addition of ribavirin to peginterferon alfa in the acute setting.

The optimum duration of therapy remains debated, but as in chronic infection viral genotype plays a critical role. A study comparing treatment duration of 8, 12 and 24 weeks using peginterferon alfa-2b monotherapy (1.5 µg/kg per week) suggested an incremental improvement in SVR rates from 67.6 to 82.4 to 91.2%, respectively. However, all genotype 2 or 3 patients achieved SVR irrespective of treatment duration, suggesting that as few as 8 weeks of therapy

could be sufficient in these genotypes. In contrast, SVR rates for genotype 1 patients were highly influenced by duration, ranging from 38 to 60 to 88% with 8, 12 and 24 weeks of therapy, respectively. Similar findings were identified in genotype 4 patients [11]. Adherence to prescribed therapy is a strong predictor of virological response [9]. The role of measuring early viral kinetics in acute HCV infection remains unclear.

The optimal timing of treatment for acute HCV infection remains controversial. Reasonably high spontaneous resolution rates make treatment unnecessary in a significant proportion of patients with acute HCV infection, but identifying such patients early in the course remains challenging. Excessive delay in initiation (> 48 weeks) clearly reduces treatment efficacy relative to early initiation of therapy (after < 12 weeks of infection). However, there are few data regarding the efficacy of therapy initiated at time points between weeks 12 and 48. Many patients who remain viraemic at week 12, but few who remain viraemic at week 24, will nonetheless resolve without therapy. Thus, some experts in the field suggest waiting for 12–24 weeks prior to initiating antiviral therapy, especially in symptomatic cases due to higher spontaneous clearance in this subgroup. Other experts recommend immediate therapy prior to 12 weeks. The authors recommend individualizing the treatment decision based on patient preference, comorbidities and early virological trends, but initiating treatment at the latest by week 24 if spontaneous resolution has not occurred [12].

Treatment in special populations

Several studies have suggested that SVR rates in patients with acute HCV co-infected with HIV are lower than in HIV-negative patients, ranging from 59 to 71%. Higher treatment response rates have been observed in patients treated for 48 weeks versus 24 weeks. Some co-infection authorities also advocate the addition of ribavirin, at a cost of increased adverse effects (anaemia and thrombocytopenia), possible interaction with antiretroviral agents, and greater pill burden. Further studies are warranted to evaluate the efficacy and safety of acute HCV therapy in patients infected with HIV and to elucidate the optimal duration of therapy in acute HCV/HIV superinfection [13].

Summary

Acute HCV infection is an under-recognized clinical entity due to its mostly asymptomatic nature and variable rates of spontaneous resolution. Symptomatic patients are more likely to spontaneously clear the virus, although approximately 70% of patients will develop chronic HCV infection. Acute HCV infection therefore represents an important window during which therapeutic intervention is highly successful. Antiviral therapy can be delayed for at least 12 weeks, possibly up to 24 weeks, from the date of exposure or onset of symptoms to allow for spontaneous resolution. Antiviral therapy with peginterferon monotherapy (for 12–24 weeks depending on genotype) achieves SVR rates over 80% in this setting. Patient adherence with therapy remains a key determinant of response rates. In acute HCV in HIV-infected persons, 48 weeks of peginterferon plus ribavirin should be considered. Further research should be directed at optimizing cost-effective methods for improving the early detection of acute HCV infection and for preventing spread of infection in high-risk populations.

References

1. Maheshwari A, Ray S, Thuluvath P. Acute hepatitis C. *Lancet* 2008;372:321–332. **Great overview of acute HCV.** 🔑

2. Armstrong GL, Wasley A, Simard EP *et al.* The prevalence of hepatitis C virus infection in the United States, 1999 through 2002. *Annals of Internal Medicine* 2006;144:705–714.

3. Kamal S. Acute hepatitis C: a systematic review. *American Journal of Gastroenterology* 2008;103:1283–1297.

4. Page-Schafer K, Pappalardo B, Tobler L *et al.* Testing strategy to identify cases of acute hepatitis C virus (HCV) infection and to project HCV incidence rates. *Journal of Clinical Microbiology* 2008;46:499–506.

5. Low E, Vogel M, Rockstroh J *et al.* Acute hepatitis C in HIV-positive individuals. *AIDS Reviews* 2008;10:245–253.

6. Gerlach JT, Deipolder HM, Zachoval R *et al.* Acute hepatitis C: high rate of both spontaneous and treatment-induced viral clearance. *Gastroenterology* 2003;125:80–88.

7. Kaplan DE, Sugimoto K, Newton K *et al.* Discordant role of CD4 T-cell response relative to neutralizing antibody and CD8 T-cell responses in acute hepatitis C. *Gastroenterology* 2007;132:654–666.

8. Jaeckel E, Cornberg M, Wedermeyer H *et al.* Treatment of acute hepatitis C with interferon alfa-2b. *New England Journal of Medicine* 2001;345:1452–1456.

9. Weigand J, Buggisch P, Boecher W *et al.* Early monotherapy with pegylated interferon alpha-2b for acute hepatitis C infection: the HEP-NET Acute-HCV-II Study. *Hepatology* 2006;43:250–256.

10. Kamal SM, Ismail A, Graham CS *et al.* Pegylated interferon α therapy in acute hepatitis C: relation to hepatitis C virus-specific T cell response kinetics. *Hepatology* 2004;39:1721–1731.

11. Kamal S, Moustafa K, Chen H *et al.* Duration of peginterferon therapy in acute hepatitis C: a randomized trial. *Hepatology* 2006;43:923–931.

12. Craxi A, Licata A. Acute hepatitis C: in search of the optimal approach to cure. *Hepatology* 2006;43:221–224. **Great overview of acute HCV.** 🔑

13. Dominguez S, Ghosn J, Valantin MA *et al.* Efficacy of early treatment of acute hepatitis C infection with pegylated interferon and ribavarin in HIV-infected patients. *AIDS* 2006;20:1157–1161.

Management of HCV genotype 1 non-responders/relapsers: a European perspective

Harald Farnik, Stefan Zeuzem

Department of Medicine, Division of Gastroenterology, Hepatology, and Endocrinology, Frankfurt University Hospital, Frankfurt am Main, Germany

LEARNING POINTS

- A large proportion of patients with genotype 1 chronic HCV infection will not respond to current therapies.

- An accurate assessment of the reasons for treatment failure and a full understanding of the nature of the virological response is essential when considering further therapy.

- For patients who have had an inadequate course of therapy, retreatment with peginterferon and ribavirin should be strongly considered.

- For patients who had a post-treatment relapse after their first course of therapy, it may be reasonable to consider a further course of therapy with prolonged duration of peginterferon and ribavirin, perhaps for 72 weeks.

- Long-term maintenance therapy with peginterferon is of no benefit for the majority of patients, although some patient subgroups may derive some benefits from this approach.

Introduction

Chronic hepatitis C virus (HCV) is a major cause of liver cirrhosis and its sequelae. The aim of antiviral therapy is a sustained virological response (SVR), defined as undetectable HCV RNA 24 weeks after the end of therapy. Sustained elimination of HCV by antiviral therapy improves liver histology and patient outcome. However, in patients with genotype 1 chronic HCV infection undergoing therapy

Clinical Dilemmas in Viral Liver Disease, 1st edition. Edited by Graham R. Foster and K. Rajender Reddy. © 2010 Blackwell Publishing.

with the current standard of care (peginterferon alfa in combination with ribavirin), almost 50% of patients fail to achieve an SVR after antiviral therapy and options for retreatment of these patients are clearly needed.

Consistent with the decline of HCV RNA during treatment, four different patterns of treatment failure can be distinguished.

1 Non-response: $< 2 \log_{10}$ IU/mL decline in HCV RNA from baseline to treatment week 12. Null response: $< 0.5 \log_{10}$ IU/mL decline in HCV RNA at any time point.
2 Partial virological response: $\geq 2 \log_{10}$ IU/mL decline in HCV RNA from baseline to treatment week 12 with detectable HCV RNA at week 24.
3 Breakthrough: detectable HCV RNA during treatment after an initial virological response.
4 Relapse: recurrence of HCV RNA after the end of therapy in patients who achieved and maintained undetectable HCV RNA during treatment.

The exact classification of these response patterns is important when retreatment is being considered as the response to subsequent courses of therapy is influenced by the initial response.

Correctable reasons for treatment failure

When assessing a patient who does not achieve SVR during the initial course of therapy, the reason for this treatment failure should be determined. Correctable reasons for treatment failure include non-compliance, medication errors, missed opportunities to manage adverse events, or treatment that has not been continued for a sufficient period of time. Patients who have a known and correctable reason for their previous treatment failure are good candidates for retreatment with peginterferon alfa and ribavirin therapy.

If patients are true non-responders with no clear correctable reasons for treatment failure, the potential success with a further course of standard peginterferon and ribavirin retreatment is much less promising and there are a number of potential treatment options, which are discussed below.

Retreatment with peginterferon and ribavirin

In the EPIC3 study, non-responders and relapsers to previous therapy with interferon alfa ($N = 1203$) or peginterferon alfa-2a/b ($N = 820$) with or without ribavirin were retreated with peginterferon alfa-2b (1.5 µg/kg per week) and ribavirin (800–1400 mg daily) [1]. The treatment duration was 48 weeks. All patients had F2 to F4 fibrosis (Metavir). The overall rate of SVR in retreated patients was 22%. The rate was higher in prior relapsers compared with prior non-responders (38% vs. 14%) and the lowest SVR rate was observed in non-responders to prior peginterferon alfa/ribavirin combination therapy (6–7%, all HCV genotypes). An early virological response at week 12 was achieved in 35% of patients. The majority of patients with an early virological response at treatment week 12 achieved SVR (56%). The results of the EPIC3 study show that retreatment of non-responders and relapsers is an option that should be considered in patients who achieve an early virological response (see also Chapters 9 and 10 for a review of the EPIC study relating to other HCV genotypes).

Increased dose of peginterferon and/or ribavirin

A small prospective study of 10 (treatment-naive) patients with HCV genotype 1 infection and high baseline viral load (> 800 000 IU/mL) showed the feasibility of treatment with even higher doses of ribavirin without major treatment interruption [2]. Ribavirin dose was calculated from a pharmacokinetic formula based on renal clearance to achieve a steady-state ribavirin concentration above 15 µmol/mL. After dose adjustments, at week 24, the average daily ribavirin dosage was 2540 mg (range 1600–3600 mg). Following this regimen, individualized ribavirin dosing with standard peginterferon alfa-2a therapy yielded SVR in 9 of 10 patients.

However, prophylactic and as-needed administration of erythropoietin and blood transfusions were required in single patients.

A recent study by Fried et al. [3] demonstrated an improvement in SVR in genotype 1-infected patients with body weight above 85 kg treated with a higher dose of ribavirin, especially in conjunction with a higher dose of peginterferon. Patients treated with peginterferon alfa-2a 270 µg and ribavirin 1600 mg daily showed an SVR of 47% compared with 28% in patients treated with the standard dosing regimen. This improvement was driven mainly by a marked reduction in relapse in the high-dose group compared with the standard-dose group (19% vs. 40% respectively). However, the use of a higher dose regimen was associated with an increased rate of haematological adverse events.

Extended treatment duration

Intensified treatment with higher fixed-dose induction of peginterferon and/or longer treatment duration may increase SVR rates in patients with prior non-response to peginterferon alfa and ribavirin treatment. The REPEAT trial compared both strategies in prior non-responders to peginterferon alfa-2b and ribavirin [4]. Patients ($N = 942$) were randomized into four arms: those in arms A and B received peginterferon alfa-2a induction (360 µg/week) for 12 weeks followed by peginterferon alfa-2a 180 µg/week for a further 60 or 36 weeks (total duration 72 and 48 weeks, respectively); those in arms C and D received peginterferon alfa-2a 180 µg/week for 72 and 48 weeks, respectively. All patients were treated with ribavirin 1000–1200 mg/day. The overall SVR rates were 16% and 7% in the peginterferon alfa-2a induction arms for 72 and 48 weeks of therapy, respectively, and 14% and 9% in the peginterferon alfa-2a non-induction arms for 72 and 48 weeks, respectively. The SVR rate was higher for pooled 72-week arms versus pooled 48-week arms ($P = 0.0006$, odds ratio 2.22), while no difference was found between the induction and non-induction arms. The results of the REPEAT trial show that retreatment of non-responders with extended treatment duration improves SVR rates while induction therapy has no beneficial effect.

In this trial the overall early virological response (EVR) rates were 62% and 58% in the peginterferon alfa-2a induction arms for 72 and 48 weeks of therapy, respectively, and 49% and 42% in the peginterferon alfa-2a non-induction arms for 72 and 48 weeks, respectively. The corresponding SVR rates were 57% and 35% in the 72-week and 48-week arms (induction, non-induction). The SVR rates in patients without EVR were 4.5% and 4.7%, respectively [5]. Multiple logistic regression analysis indicated that EVR at week 12 consistently predicts SVR regardless of favourable or unfavourable baseline prognostic factors in non-responders to peginterferon alfa-2b/ribavirin when retreated with peginterferon alfa-2a/ribavirin [5].

Maintenance therapy with low-dose peginterferon alfa

Two large multicentre trials have evaluated the potential benefits of maintenance therapy: the COPILOT (Colchicine vs. Peginterferon alfa-2b Long-Term) study [6] and the HALT-C (Hepatitis C Antiviral Long-Term Treatment Against Cirrhosis) trial [7].

The scope of the COPILOT study was to determine the effect of treatment on 4-year survival or hepatic transplantation; variceal or portal (hypertensive) bleeding; development of jaundice, ascites, encephalopathy or hepatocellular carcinoma (HCC); and deterioration of the Child–Pugh–Turcotte score. A total of 555 patients with prior failure to interferon-based antiviral therapy were randomized to peginterferon alfa-2b (0.5 µg/kg per week) ($N = 286$) or colchicine (0.6 mg twice daily) ($N = 269$); 20% of patients showed a clinical end-point within the study period. Development of HCC was more often observed in patients on peginterferon alfa-2b ($N = 26$) than in patients on colchicine ($N = 12$). Complications of portal hypertension, above all variceal haemorrhage, were more common in the colchicine ($N = 39$) than in the peginterferon alfa-2b ($N = 26$) group. Only in patients with portal hypertension was peginterferon alfa-2b superior to colchicine with respect to event-free survival at 2 and 4 years.

The HALT-C trial was a prospective, randomized, controlled study of long-term maintenance therapy with peginterferon alfa-2a in patients with chronic HCV infection and advanced fibrosis or cirrhosis (Ishak 3–6) who did not achieve SVR after treatment with interferon alfa or interferon alfa plus ribavirin [7]. A total of 1050 patients were randomly assigned to receive either peginterferon alfa-2a 90 µg/week ($N = 517$) or no treatment ($N = 533$) for 3.5 years. By the end of the study period, after 3.5 years, there was no difference between the control and treated groups in the frequencies of study end-points, such as death, hepatic decompensation or development of HCC (33.8% vs. 34.1%, respectively) [7]. Although mean serum alanine aminotransferase and HCV RNA levels decreased significantly with treatment ($P < 0.0001$), as did necroinflammatory changes on liver biopsy ($P < 0.0001$), no significant difference was observed in rates of any of the primary outcomes between the groups. The risk for development of HCC was further evaluated in a later analysis of the HALT-C study cohort [8]. The cumulative 5-year incidence was not significantly different between treated and untreated patients (5.7% and 5.1%, respectively; $P = 0.91$). Overall the COPILOT and HALT-C trials show that long-term peginterferon alfa maintenance therapy does not reduce the rate of clinical disease progression over periods of up to 4 years.

STAT-C

Studies on the structures of key replication enzymes encoded by HCV, such as NS3/4A protease and NS5B polymerase, have enabled the development of specifically targeted antiviral therapy against HCV (STAT-C). Several compounds are currently under investigation in clinical trials and show high antiviral activity in patients with chronic HCV infection [9,10]. The development of agents in different classes may allow construction of antiviral combinations that enhance the effectiveness of antiviral treatment in current non-responder patients. Safety issues and the rapid emergence of resistant mutations in monotherapy currently limit the use of anti-HCV-specific drugs [11] (see Chapter 44 for further discussion of new drugs in development for HCV).

Conclusion

Patients with treatment failure to interferon alfa-based standard therapy can be classified into non-responders, partial responders, patients with breakthrough, and relapsers. Strategies for retreatment comprise the modification of interferon alfa and ribavirin dosage and elongation of treatment duration to improve clinical outcomes. Adherence to treatment is also an important factor for attaining SVR. Failure rates after retreatment of non-responders are high for HCV genotype 1 patients, particularly those with additional poor predictive characteristics such as high baseline viraemia or advanced fibrosis. Patients with treatment failure should be carefully assessed for correctable reasons for treatment failure such as non-compliance, medication errors, missed opportunities to manage adverse events, or treatment that has not been continued for a sufficient period of time. Patients who have a correctable reason for previous treatment failure are good candidates for retreatment with peginterferon alfa and ribavirin. For patients who do not have correctable factors that may improve the response to a second course of therapy, several trials have shown that retreatment of non-responders with peginterferon/ribavirin is associated with reasonable SVR rates, particularly when patients achieve an EVR at week 12. Retreatment of non-responders with peginterferon/ribavirin for 72 weeks is associated with higher SVR rates compared with 48 weeks' retreatment and should be considered. Long-term maintenance therapy with low-dose peginterferon does not improve the clinical outcome of patients with chronic HCV infection, although some subgroups, such as patients with portal hypertension, may benefit from long-term maintenance therapy.

References

1. Poynard T, Schiff E, Terg R *et al*. Sustained viral response is dependent on baseline characteristics in the retreatment of previous alfa interferon/ribavirin nonresponders: final results from the EPIC3 program. *Journal of Hepatology* 2008;48(Suppl 2):S369.

2. Lindahl K, Stahle L, Bruchfeld A, Schwarcz R. High-dose ribavirin in combination with standard dose peginterferon for treatment of patients with chronic hepatitis C. *Hepatology* 2005;41:275–279. **A novel approach to retreatment using very high doses of ribavirin.** 🔑

3. Fried M, Jensen D, Rodriguez-Torres M *et al*. Improved sustained virological response (SVR) rates with higher, fixed doses of peginterferon alfa-2a (40KD) (PEGASYS®) plus ribavirin (RBV) (COPEGUS®) in patients with 'difficult-to-cure' characteristics. *Hepatology* 2006;44(Suppl 1):314A.

4. Jensen DM, Freilich B, Andreone P *et al*. Pegylated interferon alfa-2a (40KD) plus ribavirin (RBV) in prior non-responders to pegylated interferon alfa-2b (12KD)/RBV: final efficacy and safety outcomes of the REPEAT study. *Hepatology* 2007;46(Suppl 1):291A.

5. Marcellin P, Freilich B, Andreone P *et al*. HCV-RNA status at week 12 of treatment with PEG-Interferon alfa 2a/RBV predicts SVR in patients with prior non-respondes to pegylated interferon alfa-2b/RBV: results from REPEAT study. *Journal of Hepatology* 2008;48(Suppl 2):S301.

6. Afdhal NH, Levine R, Brown R Jr, Freilich B, O'Brien M, Brass C. Colchicine versus PEG-Interferon alfa 2b long term therapy: results of the 4 year COPILOT trial. *Journal of Hepatology* 2008;48(Suppl 2):S4.

7. Di Bisceglie AM, Shiffman ML, Everson GT *et al*. Prolonged therapy of advanced chronic hepatitis C with low-dose peginterferon. *New England Journal of Medicine* 2008;359:2429–2441. **Data from a long-term study of maintenance therapy in patients with chronic hepatitis C.** 🔑

8. Lok AS, Seeff LB, Morgan TR, Di Bisceglie AM, Sterling RK, Curto TM. Incidence rates and risk factors associated with hepatocellular carcinoma in patients with advanced liver disease due to hepatitis C: results of the HALT-C trial. *Journal of Hepatology* 2008;48(Suppl 2):S45.

9. Forestier N, Reesink HW, Weegink CJ *et al*. Antiviral activity of telaprevir (VX-950) and peginterferon alfa-2a in patients with hepatitis C. *Hepatology* 2007;46:640–648.

10. Sarrazin C, Rouzier R, Wagner F *et al*. SCH 503034, a novel hepatitis C virus protease inhibitor, plus pegylated interferon alpha-2b for genotype 1 nonresponders. *Gastroenterology* 2007;132:1270–1278.

11. Sarrazin C, Kieffer TL, Bartels D *et al*. Dynamic hepatitis C virus genotypic and phenotypic changes in patients treated with the protease inhibitor telaprevir. *Gastroenterology* 2007;132:1767–1777.

8 HCV genotype 1: how are you managing the non-responders and relapsers? A North American perspective

Michael W. Fried

University of North Carolina at Chapel Hill, Chapel Hill, North Carolina, USA

LEARNING POINTS

- Non-sustained responses to peginterferon and ribavirin comprise a heterogeneous group of antiviral responses (non-responders and relapsers). Relapsers can be further defined by the time point at which they achieved undetectable viraemia.

- Numerous fixed and correctable factors identified during the previous course of treatment must be considered when counselling about retreatment. Patients with correctable factors, such as extreme dose reductions or discontinuation of ribavirin, may be most likely to benefit from retreatment if these issues can be better managed.

- The change in HCV RNA during a prior course of therapy has important implications for the likelihood of response to retreatment.

- Optimized dosages of ribavirin and extending duration of therapy for slow virological responders may modestly improve rates of sustained virological response during retreatment.

- Preliminary data of triple combination regimens including a direct antiviral agent, such as telaprevir or boceprevir, are promising for the treatment of prior non-sustained responders but must be confirmed in Phase III clinical trials.

Introduction

The goal of antiviral therapy for chronic hepatitis C virus (HCV) infection is sustained virological response (SVR), defined as undetectable HCV RNA in serum for at least 6

Clinical Dilemmas in Viral Liver Disease, 1st edition. Edited by Graham R. Foster and K. Rajender Reddy. © 2010 Blackwell Publishing.

months after stopping therapy [1]. Non-sustained virological response encompasses a spectrum of outcomes, including relapse and non-response. Clinicians are faced with an increasing number of patients who have been previously treated with combination antiviral therapy but who have not achieved SVR. Treatment with peginterferon and ribavirin is rigorous and is associated with numerous side effects that diminish quality of life [1]. Therefore, clinicians and patients must make an informed choice about whether to repeat a course of peginterferon and ribavirin or wait until new triple-therapy regimens become available. Thus, a concise individualized strategy for managing these patients based on currently available evidence would be helpful. As discussed below, it is especially important to keep in mind that 'those who cannot remember the past are condemned to repeat it', as stated by the philosopher George Santayana.

Manage correctable factors

Numerous host and virological factors can influence the outcomes of antiviral therapy. Fixed factors are those intrinsic to HCV, such as genotype or pretreatment level of HCV RNA, or to the patient, such as race or severity of liver disease. It is well established that genotype 1 has a lower rate of virological response than other genotypes. Similarly, African-Americans and Hispanic patients have significantly lower rates of SVR compared with Caucasian patients when treated with the same medications. Other fixed factors, such as cirrhosis, hepatic steatosis and insulin resistance, can also diminish rates of SVR. Thus, it is apparent that patients with a constellation of fixed factors that negatively impact on therapeutic outcome would be at greatest disadvantage during a second course of treatment.

Correctable factors are those that occurred during initial treatment but which may be amenable to intervention during a second course of therapy. Identifying correctable factors that may have contributed to prior treatment failure can help inform decisions about retreatment and subsequent management. Thus, detailed discussion with patients about their tolerance and adherence to previous therapy and a review of past records to identify factors that may be mitigated during subsequent treatment is warranted. Transient discontinuation of ribavirin and/or peginterferon could significantly diminish rates of SVR. The most common correctable factors and potential solutions include the following.

1 Extreme dose reductions or interruptions due to side effects such as anaemia, neutropenia or depression: close monitoring, modest dose reductions earlier during treatment, the judicious use of growth factors, and other adjunctive therapies, such as prophylactic antidepressants, could minimize dose reductions and premature discontinuation of treatment.
2 Lack of adherence to the prescribed medication regimen: patients must have realistic expectations about outcomes and potential adverse events before embarking on another course of therapy. The importance of complete adherence should be stressed and a plan for monitoring adherence developed with the patient.

Definition of non-response and relapse

Patients who remain with detectable HCV RNA throughout a course of therapy are considered to be *non-responders*. Within the non-responder category, *null responders* achieve the least reduction in HCV RNA, usually less than 1-log decrease in HCV levels, and are considered the most refractory to peginterferon and ribavirin therapy. *Partial responders* may have multiple log-fold decreases in HCV

RNA in viraemia but always have detectable viraemia in serum during treatment.

In contrast, *relapsers* are those who do achieve undetectable HCV RNA during treatment, as measured by a sensitive standardized assay, but then HCV RNA again becomes measurable in serum after the end of a prescribed treatment regimen. Relapsers can be further categorized based on the time point at which they cleared virus for the first time (Table 8.1). Rapid virological responders achieve undetectable viraemia by week 4 of treatment. These patients have the highest chance of achieving an SVR (> 90%) during the initial course of therapy [2]. Patients who achieve undetectable viraemia for the first time at week 12 have had a *complete early virological response*, whereas those whose HCV RNA decreased by at least 2-logs at this point but remained detectable are considered to have had only a *partial early virological response*. Patients with a partial early virological response who then become undetectable by week 24 are considered to have a *slow virological response* (Table 8.1).

Importance of previous antiviral response

The likelihood of SVR during subsequent courses of treatment is associated with the previous response achieved by the patient during the first course of combination therapy. Therefore, it is imperative that clinicians review past records, specifically the change in HCV viraemia, to categorize patients broadly as null responders, partial responders or relapsers and further try to determine at which week of treatment they first became undetectable, according to the definitions provided above (Table 8.1). As might be expected, previous null responders are least likely to benefit from another course of therapy similar to their earlier treatment. SVR rates during retreatment rarely surpass 15% in this population, and may be lower when there are predominant unfavourable treatment factors present. Unless other compelling reasons

TABLE 8.1 Definitions of on-treatment virological response.

Response	Definition
Rapid virological response	HCV RNA negative (< 50 IU/mL) at week 4
Early virological response (EVR)	
Complete EVR	HCV RNA positive at week 4 but negative at week 12
Partial EVR	HCV RNA positive at week 4 but $\geq 2 \log_{10}$ by week 12 and undetectable by week 24
Non-EVR	$< 2 \log_{10}$ drop from baseline at week 12

exist to treat these patients (such as control of extrahepatic manifestations), the best option may be observation while waiting for triple-therapy combinations.

Prior relapsers have the best chance of achieving SVR during a second course of treatment. SVR rates as high as 50% have been reported when previous relapsers to combination therapy have been retreated with peginterferon and ribavirin. Poynard *et al.* [3] retreated over 2300 prior non-responders and relapsers (all with advanced fibrosis) with peginterferon alfa-2b and ribavirin (800–1400 mg/day) for 48 weeks. The SVR rate was 38% among prior relapsers but only 14% among prior non-responders. Genotype non-1, HCV RNA below 600 000 IU/mL, and lower fibrosis stage were associated with improved treatment response. This marked difference in success rates between relapsers and non-responders further emphasizes the importance of investigating prior treatment response.

Prolonged therapy for slow virological responders

The rationale for extending the duration of treatment in some patients has been examined in several studies [4]. Extending the duration of therapy beyond 48 weeks appears to be a promising approach for a select group of prior relapsers. Slow virological responders are those who achieve undetectable HCV RNA in serum for the first time between weeks 12 and 24 of therapy. In this group, treatment with a standard 48-week course of treatment has been associated with a high rate of virological relapse on treatment cessation. Several randomized controlled trials comparing 48 weeks of treatment to 72 weeks of treatment among those with slow virological response have been performed. While all of these studies have differed somewhat in study design, such as different doses of ribavirin and different criteria for randomization to extended treatment, the message has been very consistent: prolonged therapy can significantly improve rates of SVR, largely by decreasing the rate of relapse, among slow virological responders. In one study performed in the USA, notable for its inclusion of numerous patients with difficult-to-treat characteristics (African-Americans, high viral levels, overweight, advanced fibrosis), SVR rates for slow virological responders treated for 72 weeks was 38%, compared with only 18% for those treated for 48 weeks [5]. Relapse rates were inversely proportional to the duration of therapy (20% vs. 59% when treated for 72 or 48 weeks, respectively). Thus, one could surmise that slow virological responders who relapsed to a previous course of treatment might benefit from extend-

ing therapy to 72 weeks during a second treatment course in order to diminish the chances of relapse. However, it should be noted that one large study recently reported from Europe failed to demonstrate an advantage to prolonged combination therapy in slow responders. Furthermore, extending therapy has been regularly associated with a high rate of premature discontinuation beyond 48 weeks of treatment, which must temper this approach in many patients.

Optimizing ribavirin dosing during retreatment

The importance of ribavirin in the treatment of HCV infection has always been underestimated. Ribavirin monotherapy has negligible antiviral activity; however, when combined with peginterferon, it is critical to preventing relapse after treatment cessation. In general, higher doses of ribavirin measured on a milligram per kilogram basis are associated with improved rates of SVR. Ribavirin dosing in the range 13–15 mg/kg appears to be the best balance between optimized efficacy and intolerable haemolytic anaemia that develops at higher doses. SVR is significantly diminished when dosing is below approximately 11 mg/kg. Therefore, maximizing ribavirin dosing, particularly in overweight patients, has the potential to improve SVR during a second course of treatment and is another important factor to consider.

Similarly, numerous studies have also established that poor adherence to ribavirin significantly decreases the rate of SVR and that this effect is evident throughout the course of treatment. Reddy *et al.* [6] retrospectively analysed a large database of patients treated with peginterferon and ribavirin and demonstrated that ribavirin dose reductions generated a stepwise decrease in SVR. A cumulative ribavirin dose below 60% expected resulted in the most striking decline in SVR. As the most extreme example from a randomized trial, patients on combination therapy with undetectable HCV RNA who discontinued ribavirin in the latter 24 weeks of treatment had higher rates of virological breakthrough and relapse than those who continued on dual therapy [7]. Thus, major dose reductions or discontinuation of ribavirin during an initial course of therapy may have compromised sustained response and must be avoided, if possible, during subsequent treatment.

Increased peginterferon dose or consensus interferon

From the above discussion, it may be inferred that non-responders should be retreated with higher doses of peginterferon and ribavirin in order to maximize SVR. Unfortunately, studies of intensified regimens of combination therapy have demonstrated only modest increases in SVR. A recent four-arm study compared standard dose versus higher induction dosing of peginterferon in combination with ribavirin for either 48 or 72 weeks [8]. The highest rate of SVR was attained in the induction dose group treated for 72 weeks (16%), although a similar rate was also achieved with standard dosing of peginterferon for 72 weeks (14%), both of which were higher than the 48-week treatment arms, suggesting that the duration of therapy rather than the induction dose of peginterferon was of greater importance.

In a study of consensus interferon in previous peginterferon/ribavirin non-responders that included many patients with unfavourable treatment factors such as advanced fibrosis and high viral load, the SVR rate was 7% and 11% when patients were treated with either 9 or 15 µg of consensus interferon daily, respectively, combined with ribavirin [9]. SVR rates were higher (32%) if patients had demonstrated at least a 2-log decrease in viraemia during their previous course of peginterferon/ribavirin.

Role of maintenance therapy

Patients with advanced fibrosis who fail to respond to interferon-based therapies are at highest risk for complications of cirrhosis. The HALT-C study treated a large cohort of these patients with a low dose of peginterferon alfa-2a for 3.5 years to determine if maintenance therapy would decrease the rates of fibrosis progression, hepatic decompensation and hepatocellular carcinoma [10]. In a rigorously controlled trial, there were no differences in the rates of these events between the treated group and an observational control group. Interestingly, in a small subgroup of patients who had viral suppression from low-dose maintenance therapy, there was a suggestion of histological benefit, although the study design and small sample size precluded any meaningful post hoc analysis. At this point, maintenance therapy cannot be endorsed for prior non-responders to therapy.

Triple-combination therapies in prior non-sustained responders

The protease inhibitors telaprevir and boceprevir are direct-acting antiviral agents that have shown great promise in recent Phase II studies [11,12]. SVR rates in previously untreated patients are significantly improved when these agents are combined with peginterferon and ribavirin.

Limited data exist on their use in prior peginterferon/ribavirin non-responders but it is anticipated that SVR rates will also significantly improve. Assuming the results of Phase III trials currently underway are similar, clinicians may have additional therapeutic options to consider for their prior non-responders in the next 2–3 years, which may affect selection of candidates and the urgency for retreatment.

Practical approach to retreatment of non-sustained virological response

1 Assess patient's motivation for another course of therapy: patients must be highly motivated to undergo another treatment regimen with attendant side effects, particularly since the likelihood of SVR is substantially lower than in treatment-naïve patients.
2 Assess severity of liver disease (clinical, biochemical, histological if applicable): patients with minimal fibrosis may opt to defer treatment until triple therapies become available. It is expected that these triple regimens will improve the chance for SVR in both non-responders and relapsers.
3 Determine virological response to previous treatment course: null responders are unlikely to benefit from a second, similar treatment regimen and intensified regimens of peginterferon have demonstrated only modest improvements in SVR. Slow virological responders who have relapsed may benefit from extending the duration of therapy for up to 72 weeks.
4 Examine prior dosing regimens and adherence: optimizing ribavirin dosing on a milligram per kilogram basis, minimizing dose reductions, and avoiding interruptions to therapy are important goals during a second course of treatment.
5 Identify correctable factors and make a plan for vigilant monitoring and/or management.

References

1. Ghany MG, Strader DB, Thomas DL, Seeff LB. Diagnosis, management, and treatment of hepatitis C: an update. *Hepatology* 2009;49:1335–1374. **Comprehensive guidelines on HCV infection.** 🔑

2. Ferenci P, Fried MW, Shiffman ML *et al.* Predicting sustained virological responses in chronic hepatitis C patients treated with peginterferon alfa-2a (40 KD)/ribavirin. *Journal of Hepatology* 2005;43:425–433.

3. Poynard T, Colombo M, Bruix J *et al.* Peginterferon alfa-2b and ribavirin: effective in patients with hepatitis C who

failed interferon alfa/ribavirin therapy. *Gastroenterology* 2009;136:1618–1628.e2.

4. Sanchez-Tapias JM, Diago M, Escartin P *et al*. Peginterferon-alfa2a plus ribavirin for 48 versus 72 weeks in patients with detectable hepatitis C virus RNA at week 4 of treatment. *Gastroenterology* 2006;131:451–460.

5. Pearlman BL, Ehleben C, Saifee S. Treatment extension to 72 weeks of peginterferon and ribavirin in hepatitis C genotype 1-infected slow responders. *Hepatology* 2007;46:1688–1694.

6. Reddy KR, Shiffman ML, Morgan TR *et al*. Impact of ribavirin dose reductions in hepatitis C virus genotype 1 patients completing peginterferon alfa-2a/ribavirin treatment. *Clinical Gastroenterology and Hepatology* 2007;5:124–129.

7. Bronowicki JP, Ouzan D, Asselah T *et al*. Effect of ribavirin in genotype 1 patients with hepatitis C responding to pegylated interferon alfa-2a plus ribavirin. *Gastroenterology* 2006;131:1040–1048.

8. Jensen DM, Marcellin P, Freilich B *et al*. Re-treatment of patients with chronic hepatitis C who do not respond to peginterferon-alpha2b: a randomized trial. *Annals of Internal Medicine* 2009;150:528–540.

9. Bacon BR, Shiffman ML, Mendes F *et al*. Retreating chronic hepatitis C with daily interferon alfacon-1/ribavirin after non-response to pegylated interferon/ribavirin: DIRECT results. *Hepatology* 2009;49:1838–1846.

10. Di Bisceglie AM, Shiffman ML, Everson GT *et al*. Prolonged therapy of advanced chronic hepatitis C with low-dose peginterferon. *New England Journal of Medicine* 2008;359:2429–2441. **A large study that evaluated the role of maintenance peginterferon therapy in those who failed standard of care and had advanced fibrosis/cirrhosis. Maintenance therapy was of no benefit.** ⌐━

11. Hezode C, Forestier N, Dusheiko G *et al*. Telaprevir and peginterferon with or without ribavirin for chronic HCV infection. *New England Journal of Medicine* 2009;360:1839–1850.

12. McHutchison JG, Everson GT, Gordon SC *et al*. Telaprevir with peginterferon and ribavirin for chronic HCV genotype 1 infection. *New England Journal of Medicine* 2009;360:1827–1838.

9 Management of HCV-2 and HCV-3 non-responders and relapsers

Giada Sebastiani[1,2], Alfredo Alberti[2,3]

[1]Department of Digestive Diseases, Hepatology and Clinical Nutrition, Dell'Angelo Hospital, Venice, Italy
[2]Venetian Institute of Molecular Medicine (VIMM), Padova, Italy
[3]Department of Histology, Microbiology and Medical Biotechnologies, University of Padova, Padova, Italy

LEARNING POINTS

- Patients with HCV-2 and HCV-3 have differing outcomes from therapy.

- Treatment failure is uncommon in patients with HCV-2 and HCV-3.

- Factors that predispose to treatment failure include obesity, insulin resistance, advanced fibrosis and high pretreatment viraemia.

- Retreatment in patients with HCV-2 and HCV-3 should be considered as response rates are reasonable, particularly with prolonged duration of treatment.

Introduction

Therapy of chronic hepatitis C virus (HCV) infection is currently based on the combination of peginterferon and ribavirin [1]. The response to such treatment depends on several virus and host variables that determine the need for a more or less aggressive schedule and which are associated with a higher or lower chance of achieving a sustained virological response (SVR). Patients infected with HCV genotype 2 (HCV-2) or genotype 3 (HCV-3) have traditionally been considered easier to treat than those with HCV genotype 1 (HCV-1) or genotype 4 (HCV-4). Response rates are indeed higher in the former and, according to

current international guidelines, need shorter therapy. Most published series have reported SVR rates above 80% in HCV-2/HCV-3 infection compared with SVR rates below 60% in HCV-1 infection, and current treatment guidelines recommend 24 weeks of therapy in the former and 48 or 72 weeks in the latter [1,2]. However, a subgroup of patients with HCV-2 or HCV-3 infection do not develop an SVR and are termed 'relapser' or 'non-responder', and there is evidence that these patients behave somehow differently. In this chapter we describe the factors that have been associated with reduced response to antiviral therapy in patients with HCV-2 and HCV-3 infection and the prospects for improving response in such patients.

HCV-2 and HCV-3: the easy-to-treat HCV genotypes

In 2004, Hadziyannis *et al.* [3] provided clear evidence that HCV-2/HCV-3 infection is easier to treat than HCV-1/HCV-4 infection and requires only 24 weeks of therapy, without significant overall gain in benefit when combination therapy is given for 48–52 weeks. In most clinical trials SVR rates in patients with HCV-2/HCV-3 infection, considered as a single group, have been in excess of 80% [2]. The most recent American Association for the Study of Liver Diseases (AASLD) guidelines recommend treating patients with HCV-2 or HCV-3 infection with peginterferon for 24 weeks plus ribavirin 800 mg daily. Patients who are intolerant of a planned 24-week course of therapy can discontinue the antiviral therapy between weeks 12 and 16 if they have achieved a rapid virological response (RVR). However, patients should be informed that this schedule is associated with a higher relapse rate [1].

HCV-2 and HCV-3 have different responses to therapy

Most clinical trials have pooled treatment response rates in patients with HCV-2 and HCV-3 infection. However, in 2004 Zeuzem et al. [4] reported that SVR rates after a 24-week course of peginterferon alfa-2b plus ribavirin were 93% for HCV-2 but only 79% for HCV-3. Reduced response in HCV-3 infection was associated with a higher incidence and degree of liver steatosis and higher rates of post-treatment relapse. High viral load at baseline was also an important factor in reducing SVR in HCV-3 but not HCV-2 infection. Zeuzem and collegues calculated an overall rate of SVR as 80–89% for HCV-2 and 66–80% for HCV-3 [2]. This has been recently confirmed in a meta-analysis by Andriulli et al. [5], who estimated an 8.7% difference in SVR rates between the two genotypes after 24 weeks of treatment. The difference was not influenced by the type of peginterferon, but was significantly affected by viraemia at baseline.

Factors associated with relapse, poor response or non-response in HCV-2 and HCV-3 infection

Primary non-response to peginterferon and ribavirin is a very rare event in patients with HCV-2 and HCV-3 infection, as in the vast majority of treated patients a significant reduction in HCV RNA is usually observed with adequate therapy. On the other hand, a non-negligible subgroup of patients may show only partial response or virological relapse after therapy withdrawal. Factors that may influence the response to antiviral therapy in patients with HCV-2 and HCV-3 infection have been described in several recent studies. Baseline HCV RNA levels influence SVR rates. Indeed, patients with HCV-2 and HCV-3 infection with low viraemia respond equally well to both 12 and 24 weeks of therapy [6–10]. The ACCELERATE study has shown that high baseline viral load (> 600 000 IU/mL) is associated with a high rate of virological relapse (23%) in HCV-3 infection [7]. The NORDynamIC study found that age and HCV RNA levels on days 7 and 29 were independent predictors of SVR [8]. RVR (i.e. undetectable HCV RNA in serum 4 weeks after initiation of therapy) is a well-known predictor of virological response to antiviral therapy. Indeed,

patients with HCV-2 and HCV-3 infection who do not achieve RVR have significantly lower SVR rates with antiviral therapy. The ACCELERATE study has clearly shown that only 49% of those patients infected with HCV-2 and HCV-3 who did not achieve RVR attained an SVR [7]. In the study by Yu et al. [9], which enrolled only patients with HCV-2 infection, achievement of RVR and patient's age were independent factors associated with SVR. In the study by Dalgard et al. [10], age 40 years or less, male gender and baseline viraemia 400 000 IU/mL or less were independent predictors of RVR. Since high rates of relapse occur with 24-week therapy in HCV-2 and HCV-3 patients not achieving RVR, it is conceivable that these patients may benefit from longer therapy, but this remains to be proven in well-conducted clinical trials. Metabolic factors such as steatosis, obesity and insulin resistance have been reported to have a significant negative influence on the response to antiviral therapy in HCV infection. In the study by Zeuzem et al. [4], a significant difference in terms of SVR was observed between patients with HCV-2 and HCV-3 infection and this was associated with a higher amount of hepatic steatosis among the latter group of patients. In the study by Poustchi et al. [11] on 82 patients with HCV-2 or HCV-3 infection, the role of insulin resistance in influencing the SVR was investigated. In this study, patients able to achieve SVR had lower mean serum insulin measured by homeostasis model (HOMA) at baseline, indicating that insulin resistance was associated with reduced response. Body mass index (BMI) and fibrosis stage were independently associated with HOMA baseline values. After adjusting for fibrosis stage, patients with HOMA level less than 2 were 6.5 times more likely to achieve SVR than those with HOMA level 2 or more. Thus it is clear from these data that even in easy-to-treat HCV-2 and HCV-3 infection, insulin resistance leads to reduced response to peginterferon and ribavirin combination therapy. Since obesity and insulin resistance have been shown to have a negative impact on progression of fibrosis and on response to antiviral therapy in patients with HCV infection, including those with HCV-2 or HCV-3, it is appropriate to counsel those who are overweight about losing weight and reducing, as much as possible, insulin resistance before initiation of antiviral therapy.

A recent study by Mangia et al. [12] has investigated the determinants of relapse after a short (12-week) course of antiviral therapy in 718 patients with HCV-2 or HCV-3 infection. The RVR patients who were most likely to relapse after an abbreviated course of therapy were those with higher

BMI and lower platelet count. Indeed, a BMI of 30 or higher and a platelet count of 14×10^9/L or lower were independently associated with relapse. In this analysis, factors associated with relapse did not differ between HCV-2 and HCV-3 infection. When patients without SVR were analysed individually, at least one of the following unfavourable factors was always present: cirrhosis, age over 50 years or BMI greater than 30 kg/m^2. The authors concluded that shortening of antiviral therapy for less than 24 weeks in patients with HCV-2 or HCV-3 infection should be considered only for young patients with RVR, providing they present with no advanced fibrosis and low BMI.

The observation that patients with HCV-2 and HCV-3 infection and severe fibrosis are less likely to achieve RVR or SVR and show higher relapse rates has been described in numerous reports. In the study by Dalgard *et al.* [13], pretreatment liver histology showing no or minimal fibrosis was a solid predictor of SVR and all patients who relapsed after 14 weeks of therapy had severe fibrosis. In another study, patients with HCV-2 infection and low pretreatment levels of alanine aminotransferase were more likely to relapse following shorter treatment duration [14].

Retreatment of HCV-2 and HCV-3 infection

Several recent studies have addressed the issue of whether retreatment with peginterferon plus ribavirin could result in SVR in patients who have failed previous therapy as relapsers or non-responders (or partial responders). These studies indicate that the probability of achieving SVR with retreatment is higher in previous relapsers compared with non-responders and in HCV-2/HCV-3-infected patients compared with HCV-1-infected patients. According to available data, in patients with HCV-2/HCV-3 infection, retreatment for 48–52 weeks can achieve SVR in more than 60% of previous relapsers and in more than 30% of previous non-responders [2,3]. These figures are clearly higher than those obtained with the same retreatment schedule in patients with HCV-1 infection and mainly reflect the fact that most patients with HCV-2 and HCV-3 had received only 24 weeks of therapy during the previous unsuccessful course while those with HCV-1 had already been treated for 1 year. It is unclear whether success rates with retreatment differ between patients with HCV-2 and HCV-3 infection, as most retreatment studies pooled the two genotypes. On the basis of these findings it seems reasonable to consider retreatment with a 48–52 week course of peginterferon and

ribavirin in HCV-2 and HCV-3 patients who had been relapsers, partial responders or non-responders during previous antiviral therapy, particularly when they had received 24-week therapy. Recently, it has been suggested that patients with HCV-3 infection and advanced liver fibrosis or cirrhosis should be treated from the very beginning for at least 48 weeks, based on the observation that many of them obtain an end-of-therapy response but then relapse after therapy discontinuation when treated for only 24 weeks [2]. Further studies are needed to prove or disprove the real benefit of such approach.

STAT-C development for HCV-2 and HCV-3 infection

A number of direct antiviral agents against HCV (STAT-C) are now in the final phases of clinical development. The most promising ones include protease inhibitors and nucleoside and non-nucleoside inhibitors of the viral polymerase [2]. Most of these new compounds have been designed to target patients with HCV-1 infection, simply because this is the largest pool of individuals who fail to respond to currently available therapies. Some of these new compounds may be active on genotypes other than HCV-1; for example, telapravir has been recently shown to have significant antiviral activity against HCV-2 but not HCV-3 [15]. While there are no doubts that HCV-1 deserves priority as a target for STAT-C development, antiviral compounds active against HCV-2 and particularly HCV-3 will also need to be developed in the future, despite the more limited numbers of potential candidates.

References

1. Ghany MG, Strader DB, Thomas DL, Seeff LB. Diagnosis, management, and treatment of hepatitis C: an update. *Hepatology* 2009;49:1335–1374.
2. Zeuzem S. Interferon-based therapy for chronic hepatitis C: current and future perspectives. *Nature Clinical Practice. Gastroenterology and Hepatology* 2008;5:610–622.
3. Hadziyannis SJ, Sette H Jr, Morgan TR *et al.* Peginterferon-alpha2a and ribavirin combination therapy in chronic hepatitis C: a randomized study of treatment duration and ribavirin dose. *Annals of Internal Medicine* 2004;140:346–355. **Study demonstrating the need for different treatment durations in patients with genotype 2 and 3 HCV.** 🔑
4. Zeuzem S, Hultcrantz R, Bourliere M *et al.* Peginterferon alfa-2b plus ribavirin for treatment of chronic hepatitis C in

previously untreated patients infected with HCV genotypes 2 or 3. *Journal of Hepatology* 2004;40:993–999.

5. Andriulli A, Mangia A, Iacobellis A, Ippolito A, Leandro G, Zeuzem S. Meta-analysis: the outcome of anti-viral therapy in HCV genotype 2 and genotype 3 infected patients with chronic hepatitis. *Alimentary Pharmacology and Therapeutics* 2008;28:397–404. **Important meta-analysis of response rates in genotype 2 and 3 patients.** 🔑

6. Mangia A, Santoro R, Minerva N *et al.* Peginterferon alfa-2b and ribavirin for 12 vs. 24 weeks in HCV genotype 2 or 3. *New England Journal of Medicine* 2005;352:2609–2617.

7. Shiffman ML, Suter F, Bacon BR *et al.* Peginterferon alfa-2a and ribavirin for 16 or 24 weeks in HCV genotype 2 or 3. *New England Journal of Medicine* 2007;357:124–134.

8. Lagging M, Langeland N, Pedersen C *et al.* Randomized comparison of 12 or 24 weeks of peginterferon alpha-2a and ribavirin in chronic hepatitis C virus genotype 2/3 infection. NORDynamIC Study Group. *Hepatology* 2008;47:1837–1845.

9. Yu ML, Dai CY, Huang JF *et al.* A randomised study of peginterferon and ribavirin for 16 versus 24 weeks in patients with genotype 2 chronic hepatitis C. *Gut* 2007;56:553–559.

10. Dalgard O, Bjøro K, Ring-Larsen H *et al.* Pegylated interferon alfa and ribavirin for 14 versus 24 weeks in patients with hepatitis C virus genotype 2 or 3 and rapid virological response. *Hepatology* 2008;47:35–42.

11. Poustchi H, Negro F, Hui J *et al.* Insulin resistance and response to therapy in patients infected with chronic hepatitis C virus genotypes 2 and 3. Insulin resistance and response to therapy in patients infected with chronic hepatitis C virus genotypes 2 and 3. *J Hepatol* 2008;48:28–34.

12. Mangia A, Minerva N, Bacca D *et al.* Determinants of relapse after a short (12 weeks) course of antiviral therapy and re-treatment efficacy of a prolonged course in patients with chronic hepatitis C virus genotype 2 or 3 infection. *Hepatology* 2009;49:358–363.

13. Dalgard O, Bjøro K, Hellum KB *et al.* Treatment with pegylated interferon and ribavarin in HCV infection with genotype 2 or 3 for 14 weeks: a pilot study. *Hepatology* 2004;40:1260–1265.

14. Andriulli A, Dalgard O, Bjøro K, Mangia A. Short-term treatment duration for HCV-2 and HCV-3 infected patients. *Digestive and Liver Disease* 2006;38:741–748.

15. McHutchison JG, Everson GT, Gordon SC *et al.* Telapravir with peginterferon and ribavirin for chronic HCV genotype 1 infection. *New England Journal of Medicine* 2009;360:1827–1838.

10 Management of HCV infection in patients with thalassemia and sickle cell disease

Paul Telfer, Banu Kaya

Barts and The London NHS Trust, London, UK

LEARNING POINTS

- Chronic HCV infection is common in patients with blood dyscrasias and should be managed jointly by specialists in hepatology and haematology, preferably in a joint clinic.

- Liver biopsy is needed for histological assessment and chemical quantitation of liver iron content.

- Patients with thalassemia major should be optimally chelated before starting antiviral therapy, with liver iron maintained in the range 2–7 mg/g dry weight. Patients with sickle cell disease may require regular transfion during anti-viral therapy to reduce the risk of severe haemolysis and acute sickle crisis.

- Combination therapy with peginterferon and ribavirin induces sustained virological responses in about 50% of patients with thalassemia and should be considered if there is evidence of active inflammation or fibrosis on biopsy.

- During treatment, careful monitoring of side effects, transfusion frequency and iron chelation is required.

Introduction

Regular or intermittent red blood cell transfusion is often required for patients with inherited anaemias, and this has resulted in a proportion becoming infected with HCV as a result of receiving contaminated red cell donations. Chronic HCV infection in these patients causes particular management problems and there are no large-scale clinical trials to provide definitive guidance. Here we discuss the

Clinical Dilemmas in Viral Liver Disease, 1st edition. Edited by Graham R. Foster and K. Rajender Reddy. © 2010 Blackwell Publishing.

management options for patients who also suffer from either thalassemia major or sickle cell disease.

Thalassemia and sickle cell disease

Thalassemia major and sickle cell disease are common conditions in non-northern European populations and present particular management problems. Both are inherited as autosomal recessive conditions with mutations affecting the β-globin gene. β Thalassemia mutations reduce or abolish the production of β-globin, causing a deficiency of haemoglobin, severe anaemia and ineffective erythropoiesis with intramedullary and extramedullary erythroid marrow expansion. Patients with thalassemia major require regular transfusions for normal growth and development. In the case of sickle cell disease, there is an abnormal β-globin chain with a substitution of valine for glutamic acid at position 6. This structural haemoglobin variant tends to form polymers when deoxygenated, leading to haemolytic anaemia, acute large- and small-vessel occlusion and chronic tissue damage.

Transfusion-transmitted HCV infection

These patients require intermittent or regular transfusion therapy, and are at increased risk of infection because of exposure to multiple blood donors. The highest risk is in thalassemia major, which requires regular long-term transfusion therapy, usually given every 2–4 weeks. It is less prevalent in sickle cell disease, with about 10–20% of patients being regularly transfused, mostly in childhood for stroke prevention.

If recommended blood donor selection and screening procedures are implemented, the risk of HCV transmission is now very low. In the UK, the estimated risk of an infected unit entering the blood supply in 2002–2003 was 0.05 per million donations [1]. Most patients in the UK with persisting infection acquired HCV prior to implementation of effective HCV screening of blood donors. Some continue to be at risk through transfusion while resident in a country where exclusion of infected donors is less secure. In some multitransfused patients, there is evidence of multiple past exposures to HCV [2].

Prevalence of HCV antibody positivity in adult patients with thalassemia major varies from 30 to over 70%, with high proportions reported in Italy compared with the UK and North America. More than 50% of antibody-positive patients have evidence of chronic infection [3,4]; the remainder are persistently serum HCV RNA negative, and appear to have cleared the virus spontaneously.

Liver disease

Progression of liver disease is influenced by the pathological effects of the conditions themselves. In the case of thalassemia major, the dominant disease-altering factor is iron loading of hepatic parenchymal cells. There is increased intestinal absorption of iron in non-transfused thalassemia (thalassemia intermedia), which can result in very heavy iron loading [5]. The liver is also the major site of iron deposition in transfusion-dependent (thalassemia major) patients and hepatic iron concentration is linearly related to total body iron load [6]. Progression of hepatic fibrosis is influenced by the degree of hepatic iron overload and is most rapid in patients with heavy iron overload (> 15 mg/g dry weight) who are HCV RNA positive [7,8]. Cirrhosis and hepatocellular carcinoma are well documented, even in young patients [3,9].

Patients with sickle cell disease are also at risk of hepatic iron overload, particularly if regularly transfused. In addition, they are prone to acute and chronic hepatic complications of sickle cell disease, in part related to vaso-occlusion and sequestration of sickle haemoglobin-containing red cells in the liver [10], and it should be anticipated that chronic HCV infection will run a more severe course.

Antiviral therapy

With a combination of interferon (pegylated or standard) and ribavirin, sustained virological response (SVR) has been reported in 40–70% of patients with thalassemia, with higher rates in younger patients who have not been treated previously [11–14]. SVR can be obtained in cirrhotic patients and in those with unfavourable genotypes. The best predictor appears to be early viral clearance during therapy. Since SVR is predictable from virological response at 12 weeks, and there are potential severe long-term adverse effects of therapy in thalassemia major, it is not advisable to continue therapy beyond 12 weeks if HCV RNA is persistently positive. Hepatic iron levels are nearly always increased in these patients, and although data are conflicting on the effect of high liver iron concentration on the response to therapy, it is advisable to reduce liver iron to safe levels (2–7 mg/g dry weight) before starting therapy. The UK Thalassemia Society publishes guidelines for monitoring iron stores and for iron chelation therapy [15].

Patients with thalassemia major are at increased risk of adverse effects of interferon. The thyroid gland is vulnerable to iron overload as well as interferon-mediated autoimmune damage. Neutropenia and agranulocytosis are serious side effects of interferon as well as of deferiprone, one of the commonly used oral iron chelator drugs. Depression is a common problem in patients with long-term conditions, and severe bouts can be precipitated by interferon therapy. Ribavirin induces haemolytic anaemia, obviously undesirable in a patient with an underlying chronic anaemia. This is the reason for a specific contraindication to its use in thalassemia major and sickle cell disease (Copegus prescribing information). However, this contraindication should be reviewed, since it is unreasonable to deny patients the best means of eradicating HCV. In trials of combination therapy, transfusion requirements were increased by about 40%, mainly as a result of ribavirin-induced haemolysis. In order to maintain the recommended haemoglobin level for patients with thalassemia major (Pre- transfusion Hb 9.5–10 g/dL), transfusion volume and frequency should be increased during therapy.

For patients with thalassemia major, iron chelation needs to be continued during antiviral therapy, but the choice of drug is not straightforward. Three drugs are licensed in the European Union: desferrioxamine (given by 10–12 hour subcutaneous infusion five to six times per week), deferiprone (oral, three times daily) and deferasirox (oral, once daily). Deferiprone is best avoided because of the risk of agranulocytosis and neutropenia. Deferasirox is relatively new and has not been used in the context of antiviral therapy. Currently the best advice is for patients to be chelated with desferrioxamine during the 24–28 weeks of therapy. After completion of therapy, chelation can be modified and intensified to remove excess iron accrued during therapy as a result of increased transfusion.

There is less experience of treating patients with sickle cell disease. They may be at increased risk of complications brought about by the side effects of antiviral therapy. This may include worsening of haemolytic anaemia and induction of acute sickle cell crises. In most cases, it would seem advisable to transfuse patients with sickle cell disease regularly (additive or exchange transfusion) during therapy in order to reduce the sickle haemoglobin percentage below 30.

References

1. McClelland D. *Handbook of Transfusion Medicine*, 4th edn. http://www.transfusionguidelines.org.uk/docs/pdfs/htm_edition-4_all-pages.pdf: United Kingdom Blood Transfusion Services, 2007.

2. Lai ME, Mazzoleni AP, Argiolu F *et al.* Hepatitis C virus in multiple episodes of acute hepatitis in polytransfused thalassaemic children. *Lancet* 1994;343:388–390.

3. Cunningham MJ, Macklin EA, Neufeld EJ, Cohen AR. Complications of beta-thalassemia major in North America. *Blood* 2004;104:34–39.

4. Angelucci E, Pilo F. Treatment of hepatitis C in patients with thalassemia. *Haematologica* 2008;93:1121–1123.

5. Taher A, El Rassi F, Isma'eel H, Koussa S, Inati A, Cappellini MD. Correlation of liver iron concentration determined by R2 magnetic resonance imaging with serum ferritin in patients with thalassemia intermedia. *Haematologica* 2008;93:1584–1586.

6. Angelucci E, Brittenham GM, McLaren CE *et al.* Hepatic iron concentration and total body iron stores in thalassemia major. *New England Journal of Medicine* 2000; 343:327–331.

7. Di Marco V, Capra M, Gagliardotto F *et al.* Liver disease in chelated transfusion-dependent thalassemics: the role of iron overload and chronic hepatitis C. *Haematologica* 2008;93:1243–1246.

8. Angelucci E, Muretto P, Nicolucci A *et al.* Effects of iron overload and hepatitis C virus positivity in determining progression of liver fibrosis in thalassemia following bone marrow transplantation. *Blood* 2002;100:17–21. **Pivotal study outlining the deleterious effects of HCV in patients with iron overload.** ⚷

9. Borgna-Pignatti C, Vergine G, Lombardo T *et al.* Hepatocellular carcinoma in the thalassaemia syndromes. *British Journal of Haematology* 2004;124:114–117.

10. Berry PA, Cross TJ, Thein SL *et al.* Hepatic dysfunction in sickle cell disease: a new system of classification based on global assessment. *Clinical Gastroenterology and Hepatology* 2007;5:1469–1476.

11. Telfer PT, Garson JA, Whitby K *et al.* Combination therapy with interferon alpha and ribavirin for chronic hepatitis C virus infection in thalassaemic patients. *British Journal of Haematology* 1997;98:850–855. **Early study of combination therapy illustrating the use of ribavirin in patients with severe anaemia.** ⚷

12. Harmatz P, Jonas MM, Kwiatkowski JL *et al.* Safety and efficacy of pegylated interferon alpha-2a and ribavirin for the treatment of hepatitis C in patients with thalassemia. *Haematologica* 2008;93:1247–1251.

13. Li CK, Chan PK, Ling SC, Ha SY. Interferon and ribavirin as frontline treatment for chronic hepatitis C infection in thalassaemia major. *British Journal of Haematology* 2002;117: 755–758.

14. Inati A, Taher A, Ghorra S *et al.* Efficacy and tolerability of peginterferon alpha-2a with or without ribavirin in thalassaemia major patients with chronic hepatitis C virus infection. *British Journal of Haematology* 2005;130:644–646.

15. UK Thalassaemia Society. *Standards for the Clinical Care of Children and Adults with Thalassaemia in the UK*, 2nd edn, 2008. Available at http://www.ukts.org/pdfs/awareness/ukts-standards-2008.pdf

Management of HCV in dialysis patients

Fabrizio Fabrizi, Paul Martin

Division of Hepatology, School of Medicine, University of Miami, Miami, FL, USA

LEARNING POINTS

- HCV infection remains frequent in patients on maintenance haemodialysis.

- HCV infection plays a detrimental role on survival in haemodialysis patients and renal transplant recipients.

- No optimal antiviral therapy of chronic HCV infection in dialysis populations exists.

Introduction

Chronic hepatitis C virus (HCV) infection remains prevalent in the haemodialysis population despite elimination of HCV from the blood supply, partly reflecting nosocomial spread within haemodialysis units [1,2]. Although there is increasing information on the detrimental impact of HCV on survival in patients with chronic kidney disease (CKD), the treatment of HCV infection in this population remains a challenge to clinicians.

The treatment of HCV infection in patients on chronic haemodialysis is predicated on the premise that HCV is associated with decreased patient survival. Some information on the association between positive anti-HCV serological status and survival in dialysis populations already exists [3], even if an accurate assessment of the natural history of HCV in dialysis patients is difficult [1]. A recent meta-analysis on the impact of HCV on mortality (seven observational studies enrolling 11 589 unique patients on maintenance haemodialysis) showed that the summary

Clinical Dilemmas in Viral Liver Disease, 1st edition. Edited by Graham R. Foster and K. Rajender Reddy. © 2010 Blackwell Publishing.

estimate for adjusted relative risk (RR) of all-cause mortality with anti-HCV was 1.34 (95% CI 1.13–1.59) [3]. Liver dysfunction has been implicated in lower survival of seropositive patients; the summary estimate for RR of liver-related mortality with anti-HCV was 3.75 (95% CI 1.93, 17.99) [3]. These results are consistent with evidence from other sources. A large survey (DOPPS) of patients on long-term dialysis in three continents reported an independent and significant association between positive anti-HCV serological status and mortality (RR 1.17; $P < 0.02$) (reviewed in ref. 4).

Antiviral therapy of HCV in dialysis patients: rationale

The information in the literature on the antiviral therapy of HCV in dialysis populations is not abundant. Clinicians have so far been reluctant to offer interferon-based therapy for HCV infection in dialysis populations as it was felt to be too toxic in this setting. The immunomodulatory activity of interferon supports a large spectrum of side effects in patients with chronic HCV infection and normal renal function, including alopecia, depression, fever/flu-like syndrome, and infections. Dialysis patients are typically older and have several comorbidities (including cardiomyopathy, malnutrition and gastrointestinal abnormalities).

The decision to treat HCV infection in the CKD patient should be based on liver histology, age, comorbidities, and ability to tolerate therapy. Potential benefits of successful therapy include aborting the progression of liver disease and reducing the risk of post-transplant complications associated with HCV. Positive anti-HCV serological status after kidney transplantation is implicated in the pathogenesis of acute glomerulopathy, *de novo* graft-associated nephropathy, new-onset diabetes mellitus after transplantation, and increased incidence of infections. In some patients, there are good data to support antiviral treatment, for example in the pretransplant patient. For HCV-infected dialysis patients who are kidney transplant candidates, antiviral therapy is suggested in order to prevent extrahepatic complications even in those with a pattern of histological injury that does not meet the recommended degree of fibrosis to qualify for therapy in the general population (i.e. Metavir score < 2 and Ishak score < 3) [4]. Given the generally indolent progression of HCV, treatment is not recommended for the dialysis patient with less than a 5-year estimated survival due to comorbidities such as cardiovascular disease. This is particularly the case if liver histology shows an absence of extensive fibrosis. The decision to treat an HCV-infected patient on regular dialysis must be made in the context of the patient's clinical situation. The patient should be appropriately informed of the risks and benefits of antiviral therapy and should also participate in the decision-making process.

With regard to the question of liver biopsy prior to treatment, the information derived from a liver biopsy in haemodialysis patients may be particularly useful, as clinical and biochemical findings may underestimate severity of liver disease. Pretransplant liver biopsy provides useful prognostic information. Staging of disease severity may guide considerations for antiviral therapy as patients identified with advanced fibrosis should be considered for liver–kidney transplantation.

Although genotype does not predict the outcome of infection, it has been shown to predict the probability of response to, and determine the necessary duration of, therapy. Infections with HCV genotypes 1 and 4 are less responsive to interferon-based therapy and require 48 weeks of treatment. In contrast, genotypes 2 and 3 are far more responsive to treatment and require only 24 weeks of therapy to achieve a sustained virological response (SVR). HCV genotype 5 appears to have a response similar to genotypes 2 and 3 but requires 48 weeks of therapy. Genotype 6 responds better than genotype 1 but not so well as genotypes 2 and 3. These results have been obtained in patients with HCV infection and normal kidney function. In a meta-analysis of patients on maintenance haemodialysis, the overall summary estimate for SVR was 37% in the whole group and 30% in those patients with HCV genotype 1 [5]. In another review, the pooled SVR rate was 33% in the whole group and 26% in those with HCV genotype 1 [6].

Interferon monotherapy

Numerous clinical trials have been published on antiviral therapy (conventional or pegylated interferon alone) for chronic HCV infection in dialysis populations but most of these have an uncontrolled design; also, the size of the study groups is rather small. At this time, there are data, albeit very limited, supporting peginterferon as monotherapy for the treatment of HCV infection in patients receiving long-term dialysis [7–21].

A recent meta-analysis identified 24 clinical trials enrolling 429 unique patients on maintenance dialysis who received conventional interferon monotherapy; the summary estimate for SVR rate was 39% (95% CI 32, 46) and the drop-out rate was 19% (95% CI 13, 26) [5]. The most frequent side effects requiring interruption of treatment were flu-like symptoms and gastrointestinal and haematological changes. A relationship between age and drop-out rate was found, even if no statistical significance was reached ($P = 0.064$). The studies were heterogeneous with regard to SVR and drop-out rate. No publication bias was found. The conclusion of the authors was that one-third of dialysis patients with chronic HCV infection were successfully treated with conventional interferon monotherapy.

The viral response to monotherapy with standard interferon in maintenance haemodialysis patients (summary estimate of 39%) is higher than that observed in patients with chronic HCV infection and normal kidney function (7–16%) who received conventional interferon monotherapy. Several mechanisms account for the relatively higher response to interferon in subjects receiving regular haemodialysis: dialysis patients with HCV infection usually have a lower viral load; the infection is frequently associated with milder forms of histological liver disease; clearance of interferon is lower in dialysis than in non-CKD patients; and an increase in endogenous interferon release from circulating white blood cells during haemodialysis procedures has been reported. Marked and prolonged synthesis of hepatocyte growth factor (or other cytokines) caused by haemodialysis could play an additional role [4].

Although response rates to conventional interferon are better in the dialysis population, tolerance to interferon monotherapy appears lower in patients on maintenance haemodialysis than in non-CKD individuals. The summary estimate for drop-out rate was 19% in dialysis patients who received standard interferon monotherapy, whereas the frequency of side effects requiring interferon discontinuation ranged between 5 and 9% in non-CKD patients with chronic HCV infection who received a usual dose of standard interferon monotherapy (3 million units thrice weekly for 6 months). The altered pharmacokinetic parameters of interferon in the haemodialysis population may, to some extent, explain the higher frequency of side effects leading to interferon discontinuation. The interferon alfa half-life was longer in dialysis than in normal controls (9.6 vs. 5.3 hours; $P = 0.001$) and the area under the curve was twice that seen in patients with normal kidney function. Additional mechanisms were older age and high rate of comorbid conditions in haemodialysis populations [5].

Combination therapy

The information on combined antiviral therapy (i.e. conventional interferon plus ribavirin) in the CKD population is preliminary in nature [22] and the data on peginterferon plus ribavirin are even more sparse [23–27]. The quality of evidence on this issue is very low. The results provided in some trials have been encouraging in terms of efficacy and safety, but the limited size of the study groups does not allow definitive recommendations (Table 11.1). Very little ribavirin is removed via dialysis so there is a propensity for the drug to accumulate, exacerbating haemolysis in the dialysis population already at significant risk for anaemia. Ribavirin therapy in this setting is not recommended.

We feel that if a decision is made to use ribavirin in patients on maintenance haemodialysis, it should be used very cautiously and only after the implementation of several precautions, including (i) very low doses of ribavirin (200 mg thrice weekly), (ii) weekly monitoring of haemoglobin levels, and (iii) high doses of erythropoietin to treat anaemia. This will typically be performed at specialized centres [4].

Limitations and research recommendations

There is still concern about the applicability of the results of these studies to all dialysis patients, as most of the subjects included were on the waiting list for kidney transplantation and were younger and probably healthier than the general dialysis population. Furthermore, only a few studies were from North America, where many CKD patients are African-American. This is of special relevance, as there are racial differences in the response to interferon therapy in subjects with normal kidney function.

Early virological response (i.e. virological response obtained 12 weeks after initiation of antiviral therapy with at least a 2-log fall in the HCV viral titre) has been demonstrated to be highly predictive of SVR in HCV-infected patients with normal kidney function. There are studies which have formally addressed the predictive value of early viral response in evaluating the response of HCV-infected CKD patients to antiviral therapy. Many dialysis patients who receive antiviral therapy are potential renal transplant candidates, but they cannot be assigned to a transplant waiting list while receiving antiviral therapy. Thus, the failure to achieve a virological response 12 weeks after the initiation of antiviral therapy can support an early interruption of antiviral treatment, giving the patient the possibility of rapid inclusion in the waiting list for transplantation. Prospective studies on the clinical utility of early changes in the viral load, measured as absolute viral loads or change in viral load from baseline, are required in CKD-infected patients who receive antiviral therapy.

Information on the rate of adverse effects during interferon therapy in dialysis patients is unsatisfactory. It remains unclear whether the adverse effects in dialysis patients with

Reference	SVR	Antiviral agent
Bruchfeld et al. 2006 [23]	50% (3/6)	Peginterferon alfa-2a ($N = 2$) or peginterferon alfa-2b ($N = 4$) plus ribavirin
Rendina et al. 2007 [24]	97% (34/35)	Peginterferon alfa-2a plus ribavirin
Schmitz et al. 2007 [25]*	50% (3/6)	Peginterferon alfa-2b plus ribavirin
van Leusen et al. 2008 [26]	71% (4/7)	Peginterferon alfa-2a plus ribavirin
Carriero et al. 2008 [27]	29% (4/14)	Peginterferon alfa-2a plus ribavirin

TABLE 11.1 Peginterferon in combination with ribavirin in patients with chronic HCV infection on maintenance haemodialysis: clinical trials.

Results have been calculated according to an intention to-treat analysis.
* This study concerned liver–kidney transplant recipients.

HCV are related to interferon activity *per se* or to the high prevalence of comorbid conditions typical of dialysis patients. Prospective controlled studies in dialysis patients are required to compare the rate of adverse effects during interferon-based therapy with those patients who do not receive antiviral therapy. Prospective trials involving the treatment of HCV-infected patients on peritoneal dialysis are needed. Essentially, all information available on the treatment of dialysis patients comes from studies in haemodialysis patients.

The higher efficacy of combined antiviral therapy compared with interferon monotherapy for HCV infection in patients with normal renal function is likely related to the synergistic activity played by ribavirin. However, the activity of ribavirin appears to be dose-dependent, and the effective role of low-dose ribavirin in enhancing the antiviral activity of interferon in dialysis patients remains to be determined. Controlled studies designed to answer this question should be performed.

Prospective studies are needed to assess whether the benefit of therapy in terms of lower mortality is realized in a patient population with significantly reduced long-term survival.

Conclusions

Combined therapy with peginterferon and ribavirin is the gold standard of treatment in the general population. However, ribavirin is not recommended in those patients with glomerular filtration rate less than 50 mL/min per 1.73 m^2. We recommend that standard interferon (3 million units thrice weekly subcutaneously) be used for the treatment of HCV-infected maintenance haemodialysis patients. For the kidney transplant candidate with HCV, we suggest a liver biopsy. For HCV-infected dialysis patients who are kidney transplant candidates, antiviral therapy is recommended even for those with a lesser degree of fibrosis on biopsy than is generally recommended for the non-CKD population. The data on combined antiviral therapy (standard or pegylated interferon plus ribavirin) in patients undergoing regular dialysis appear encouraging but more studies are needed to confirm these early findings before clear recommendations can be made.

Acknowledgements

This work has been supported in part by the grant 'Project Glomerulonephritis' in memory of Pippo Neglia.

References

1. Fabrizi F, Lunghi G, Ganeshan V *et al.* Hepatitis C virus infection and the dialysis patient. *Seminars in Dialysis* 2007;20:416–422.

2. Finelli L, Miller JT, Tokars JI *et al.* National surveillance of dialysis-associated diseases in the United States, 2002. *Seminars in Dialysis* 2005;18:52–61.

3. Fabrizi F, Takkouche B, Lunghi G *et al.* The impact of hepatitis C virus infection on survival in dialysis patients: meta-analysis of observational studies. *Journal of Viral Hepatitis* 2007;14:697–703.

4. Kidney Disease: Improving Global Outcomes. KDIGO clinical practice guidelines for the prevention, diagnosis, evaluation, and treatment of hepatitis C in chronic kidney disease. *Kidney International Supplement* 2008;109:S1–S99. **A comprehensive guideline on various aspects of HCV infection in chronic kidney disease. This was developed by experts based on evidence in the literature and on expert opinion.** 🔑

5. Fabrizi F, Dixit V, Messa P, Martin P. Interferon monotherapy of chronic hepatitis C in dialysis patients: meta-analysis of clinical trials. *Journal of Viral Hepatitis* 2008;15:79–88.

6. Russo MW, Goldsweig C, Iacobson M *et al.* Interferon monotherapy for dialysis patients with chronic hepatitis C: an analysis of the literature on efficacy and safety. *American Journal of Gastroenterology* 2003;98:1610–1615.

7. Annichiarico BE, Siciliano M. Pegylated interferon alpha-2b monotherapy for hemodialysis patients with chronic hepatitis C. *Alimentary Pharmacology and Therapeutics* 2004;20:123–127.

8. Teta D, Luscher BL, Gonvers JJ *et al.* Pegylated interferon for the treatment of hepatitis C virus in haemodialysis patients. *Nephrology, Dialysis, Transplantation* 2005;20:901–903.

9. Mukherjee S, Gilroy RK, McCashland TM *et al.* Pegylated interferon for recurrent hepatitis C in liver transplant recipients with renal failure: a prospective cohort study. *Transplantation Proceedings* 2003;35:1478–1479.

10. Covic A, Maftei ID, Mardare NGI *et al.* Analysis of safety and efficacy of pegylated-interferon alpha-2a in hepatitis C virus positive hemodialysis patients: results from a large, multicenter audit. *Journal of Nephrology* 2006;19:794–801.

11. Russo MW, Ghalib R, Sigal S *et al.* Randomized trial of pegylated interferon alpha-2b monotherapy in hemodialysis patients with chronic hepatitis C. *Nephrology, Dialysis, Transplantation* 2006;21:437–443.

12. Kokoglu OF, Ucmak H, Hosoglu S *et al.* Efficacy and tolerability of pegylated-interferon alpha-2a in hemodialysis patients with chronic hepatitis C. *Journal of Gastroenterology and Hepatology* 2006;21:575–580.

13. Sporea I, Popescu A, Sirli R *et al*. Pegylated interferon alpha2a treatment for chronic hepatitis C in patients on chronic hemodialysis. *World Journal of Gastroenterology* 2006;16:4191–4194.

14. Casanovas-Taltavull T, Baliellas C, Llobet M *et al*. Preliminary results of treatment with pegylated interferon alpha2a for chronic hepatitis C virus in kidney transplant candidates on hemodialysis. *Transplantation Proceedings* 2007;39:2125–2127.

15. Chan TM, Ho SKN, Tang CSO *et al*. Pilot study of pegylated interferon-alpha 2a in dialysis patients with chronic hepatitis C virus infection. *Nephrology* 2007;12:11–17.

16. Amarapurkar DN, Patel ND, Kirpalani AL. Monotherapy with peginterferon alpha-2b (12kDA) for chronic hepatitis C infection in patients undergoing haemodialysis. *Tropical Gastroenterology* 2007;28:16–18.

17. Liu CH, Liang CC, Lin JW *et al*. Pegylated interferon alfa-2a versus standard interferon alfa-2a for treatment-naïve dialysis patients with chronic hepatitis C: a randomised study. *Gut* 2008;57:525–530.

18. Ayaz C, Celen MK, Yuce UN *et al*. Efficacy and safety of pegylated-interferon alpha-2a in hemodialysis patients with chronic hepatitis C. *World Journal of Gastroenterology* 2008;14:255–259.

19. Akhan SC, Kalender B, Ruzgar M. The response to pegylated interferon alpha 2a in haemodialysis patients with hepatitis C virus infection. *Infection* 2008;36:341–344.

20. Ucmak H, Kokoglu OF, Hosoglu S *et al*. Long-term efficacy of pegylated interferon alpha-2a in HCV-positive hemodialysis patients. *Renal Failure* 2008;30:227–232.

21. Sikole A, Dzekova P, Selja N *et al*. Treatment of hepatitis C in haemodialysis patients with pegylated interferon alpha2a as monotherapy. *Renal Failure* 2007;29:961–966.

22. Mousa DH, Abdalla AH, Al-Shoail G *et al*. Alpha-interferon with ribavirin in the treatment of hemodialysis patients with hepatitis C. *Transplantation Proceedings* 2004;36:1831–1834.

23. Bruchfeld A, Lindahl K, Reichard O *et al*. Pegylated interferon and ribavirin treatment for hepatitis C in hemodialysed patients. *Journal of Viral Hepatitis* 2006;13:316–321. **A paper describing the experience with pegylated interferon and low-dose ribavirin in haemodialysis patients with chronic HCV infection.** ⚷

24. Rendina M, Castellaneta NM, Castellaneta A *et al*. The treatment of chronic hepatitis C with peginterferon alpha2a (40 kDA) plus ribavirin in hemodialysed patients awaiting renal transplant. *Journal of Hepatology* 2007;46:764–768.

25. Schmitz V, Kiessling A, Bahra M *et al*. Peginterferon alfa-2b plus ribavirin for the treatment of hepatitis C recurrence following combined liver and kidney transplantation. *Annals of Transplantation* 2007;12:22–27.

26. van Leusen R, Adang RP, de Vries RA *et al*. Pegylated interferon alfa-2a (40kD) and ribavirin in haemodialysis patients with chronic hepatitis C. *Nephrology, Dialysis, Transplantation* 2008;23:721–725.

27. Carriero D, Fabrizi F, Uriel A *et al*. Treatment of dialysis patients with chronic hepatitis C using pegylated-interferon and low dose ribavirin. *International Journal of Artificial Organs* 2008;31:295–302.

12 Management of HCV in patients with a renal transplant

Richard Marley, Janet Dearden

Department of Hepatology, The Royal London Hospital, London, UK

> **LEARNING POINTS**
>
> - HCV infection reduces both graft and patient survival in recipients of renal transplants.
>
> - Progression of liver disease after renal transplantation is unpredictable, but liver disease remains a major cause of death.
>
> - New-onset diabetes and renal lesions are both common after transplantation in patients infected with HCV.
>
> - Historically, antiviral therapy has been avoided after renal transplantation due to risks of precipitating graft rejection. Recent small studies have challenged this dogma.

Background

The prevalence of antibodies against hepatitis C virus (HCV) varies between 10 and 49% in patients who have undergone kidney transplantation. Country, race and mode of dialysis treatment (haemodialysis vs. peritoneal dialysis) all have effects on this figure [1]. The frequency of HCV infection has steadily declined in patients on haemodialysis, and so has the prevalence of HCV infection in transplant recipients. A retrospective study of patients receiving allografts in Spain during 1990, 1994 and 1998 demonstrates a progressive decline in prevalence of HCV antibody, from 29.5% in 1990, 19% in 1994 to 10% in 1998 [2].

Although HCV infection influences graft and patient survival, it should not be considered a contraindication to renal transplantation. Sezer *et al.* [3] showed that the 5-year survival rates for HCV antibody-positive patients are significantly better if they receive a transplant rather than remaining on haemodialysis (85.2% vs. 74.5%).

The KDIGO (Kidney Disease: Improving Global Outcomes) clinical guidelines for HCV infection in chronic kidney disease recommend that antiviral therapy should be given to patients, even with mild fibrosis, who are being considered for renal transplantation [4]. This is discussed in Chapter 11. In those patients for whom therapy is inappropriate or for those who fail to respond to therapy, HCV infection can lead to potential complications in the renal allograft, the development of liver disease, and other health consequences (Table 12.1). These areas are discussed below.

Effect of HCV on graft and patient survival

HCV infection adversely affects both graft and patient survival. The increase in mortality has been demonstrated in many studies and appears to be a delayed effect, occurring between 5 and 10 years after transplantation [1]. Mathurin

TABLE 12.1 HCV-related complications after renal transplantation.

General
Reduced allograft survival
Reduced patient survival

Liver
Liver failure
Hepatocellular carcinoma
Fibrosing cholestatic hepatitis

Renal
Membranoproliferative glomerulonephritis
Membranous glomerulonephritis

Other
New-onset diabetes after transplantation

Clinical Dilemmas in Viral Liver Disease, 1st edition. Edited by Graham R. Foster and K. Rajender Reddy. © 2010 Blackwell Publishing.

et al. [5] published a case–control study in which 10-year survival was significantly lower in HCV-positive recipients compared with HCV-negative ones (63.5% vs. 85.3%; *P* < 0.001). Similarly, delayed effects on graft survival have been shown in many studies. Morales *et al.* [2] compared 10-year graft survival between the two groups and demonstrated a significant reduction (69% vs. 79%; *P* < 0.0001) in the HCV-positive patients.

Effects of transplantation on HCV-related liver disease

The increase in patient mortality is predominantly liver related. Death from hepatocellular carcinoma and liver failure is significantly higher in HCV-positive recipients than HCV-negative recipients [6]. However, the rate of fibrosis progression after transplantation is unclear. One case–control study of serial biopsies has shown a slower rate of progression compared with immunocompetent controls [7], whereas another matched study has shown a faster rate of fibrosis [8]. It is not clear whether different immuno-suppression regimens alter fibrosis progression. With the increasing availability of non-invasive markers of fibrosis, such as liver stiffness measurement, it will become easier to assess fibrosis progression and the risk of end-stage liver disease in individual patients.

The time of acquisition of HCV influences the natural history of the associated liver disease. Although uncommon because of effective screening of donor blood and renal graft, infection at or around the time of renal transplantation is associated with a rapidly progressive course, leading to a 20% rate of hepatic decompensation within 7 years [9]. The reasons behind this observation remain unclear, but might relate to the level of immunosuppression in the early stages of the infection. Another small series describes how the rapidly progressive lesion, fibrosing cholestatic hepatitis, evolves more commonly in patients who acquire the virus at the time of transplantation. In a small series of four such patients, two died of liver failure within 18 months and two survived following dramatic reductions in immunosuppression [10].

Non-hepatic effects of HCV following renal transplantation

In addition to problems with liver disease, patients with HCV infection undergoing renal transplantation are at increased risk of developing new-onset diabetes and have a higher incidence of severe septic episodes. As in non-transplanted patients, renal lesions are common in the allograft and include both acute glomerulopathy and *de novo* immune complex glomerulonephritis.

The rates of new-onset diabetes after transplantation in HCV-positive recipients are threefold to fivefold higher than non-infected recipients, with an overall prevalence of 10–65%. It typically occurs within 3 months of transplantation and the risk of diabetes appears to be higher in tacrolimus-based immunosuppression regimens [4]. New-onset diabetes is a significant risk factor for major cardiac events and mortality following renal transplantation [11].

Renal lesions and proteinuria are more common in allografts in HCV antibody-positive recipients. Membrano-proliferative glomerulonephritis (MPGN) is commonly observed in kidney allograft biopsies in HCV-infected patients with proteinuria and may be associated with both chronic allograft nephropathy and either *de novo* disease or post-transplant recurrence of the native kidney lesion [12]. Thus a biopsy of the kidney allograft should be performed in HCV-infected patients with proteinuria to look for evidence of cryoglobulinaemic MPGN [4], as there might be a role for rituximab therapy in such cases to rescue declining renal function [13].

Antiviral therapy after renal transplantation

Treatment of HCV infection in renal transplant patients remains controversial. Historically, it has been associated with both poor efficacy and an increased risk of interferon-induced allograft rejection. Interferon-based therapy has only been advocated in fibrosing cholestatic hepatitis where the potential benefits of treatment outweigh the risks of graft loss. Trials of monotherapy with ribavirin or amantadine have been disappointing and have shown no benefit in either reducing viral load or halting fibrosis.

The majority of the published studies of interferon-based treatment of HCV infection in renal transplant recipients have been observational studies of small patient numbers. It is therefore difficult to draw conclusions as to both efficacy of therapy and associated risks. A meta-analysis published in 2004 included 12 interferon-based treatment trials comprising 102 patients [14]. Treatment was discontinued in 35% of these patients, the majority due to graft dysfunction, and only 18% of them obtained a sustained virological response (SVR). In nine of the trials, interferon was used as monotherapy, mainly at very high doses. Of the three trials that used interferon and ribavirin, one looked at acute HCV infection acquired at the time of transplantation and the other two included only 23 patients of whom seven had an SVR and three had graft dysfunction.

More recently, two studies have reported treatment with peginterferon and ribavirin, one in combined liver and kidney transplant recipients and the other in renal transplant alone. Both studies are small (six and eight patients respectively), and in both 50% obtained an SVR [15,16]. Appropriate dose reductions and use of growth factors were employed. Most importantly, there was no renal graft rejection reported in any of the patients included, although one patient developed haemolytic–uraemic syndrome.

The timing of treatment is also likely to be of importance. There appears to be an inverse relationship between the median time therapy is commenced after transplant and the risk of precipitating graft rejection. Although later treatment might not be as beneficial to the underlying liver disease or HCV-related renal disease, it may prove safer in terms of allograft survival.

In the future, STAT-C therapy will be valuable in the post-renal transplant patient with HCV infection. The side-effect profiles and interaction with immunosuppressant drugs will be a challenge and lessons are likely to be learned from the management of HCV recurrence after liver transplantation.

References

1. Dominguez-Gil B, Morales JM. Transplantation in the patient with hepatitis C. *Transplant International* 2009 [Epub ahead of print]. **Excellent article comprehensively reviewing the hepatic and non-hepatic manifestations of HCV infection following renal transplantation.** 🔑

2. Morales JM, Domínguez-Gil B, Sanz-Guajardo D *et al.* The influence of hepatitis B and hepatitis C virus infection in the recipient on late renal allograft failure. *Nephrology, Dialysis, Transplantation* 2004;19(Suppl 3):72–76.

3. Sezer S, Ozdemir FN, Akcay A *et al.* Renal transplantation offers a better survival in HCV-infected ESRD patients. *Clinical Transplantation* 2004;18:619–623.

4. Kidney Disease: Improving Global Outcomes. KDIGO clinical practice guidelines for the prevention, diagnosis, evaluation and treatment of hepatitis C in chronic kidney disease. *Kidney International Supplement* 2008;109;S1–S99. **Clear practice guidelines from the KDIGO working group on management of HCV before and after transplantation in patients with chronic kidney disease.** 🔑

5. Mathurin P, Mouquet C, Poynard T *et al.* Impact of hepatitis B and C virus on kidney transplantation outcome. *Hepatology* 1999;29:257–263.

6. Fabrizi F, Martin P, Dixit V *et al.* Hepatitis C virus antibody status and survival after renal transplantation: meta-analysis of observational studies. *American Journal of Transplantation* 2005;5:1452–1461.

7. Alric L, Di Martino V, Selves J *et al.* Long-term impact of renal transplantation on liver fibrosis during hepatitis C virus infection. *Gastroenterology* 2002;123:1494–1499.

8. Zylberberg H, Naplas B, Carnot F *et al.* Severe evolution of chronic hepatitis C in renal transplantation: a case controlled study. *Nephrology, Dialysis, Transplantation* 2002;17:129–133.

9. Toz H, Nart D, Turan I *et al.* The acquisition time of infection: a determinant of the severity of hepatitis C virus-related liver disease in renal transplant patients. *Clinical Transplantation* 2009;23:723–731.

10. Delladetsima JK, Boletis JN, Makris F *et al.* Fibrosing cholestatic hepatitis in renal transplant recipients with hepatitis C virus infection. *Liver Transplantation and Surgery* 1999;5:294–300.

11. Hjelmesaeth J, Hartmann A, Leivestad T *et al.* The impact of early-diagnosed new-onset post-transplantation diabetes mellitus on survival and major cardiac events. *Kidney International* 2006;69:588–595.

12. Morales JM. Hepatitis C virus infection and renal disease after renal transplantation. *Transplantation Proceedings* 2004;36:760–762.

13. Basse G, Ribes D, Kamar N *et al.* Rituximab therapy for mixed cryoglobulinemia in seven renal transplant patients. *Transplantation Proceedings* 2006;38:2308–2310.

14. Fabrizi, F, Lunghi G, Dixit V *et al.* Meta-analysis: anti-viral therapy of hepatitis C virus-related liver disease in renal transplanted patients. *Alimentary Pharmacology and Therapeutics* 2006;24:1413–1422. **The only published meta-analysis of the early trials of antiviral therapy for HCV infection in recipients of renal transplants.** 🔑

15. Pageaux G, Hilleret MN, Garrigues V *et al.* Pegylated interferon-α-based treatments for chronic hepatitis C in renal transplant recipients: an open pilot study. *Transplant International* 2009;22:562–567. **A small but important study demonstrating successful treatment of HCV infection without precipitating graft dysfunction following renal transplantation.** 🔑

16. Schmitz V, Kiessling A, Bahra M *et al.* Peginterferon alfa-2b plus ribavirin for the treatment of hepatitis C recurrence following combined liver and kidney transplantation. *Annals of Transplantation* 2007;12:22–27.

13 Management of HCV in patients with psychiatric comorbidity

Alexander Evans, William Rosenberg

UK Clinical Research Network, University College London, London, UK

LEARNING POINTS

- Psychiatric comorbidity is common in patients with chronic HCV infection.

- Psychiatric side effects are common following treatment with interferon alfa therapy.

- Treatment of patients with HCV infection and psychiatric comorbidity requires an interdisciplinary team approach including hepatologists and psychiatrists.

- Prospective clinical trials suggest that within an interdisciplinary team approach, patients with HCV infection and psychiatric comorbidity can be safely and effectively treated with antiviral regimens including interferon alfa.

- Early intervention with antidepressant therapy may attenuate/prevent major depressive episodes in those patients at risk of worsening depressive symptoms.

Introduction

One of the commonest challenges in the treatment of hepatitis C virus (HCV) infection is the management of a patient presenting with current or a past mental illness. Interferon, with its known neuropsychiatric side effects, is relatively contraindicated in these patients. However, this recommendation is based on the reporting of adverse events, as opposed to robust clinical trials conducted with patients suffering from psychiatric comorbidity. The occurrence of neuropsychiatric illness in patients with HCV infection is common; various studies have reported a prevalence of up to 60% of infected patients having concurrent significant

Clinical Dilemmas in Viral Liver Disease, 1st edition. Edited by Graham R. Foster and K. Rajender Reddy. © 2010 Blackwell Publishing.

psychiatric comorbidity [1,2]. This is perhaps unsurprising in view of the association between HCV and intravenous drug use, which is independently associated with a high prevalence of psychiatric comorbidity [3].

By inference patients with psychiatric illness represent an important reservoir of undiagnosed and untreated HCV infection [4]. One study reported the prevalence of HCV in patients with severe mental illness to be 20%, while half of those studied with both a substance use disorder and a psychiatric disorder were seropositive for exposure to HCV [1,5].

Neuropsychiatric side effects of Interferon therapy

The standard of care for the treatment of chronic HCV infection is currently a combination of peginterferon (alfa-2a or alfa-2b) and ribavirin. Importantly, emerging studies suggest that interferon-alfa will remain a key component of regimens incorporating the new HCV protease inhibitors [7]. The established psychiatric side effects of interferon therapy increase the complexity of treating patients with mental health problems as interferon may both exacerbate underlying symptoms and trigger new ones. Interferon alfa therapy has been associated with many neuropsychiatric side effects, including psychosis, mania, anxiety, suicidal ideation leading to suicide, anhedonia, irritability, cognitive disturbances, delirium and depression [8,9]. Studies estimate that neuropsychiatric side effects occur in up to 50% of all patients receiving treatment with peginterferon alfa and ribavirin, the commonest of which is depression. In trials from which subjects with significant unstable psychiatric illness were excluded, reported rates of depression vary widely, with up to 41% described in some series [6]. Mania and psychosis are much less common side effects of therapy; one study reported that 9 of 121 patients (7%) treated with interferon alfa developed these side effects. Importantly none of these patients had previous psychiatric illness and all their symptoms resolved with cessation of therapy.

Previous guidelines on the treatment of HCV infection in patients with psychiatric comorbidity

In view of these established neuropsychiatric side effects, many hepatologists are understandably reluctant to provide interferon to patients with HCV infection and psychiatric comorbidity despite the relatively high prevalence of HCV in this patient group. Indeed, consensus opinion from both the European Association for the Study of the Liver and the National Institutes of Health (NIH) in the 1990s recommended that pre-existing mental disorders were a contraindication to antiviral therapy [10,11]. However, in the last decade recognition of the prevalence of psychiatric comorbidity in patients with HCV infection allied to a desire to improve access to treatment has led to clinical trials for these patients. This shift in emphasis was reflected in the NIH consensus statement of 2002, which stated that efforts should be made to increase availability of best current treatment for patients with chronic HCV infection who were ineligible for trials because of neuropsychiatric comorbidity [12]. This statement also encouraged collaboration between hepatologists and mental health clinicians as a means of coordinating treatment for these patients.

Treatment of HCV infection in patients with psychiatric illness: the evidence

It is not surprising that there are few clinical trials which prospectively address the issue of interferon alfa therapy in patients with pre-existing psychiatric comorbidity. The published trials are prone to limitations of small sample size, heterogeneous patient populations and high drop-out rates. However two small, prospective, controlled clinical trials published in 2003 and 2007 showed that both controls and patients who had pre-existing psychiatric comorbidity experienced comparable rates of neuropsychiatric side effects, adherence to treatment and sustained virological response (SVR) in response to standard or pegylated interferon and ribavirin [3,13]. These publications also describe no difference in the rates of new major depressive episodes during treatment in these groups. Although these trials recruited relatively small numbers of subjects (81 and 100), they challenge the preconception that patients with psychiatric comorbidity are at increased risk of severe psychiatric side

effects during therapy. The more recent of these trials, which treated patients with peginterferon, used a structured clinical interview for *Diagnostic and Statistical Manual of Mental Disorders* (DSM)-IV diagnoses. The scale used for assessment of depression (Montgomery–Asberg Depression Scale, MADRS) and that used for assessment of psychosis (Brief Psychiatric Rating Scale, BPRS) are among the most widely used and psychometrically validated in psychiatric research, enhancing the impact of this paper. The authors of this study emphasize the importance of an interdisciplinary team approach involving hepatologists and mental health physicians in the successful treatment of these patients. Indeed, in this study all patients had at least three appointments with hepatologists and three appointments with psychiatrists prior to commencing interferon alfa-based therapy. Other studies have highlighted the importance of close collaboration between HCV specialists and psychiatrists in the treatment of patients with significant psychiatric comorbidity [4,14]. While these results support the widening of access to treatment for patients with mental health problems, it is important to note that patients who were deemed to have an unstable psychiatric disorder were appropriately excluded from these trials. Furthermore, those included had been subjected to extensive psychiatric assessment.

Schaefer *et al.* [3] reported an interesting observation which indicated that there was no increased incidence of depression in patients with psychiatric comorbidity compared with controls, during treatment with peginterferon alfa therapy. This was despite higher baseline depression scores in patients with psychiatric comorbidity at treatment initiation. One of the explanations for this was intervention with antidepressants prior to and during treatment, which may prevent or attenuate depressive reactions. This theory is supported by other studies. A stepwise logistic regression performed in this study suggested that genotype alone was predictive of SVR and the factors influencing response did not differ between patients with psychiatric comorbidity and the controls. This study supports other work suggesting that stable treated psychiatric comorbidity does not impact on adherence to antiviral therapy or rates of SVR [15].

Because patients with psychiatric comorbidity are common among those with chronic HCV infection, their treatment is crucial if the incidence and prevalence of HCV are to be reduced long term. It is also clear that patients with psychiatric comorbidity suffer significant morbidity and mortality from their untreated HCV infection, supporting the need for these patients to receive treatment wherever possible.

Conclusions

Psychiatric comorbidity is common in patients with chronic HCV infection. A formal psychiatric assessment requires expertise and is an important step prior to reaching decisions about the management of patients in whom psychiatric illness is suspected. Ideally, all patients with known psychiatric comorbidity should be assessed by a healthcare professional trained in psychiatric assessment who understands both the impact of HCV infection and the benefits and adverse effects of interferon-based regimens. Where this is not possible, hepatologists and clinical nurse specialists should receive training in the assessment of these patients. The use of formal psychometrically validated tools such as MADRS or BPRS will standardize and objectify assessment and improve the ability of the hepatologist to assess these patients.

In the absence of adequate psychiatric assessment and support for these patients, many of them will be excluded from access to interferon alfa-based therapy due to the fear of exacerbating or inducing severe psychiatric illnesses. While this prudent approach is entirely appropriate, it has long-term implications, not just for the individual patients who are denied access to effective treatment but also for the long-term prevalence and incidence of chronic HCV infection in the population. It is clear from the limited evidence available that a significant proportion of patients with chronic HCV infection and stable psychiatric comorbidity can be safely and effectively treated with antiviral regimens that include interferon alfa therapy.

Following assessment, patients who are deemed suitable to receive therapy with interferon should be closely followed through a course of antiviral therapy by both hepatologists and mental health professionals as part of a multidisciplinary team. Specialist clinics for patients with chronic HCV infection should ideally have a named psychiatrist with experience in this field attached to the team with regular scheduled multidisciplinary meetings to discuss the care of individual patients. Through close collaboration between hepatologists and mental health professionals, those patients with stable, well controlled, psychiatric comorbidity can be treated for their HCV infection safely and effectively.

References

1. Rosenberg SD, Swanson JW, Wolford GL *et al*. The five-site health and risk study of blood-borne infections among persons with severe mental illness. *Psychiatric Services* 2003;54:827–835.

2. El-Serag HB, Kunik M, Richardson P *et al*. Psychiatric disorders among veterans with hepatitis C infection. *Gastroenterology* 2002;123:476–482.

3. Schaefer M, Hinzpeter A, Mohmand A *et al*. Hepatitis C treatment in 'difficult-to-treat' psychiatric patients with pegylated interferon-alpha and ribavirin: response and psychiatric side-effects. *Hepatology* 2007;46:991–998. **One of several studies showing that patients with HCV infection and psychiatric problems can be successfully treated.** ⚷

4. Geppert CM, Arora S. Ethical issues in the treatment of hepatitis C. *Clinical Gastroenterology and Hepatology* 2005;3:937–944.

5. Rifai MA, Rosenstein DL. Hepatitis C and psychiatry. *Focus* 2005;3:194–202.

6. Crone C, Gabriel G. Comprehensive review of hepatitis C for psychiatrists: risks, screening, diagnosis, treatment, and interferon-based therapy complications. *Journal of Psychiatric Practice* 2003;9:93–110.

7. Davis GL. New therapies: oral inhibitors and immune modulators. *Clinics in Liver Disease* 2006;10:867–880.

8. Hosoda S, Takimura H, Shibayama M, Kanamura H, Ikeda K, Kumada H. Psychiatric symptoms related to interferon therapy for chronic hepatitis C: clinical features and prognosis. *Psychiatry and Clinical Neurosciences* 2000;54:565–572.

9. Schaefer M. Engelbrecht MA, Gut O *et al*. Interferon alpha (IFNalpha) and psychiatric syndromes: a review. *Progress in Neuropsychopharmacology and Biological Psychiatry* 2002;26:731–746.

10. European Association for the Study of the Liver. EASL consensus statement: International Consensus Conference on Hepatitis C. *Journal of Hepatology* 1999;30:956–961.

11. National Institutes of Health. Management of hepatitis C. *NIH Consensus Statement* 1997;15(3):1–41.

12. National Institutes of Health. National Institutes of Health Consensus Development Conference Statement. Management of hepatitis C 2002. *Hepatology* 2002;36(Suppl):S3–S20.

13. Schaefer M, Schmidt F, Folwaczny C *et al*. Adherence and mental side effects during hepatitis C treatment with interferon alfa and ribavirin in psychiatric risk groups. *Hepatology* 2003;37:443–451.

14. Knott A, Dieperink E, Willenbring ML *et al*. Integrated psychiatric/medical care in a chronic hepatitis C clinic: effect on antiviral treatment evaluation and outcomes. *American Journal of Gastroenterology* 2006;101:2254–2262. **The value of multidisciplinary care for patients with psychiatric comorbidities.** ⚷

15. Dollarhide AW, Loh C, Leckband SG, Endow-Eyer R, Robinson S, Meyer J. Psychiatric comorbidity does not predict interferon treatment completion rates in hepatitis C seropositive veterans. *Journal of Clinical Gastroenterology* 2007;41:322–328.

14 Morbid obesity and HCV: management strategies

Venessa Pattullo[1,2], Jenny Heathcote[1]

[1]Division of Gastroenterology, Toronto Western Hospital, University Health Network, University of Toronto, Toronto, Ontario, Canada
[2]Faculty of Medicine, University of Sydney at Westmead Hospital, Sydney, Australia

Introduction

Obesity – a body mass index (BMI) of 30 kg/m^2 or above – is a global health problem affecting approximately 300 million people worldwide. Obese individuals with a BMI of 40 or above (World Health Organization class III obesity) are considered morbidly obese. The prevalence of obesity in patients with chronic hepatitis C virus (HCV) infection attending a single tertiary hospital setting has been estimated as 28.8% [1]. Obesity promotes hepatic fibrosis and is associated with more rapid progression to advanced liver disease, liver failure and hepatocellular carcinoma [2]. Higher morbidity and mortality is also demonstrated in the obese compared with non-obese in the liver transplant setting [3].

Clinical Dilemmas in Viral Liver Disease, 1st edition. Edited by Graham R. Foster and K. Rajender Reddy. © 2010 Blackwell Publishing.

Obese individuals with HCV infection have a lower chance of clearing the virus with antiviral therapy compared with individuals whose BMI is in the normal range when matched for genotype, viral load and severity of liver disease [4]. Obesity is independently associated with insulin resistance (IR) in patients with HCV infection who do not have cirrhosis. Obesity and IR predispose patients to the non-hepatic health problems of the metabolic syndrome and diabetes, and the latter is also associated with increased risk of hepatocellular carcinoma in HCV infection. The prevalence of IR increases with higher BMI and is associated with reduced response to antiviral therapy [5]. Thus, obesity in patients with HCV infection needs to be addressed prior to the start of antiviral therapy.

Obesity and sustained virological response

Three main mechanisms for the poor response to antiviral therapy in obese individuals with chronic HCV infection have been proposed: the actions of inflammatory cytokines (adipokines), IR and reduced interferon bioavailability.

Inflammatory cytokines

Central obesity is now recognized as a low-grade proinflammatory condition as evidenced by elevation in serum levels of inflammatory cytokines (adipokines) such as tumour necrosis factor (TNF)-α and interleukin (IL)-6 produced by adipocytes and stimulated macrophages and biologically active proteins (or hormones) including adiponectin and leptin. TNF-α induces suppression of SOCS3 (cytokine signaling protein 3), leading to reduced interferon signalling and thereby interfering with treatment efficacy in the obese with chronic HCV infection [6]. There is a reciprocal association between BMI and adiponectin; low levels of adiponectin are associated with reduced HCV-specific CD4 and CD8 T-cell responses in patients with chronic HCV infection [7]. Leptin induces the production of TNF-α, IL-6, IL-12 and IL-1β, stimulating the Th1 immune response through which interferon mediates some of its antiviral effects. Although obese individuals have high circulating leptin levels, it has been suggested that leptin resistance contributes to a failure of Th1 immune stimulation; this may account for the poor response to interferon in obese patients with chronic HCV infection [8].

Insulin resistance

IR is associated with a lower rate of treatment-induced viral clearance [5]. The HCV core and NS5A proteins act directly to mediate IR [9]. Both obesity and HCV-induced TNF-α production induce IR through serine phosphorylation of the insulin receptor substrate subunit of the insulin receptor by c-jun terminal amino kinase (JNK) and IKβ/NF-κB, by acting directly on pancreatic β cells and via increased expression of SOCS3 [10]. While upregulation of SOCS3 may be partly genotype dependent, it may be that all obese individuals with HCV have increased expression of SOCS3 compared with their lean counterparts, accounting for the higher rate of IR and lower rates of sustained virological response (SVR) in obese patients independent of genotype effects [6].

Interferon bioavailability

Absorption of high-molecular-weight compounds occurs predominantly via the lymphatics as opposed to via capillaries [11]. Obese individuals may have impaired lymphatic drainage, potentially resulting in lower drug bioavailability and reduced access to the vascular space.

Management of obesity and insulin resistance in chronic HCV infection

An instinctive approach to the management of HCV infection in the obese is to target weight loss through lifestyle intervention, thereby potentially enhancing response to antiviral therapy. A collateral benefit of such interventions may be a reduction in the prevalence of metabolic syndrome (and therefore vascular risk). Modest weight loss achieved by diet and exercise in overweight patients with chronic HCV infection improves liver histology and fasting insulin levels [12]. An important future direction of the management of HCV in the obese will be to evaluate the rate of SVR following antiviral therapy in obese and/or insulin-resistant subjects with chronic HCV infection who have lost weight and/or reduced their IR through pretreatment lifestyle intervention.

Insulin-sensitizing agents have been used in attempts to both reduce IR and improve response to antiviral therapy; however, limited efficacy and side effects may preclude their use in chronic HCV infection. Metformin successfully improved (but did not reverse) IR in genotype 1 infected patients being treated concurrently with peginterferon and ribavirin, although no significant difference was achieved in rate of negative HCV PCR at weeks 12, 24, 48 or 72 compared with the patients not receiving metformin [13]. Similarly, while pioglitazone (a thiazolidinedione) improved IR in 3 of 5 non-responders to prior antiviral therapy, no patient achieved an early virological response at week 12 [14]. The use of insulin-sensitizing medications to enhance antiviral treatment response cannot be universally recommended at this time, but this is certainly an area for further study.

Management of HCV in the obese

Tailored antiviral therapy using weight-based dosing algorithms may overcome the problems with reduced drug delivery in the morbidly obese. Morbidly obese individuals at the extreme of body weight are unlikely to be receiving equivalent systemic drug dosages (particularly agents distributed outside the vascular space) when compared with their lean counterparts.

Of the two commercially available drugs, peginterferon alfa-2b is dosed by weight because, due to the 12-kDa polyethylene glycol (PEG) moiety, its volume of distribution varies substantially according to body weight; this is in contrast to peginterferon alfa-2a which has a molecular mass of 60 kDa (40-kDa PEG moiety) and therefore a volume of distribution that is not affected by body weight [8]. Both peginterferon alfa-2a and alfa-2b are coadministered with ribavirin, which although already dosed on weight category to some degree, may be limited by the dose that is prepackaged with peginterferon.

A handful of studies have investigated the role of weight-based dosing regimens in patients with HCV (Table 14.1).

TABLE 14.1 Outcomes of studies examining effects of weight-based antiviral therapy dosing on SVR and relapse rates.

Study population	Treatment regimen		Treatment duration	Outcomes (%)	
	Peginterferon (µg/week)	Ribavirin (mg/day)		SVR	Relapse
Shiffman et al. [15] Genotype 1	Peg-IFN alfa-2b 1.5 µg/kg	13.3 mg/kg	48 weeks	29	36
		13.3 mg/kg + EPO		19	40
		15.2 mg/kg + EPO		49*	8*
Jacobson et al. [16] Genotype 1	Peg-IFN alfa-2b 1.5 µg/kg	FD	48 weeks	28.9	29.6
		WBD		34†	23.0
Genotype 2/3	Peg-IFN alfa-2b 1.5 µg/kg	FD	24 or 48 weeks	59.5	8.3
		WBD		61.9‡	7.0
Fried et al. [17] Genotype 1, weight > 85 kg, high viral load (> 8 × 10^6 IU/mL)	Peg-IFN alfa-2a 180 µg	1200 mg	48 weeks	28.3	40
	Peg-IFN alfa-2a 180 µg	1600 mg		31.9	42
	Peg-IFN alfa-2a 270 µg	1200 mg		36.2	46
	Peg-IFN alfa-2a 270 µg	1600 mg		46.8§	19¶

* Significant compared with ribavirin 13.3 mg/kg ± EPO.
† $P = 0.005$ compared with FD group.
‡ $P = 0.252$ compared with FD group.
§ $P = 0.09$ compared with Peg-IFN alfa-2a 180 µg + RBV 1200 mg group.
¶ $P = 0.0001$ compared with Peg-IFN alfa-2a 180 µg + RBV 1200 mg group.
Peg-IFN, peginterferon; EPO, epoetin alfa.
FD, flat dose: 65–125 kg, ribavirin 800 mg.
WBD, weight-based dose: < 65 kg, ribavirin 800 mg; 65–85 kg, ribavirin 1000 mg; 85–105 kg, ribavirin 1200 mg; 105–125 kg, ribavirin 1400 mg.

Peginterferon in combination with high-dose ribavirin (15.2 mg/kg) with the support of epoetin alfa reduced relapse rates and increased the rate of SVR compared with low-dose ribavirin (13.3 mg/kg) [15]. There is evidence to suggest that weight-based dosing of ribavirin (800 mg for patients weighing < 65 kg, 1000 mg for patients weighing 65–85 kg, 1200 mg for patients weighing 85–105 kg, and 1400 mg for patients weighing > 105 but < 125 kg) is safe, and leads to higher rates of SVR compared with flat-dosed ribavirin in genotype 1 (but not genotype 2 or 3) patients [16]. The use of high-dose peginterferon alfa-2a (270 µg weekly) and ribavirin (up to 1600 mg daily) in difficult-to-treat patients with chronic HCV infection (genotype 1, high viral load, weight > 85 kg) leads to a numerically higher SVR rate (47% vs. 28%; $P = 0.09$) and lower relapse rate (19% vs. 40%; $P = 0.0001$) compared with patients receiving standard-dose regimens; however, high-dose treatment was less well tolerated, which may limit its universal use [17]. Most studies evaluating the efficacy of antiviral therapy have only a small proportion of obese patients, and even fewer who are morbidly obese. It is therefore not possible to provide evidence-based algorithms for antiviral therapy in the morbidly obese and it is clearly important that the optimum treatment regimen for these individuals is further investigated. Considerations for further investigation may include (i) the assessment of the safety of higher ribavirin dosages in individuals with body weight in excess of 125 kg and the efficacy of such doses in combination with peginterferon and (ii) drug dosage and/or duration of therapy based on presence and degree of IR.

Summary

Obesity impacts adversely on overall survival in patients chronically infected with HCV, because they are less likely to achieve SVR with antiviral therapy, disease progression is more rapid (therefore risk of liver failure and hepatocellular carcinoma higher) and the outcome following liver transplant is worse. Obesity (and concomitant IR) may be managed with lifestyle interventions (including diet and physical activity) and/or insulin-sensitizing medications; however, the benefits of these approaches remain unproven. Further research is required to develop evidence-based antiviral treatment algorithms for such patients at the extreme of body weight and BMI.

References

1. Chen W, Wong T, Tomlinson G, Krahn M, Heathcote EJ. Prevalence and predictors of obesity among individuals with positive hepatitis C antibody in a tertiary referral clinic. *Journal of Hepatology* 2008;49:711–717.

2. Missiha SB, Ostrowski M, Heathcote EJ. Disease progression in chronic hepatitis C: modifiable and nonmodifiable factors. *Gastroenterology* 2008;134:1699–1714.

3. Thuluvath PJ. Morbid obesity with one or more other serious comorbidities should be a contraindication for liver transplantation. *Liver Transplantation* 2007;13:1627–1629.

4. Bressler BL, Guindi M, Tomlinson G, Heathcote J. High body mass index is an independent risk factor for nonresponse to antiviral treatment in chronic hepatitis C. *Hepatology* 2003;38:639–644. **Impact of BMI on response to therapy in HCV infection.** ⚷

5. Romero-Gomez M, Del Mar Viloria M, Andrade RJ *et al.* Insulin resistance impairs sustained response rate to peginterferon plus ribavirin in chronic hepatitis C patients. *Gastroenterology* 2005;128:636–641.

6. Walsh MJ, Jonsson JR, Richardson MM *et al.* Non-response to antiviral therapy is associated with obesity and increased hepatic expression of suppressor of cytokine signalling 3 (SOCS-3) in patients with chronic hepatitis C, viral genotype 1. *Gut* 2006;55:529–535.

7. Palmer C, Hampartzoumian T, Lloyd A, Zekry A. A novel role for adiponectin in regulating the immune responses in chronic hepatitis C virus infection. *Hepatology* 2008;48:374–384.

8. Charlton MR, Pockros PJ, Harrison SA. Impact of obesity on treatment of chronic hepatitis C. *Hepatology* 2006;43:1177–1186.

9. Shintani Y, Fujie H, Miyoshi H *et al.* Hepatitis C virus infection and diabetes: direct involvement of the virus in the development of insulin resistance. *Gastroenterology* 2004;126:840–848.

10. Harrison SA. Insulin resistance among patients with chronic hepatitis C: etiology and impact on treatment. *Clinical Gastroenterology and Hepatology* 2008;6:864–876.

11. Porter CJ, Charman SA. Lymphatic transport of proteins after subcutaneous administration. *Journal of Pharmaceutical Sciences* 2000;89:297–310.

12. Hickman IJ, Clouston AD, Macdonald GA *et al.* Effect of weight reduction on liver histology and biochemistry in patients with chronic hepatitis C. *Gut* 2002;51:89–94.

13. Romero-Gomez M, Diago M, Andrade RJ *et al.* Treatment of insulin resistance with metformin in naive genotype 1 chronic hepatitis C patients receiving peginterferon alfa-2a plus ribavirin. *Hepatology* 2009;50:1702–1708.

14. Overbeck K, Genne D, Golay A, Negro F. Pioglitazone in chronic hepatitis C not responding to pegylated interferon-alpha and ribavirin. *Journal of Hepatology* 2008;49:295–298.

15. Shiffman ML, Salvatore J, Hubbard S *et al.* Treatment of chronic hepatitis C virus genotype 1 with peginterferon, ribavirin, and epoetin alpha. *Hepatology* 2007;46:371–379.

16. Jacobson IM, Brown RS Jr, Freilich B *et al.* Peginterferon alfa-2b and weight-based or flat-dose ribavirin in chronic hepatitis C patients: a randomized trial. *Hepatology* 2007;46:971–981.

17. Fried MW, Jensen DM, Rodriguez-Torres M *et al.* Improved outcomes in patients with hepatitis C with difficult-to-treat characteristics: randomized study of higher doses of peginterferon alpha-2a and ribavirin. *Hepatology* 2008;48:1033–1043. **Attempts to improve response to therapy by increasing the dose of ribavirin.** ⚷

15 Management of cytopenias during chronic hepatitis C therapy

Alyson N. Fox[1], Vinod K. Rustgi[2]

[1]Hospital of the University of Pennsylvania, Division of Gastroenterology, Philadelphia, Pennsylvania, USA
[2]Georgetown University Medical Center, Fairfax, Virginia, USA

LEARNING POINTS

- Clinical trials suggest that the use of erythrocyte colony-stimulating growth factors is efficacious in raising the haemoglobin concentration, maintaining ribavirin doses and improving quality of life. However, a favourable impact on SVR has not been observed.

- If used, the goal of erythropoietin therapy should be to maintain haemoglobin in the range 11–12 g/dL.

- G-CSF has been shown to be successful at maintaining neutrophil counts and avoiding dose reduction of peginterferon.

- Given the importance of therapy adherence for maximal virological response, it is appropriate to use G-CSF as an adjuvant therapy in order to allow the continuation of antiviral therapy. However, there is no consensus on the absolute neutrophil count (ANC) threshold at which it should be used. An ANC threshold of 500×10^6/L for the use of G-CSF appears reasonable.

- Thrombocytopenia exacerbated by interferon therapy is managed by dose reduction or discontinuation of interferon. The threshold for the platelet count for dose modification or drug discontinuation is dependent on the experience of the treating physician. Bleeding rarely evolves at platelet counts above 20×10^9/L.

- Thrombopoietin receptor agonists may provide an alternative to medication reduction or cessation but are currently under investigational use only.

Clinical Dilemmas in Viral Liver Disease, 1st edition. Edited by Graham R. Foster and K. Rajender Reddy. © 2010 Blackwell Publishing.

Introduction

The current standard of care for the treatment of chronic hepatitis C virus (HCV) infection focuses on treatment with peginterferon alfa and ribavirin [1,2]. The combination of these agents has been shown to produce a sustained virological response (SVR) in up to 46% (range 34–46%) of those with genotype 1 disease [1,2]. It has also been demonstrated that the chances of achieving an early and sustained virological response are higher when patients receive at least 80% of both their total interferon and ribavirin doses for at least 80% of the duration of therapy [3]. Recently, it has been established that maintenance of an adequate ribavirin dose throughout the entire treatment course may be the pivotal factor in the achievement of high SVR rates [4].

Despite this knowledge, our use of combination therapy for HCV infection is often limited by the development of adverse effects. Chief among these are the development of cytopenias, which can lead to dose reductions in up to 25% of patients [1,2].

Anaemia

The anaemia that develops as a result of treatment with peginterferon and ribavirin is primarily mediated by ribavirin-induced haemolysis and secondarily by interferon-mediated bone marrow suppression. The mechanism for ribavirin-induced red cell haemolysis is the accumulation of phosphorylated ribavirin within erythrocytes. The red cells are unable to break down these phosphates, which accumulate and lead to oxidative injury and cell lysis [5]. Concurrent bone marrow suppression from interferon treatment renders the bone marrow unable to compensate for this haemolysis. Typically, the anaemia occurs within the first few weeks of therapy initiation [6].

It has been observed that median haemoglobin decreases seen with combination therapy are around 2.5 g/dL [1,2]. Likewise, significant anaemia (< 10 g/dL) has been reported in up to 13% of patients receiving combination therapy [1]. The package insert from the manufacturer of ribavirin recommends a dose reduction when the haemoglobin falls below 10 g/dL and discontinuation when it falls below 8.5 g/dL [7].

Since the anaemia experienced while on combination therapy is dose dependent, dose reduction of ribavirin has been a primary tactic to combat unacceptable levels of anaemia. However, we know that full-dose therapy yields maximal results. Therefore, the goal of the prescribing practitioner should be to maintain ribavirin and peginterferon doses for the duration of therapy. To that end, the use of recombinant human erythropoietin has been evaluated in the management of anaemia.

Epoetin alfa

Epoetin alfa is a recombinant form of erythropoietin, a glycoprotein normally produced by the kidney to stimulate red blood cell production by the bone marrow. The role of epoetin alfa has been established in the management of anaemia due to chronic renal disease, in HIV patients treated with zidovudine and in those who receive chemotherapy [8]. Given its efficacy in improving anaemia in these populations, its use has been evaluated in the management of anaemia due to treatment with interferon and ribavirin.

The use of epoetin alfa in the management of ribavirin-induced anaemia was evaluated in 185 patients with haemoglobin of 12 g/dL or less undergoing treatment with combination therapy for chronic HCV infection [9]. The authors found that in those patients randomized to receive weekly subcutaneous erythropoietin injections, the average haemoglobin increased by 2.2 g/dL and ribavirin doses were maintained in 88% of patients versus only 60% in the placebo group. Quality of life was also assessed and found to be significantly better in the group receiving epoetin alfa. Clearly, an improved perception of quality of life has implications for therapy maintenance and achievement of an SVR.

Most recently, Shiffman *et al.* [10] examined the rates of virological response in treatment-naive genotype 1 patients treated with combinations of peginterferon alfa-2b, weight-based ribavirin and epoetin at the outset of therapy. While there were no significant differences in rapid, early or end-of-treatment responses between groups, there were differences in the sustained responses. The group treated with high-dose weight-based ribavirin (15.2 mg/kg body weight daily), peginterferon and epoetin alfa had a significantly lower relapse rate and thus improved SVR. These results suggest that although epoetin alfa co-therapy is costly, it may improve our ability to treat with high-dose ribavirin and achieve improved SVR.

Of note, while adjuvant therapy with epoetin alfa is generally thought to be safe, there are potentially serious side effects associated with its use, including a risk of hypertension, thrombosis and cardiovascular events [8]. There have also been reports of pure red cell aplasia in conjunction with antibodies to erythropoietin in those treated for chronic HCV infection [11].

Darbepoetin

Darbepoetin is an erythropoiesis-stimulating protein that has effects similar to those of epoetin alfa. The advantage of darbepoetin is that it has a longer half-life and is given as a weekly or biweekly drug. It is currently indicated in the treatment of anaemia due to chronic renal disease and chemotherapy [12]. A 2007 Phase II study examined the role of darbepoetin and a granulocyte colony-stimulating factor (G-CSF) in the outcome of combination therapy for chronic HCV infection [13]. Darbepoetin was given on a biweekly basis to patients who developed haemoglobin concentrations less than 10.5 g/dL. Of the patients who received darbepoetin, 58% achieved SVR compared with 37% of those who did not receive darbepoetin. These findings suggest that the use of growth factors may improve our ability to maintain treatment, thereby improving rates of SVR. However, other studies have not demonstrated such benefit [14].

Iron supplementation

Iron supplementation in the presence of HCV infection may have harmful effects on hepatic fibrosis [15]. Early studies have even used iron reduction successfully as an adjuvant therapy in the treatment of chronic hepatitis [16]. There are currently no data to support or refute the use of iron supplementation in patients with ribavirin-mediated anaemia who are treated with epoetin alfa. Given its potentially deleterious effects on the course of chronic liver disease, iron supplementation is not recommended.

Recommendations

Currently, recombinant erythropoietin is not approved by the Food and Drug Administration to treat interferon- and ribavirin-mediated anaemia. Clinical trials suggest that the use of erythrocyte colony-stimulating growth factors is efficacious in raising haemoglobin concentrations, maintaining ribavirin doses and improving quality of life. We recommend initiation of epoetin alfa (40 000 units/week) or darbepoetin (3 μg/kg every other week) when haemoglobin levels fall to less than 10 g/dL. If they are used, the goal of erythropoietin therapy should be to maintain haemoglobin in the range 11–12 g/dL. In an effort to maintain these levels, the growth factors should be titrated accordingly.

Neutropenia

The neutropenia that accompanies combination therapy with peginterferon and ribavirin is thought to be due to interferon-related bone marrow toxicity. In the initial trials that established the efficacy of combination therapy, up to 18% of subjects underwent dose reductions of peginterferon for neutropenia [1,2]. Typically, neutropenia occurs within the first 3–4 months of therapy. The perceived concern of neutropenia is the development of infection. In an effort to evaluate the relationship between neutropenia and risk of infection during peginterferon and ribavirin treatment, Antonini et al. [17] found that the incidence of infection was 41 per 100 patient-years and the development of infection had a greater association with age than with severity of neutropenia. These findings suggest that interferon-mediated neutropenia does not confer increased risk of sepsis events. Despite our seeming lack of evidence for infection risk in the presence of interferon-mediated neutropenia, the manufacturers of both peginterferon alfa-2a and alfa-2b recommend dose reductions when the ANC falls below 750×10^6/L and discontinuation when it falls below 500×10^6/L [18,19]. In clinical practice, however, the threshold is 500×10^6/L and this serves as a balance between the maintenance of adequate doses of peginterferon and an acceptable risk of infection.

Filgrastim

Filgrastim (recombinant G-CSF) is indicated in the treatment of neutropenia for those with cancer receiving myelosuppressive chemotherapy or bone marrow transplants, those undergoing peripheral progenitor cell collection and those with severe chronic neutropenia. G-CSF has been studied in patients undergoing therapy for HCV infection in an effort to maintain peginterferon therapy.

Koirala et al. [20] examined a group of 60 patients being treated for HCV infection with peginterferon and ribavirin to determine the appropriate dose of G-CSF and timing of administration. In this observational study, 30 of 60 subjects developed neutropenia (ANC < 1000×10^6/L) and were started on weekly G-CSF. While G-CSF improved neutrophil counts in those who received it, there was no difference in SVR rates between those who were treated and those who were not. An important finding of the study was that most patients who developed neutropenia were successfully maintained on a filgrastim dose of 300 μg per week, although a few patients received higher or lower doses as needed. The only adverse effect reported was bone pain, which was reduced when filgrastim was given 2 days apart from interferon.

Koskinas et al. [21] performed a retrospective study to examine the safety and efficacy of G-CSF in patients undergoing combination therapy and the virological outcomes. They found that adherence to antiviral therapy was 95% in the group treated with G-CSF as compared with 73.1% in the group who underwent standard dose reductions for neutropenia (ANC < 800×10^6/L). Furthermore, none in the G-CSF group required dose reductions. There was no difference in SVR between the group receiving G-CSF and the group that did not. The authors concluded that G-CSF therapy represented an important agent in the maintenance of antiviral dose and has promise in showing improvement in virological outcomes in a randomized controlled trial.

Recommendations

The data regarding the use of G-CSF is limited by the fact that these are observational studies. G-CSF has been shown to be successful at maintaining neutrophil counts and avoiding dose reduction of peginterferon. Given the importance of therapy adherence for maximal virological response, it is appropriate to use G-CSF as adjuvant therapy in order to allow the continuation of antiviral therapy. Likewise, an association between the development of significant infection and level or duration of neutropenia has not been observed in clinical trials [17]. We recommend initiating adjuvant therapy with G-CSF 300 μg weekly when ANC falls below 500×10^6/L. The dose and frequency of G-CSF administration should be tailored to the patient's ANC response.

Thrombocytopenia

Thrombocytopenia is a common complication of chronic HCV infection and is multifactorial in nature. Direct virus-mediated bone marrow inhibition, splenic sequestration of platelets and decreased hepatic production of thrombopoietin are all contributors. Approximately 13% of patients with cirrhosis have moderate thrombocytopenia (platelet count 50–75 × 10^9/L) [22]. Many patients with HCV infection and concurrent thrombocytopenia are excluded from treatment consideration due to the presence of thrombocytopenia, since it can be exacerbated by interferon-related marrow suppression. Typically, thrombocytopenia occurs within the first 8 weeks of therapy and is managed by peginterferon dose reduction or discontinuation depending on the severity of thrombocytopenia. The manufacturers of peginterferon alfa-2a and alfa-2b have recommended dose reduction for platelet counts less than 50 × 10^9/L and discontinuation for platelet counts less than 25 × 10^9/L [18,19].

Interleukin-11

Oprelvekin is a recombinant human interleukin-11 that is approved for the prevention of thrombocytopenia in patients receiving chemotherapy. Oprelvekin was evaluated in 13 patients with platelet counts of less than 100 × 10^9/L undergoing therapy with standard interferon and ribavirin [23]. Although platelet counts improved in those who received oprelvekin, the major side effect of water retention resulted in diuretic use in most patients. Given the serious side-effect profile, the use of oprelvekin is limited.

Eltrombopag

Eltrombopag is an oral thrombopoietin receptor agonist approved for use in refractory idiopathic thrombocytopenic pupura. Given the potential of other haematological growth factors in the management of treatment-related cytopenias, it has been considered in the management of patient with HCV infection. Recently, McHutchison et al. [24] evaluated the efficacy of eltrombopag in patients with HCV-related cirrhosis and platelet counts between 20 and 70 × 10^9/L [24]; 74 patients were randomized to receive placebo or three graduated doses of eltrombopag. At 4 weeks of treatment, 95% of those receiving the highest dose of eltrombopag (75 mg) had platelet counts of 100 × 10^9/L or greater, while none of the patients in the placebo arm had platelet counts greater than 100 × 10^9/L. Antiviral combination therapy was then commenced for 12 weeks in those with platelet counts greater than 70 × 10^9/L. Although platelet counts were found to decrease during antiviral therapy, those receiving concurrent eltrombopag maintained higher platelet counts than those in the placebo group. The authors concluded that therapy with eltrompobag increased platelet counts sufficiently to allow the initiation of combination therapy for HCV infection.

Recommendations

We recommend that thrombocytopenia that is exacerbated by interferon therapy should be managed by dose reduction or discontinuation of interferon. Thrombopoietin receptor agonists may provide an alternative to medication reduction or cessation but are currently under investigational use only.

Summary

Table 15.1 shows the recommended course of action when cytopenias occur during the treatment of HCV infection.

TABLE 15.1 Summary of recommendations.

Anaemia	
Haemoglobin ≤ 10 g/dL	Initiate therapy with epoetin alfa 40 000 units/week or darbepoetin 3 µg/kg biweekly
	Goal: haemoglobin 11–12 g/dL. Titrate growth factors as necessary
Neutropenia	
ANC ≤ 500 × 10^6/L	Initiate therapy with G-CSF 300 µg weekly
	Goal: ANC > 1500 × 10^6/L
Thrombocytopenia	
Platelet count ≤ 50 × 10^9/L	Dose reduction of peginterferon. Some clinicians may not reduce at this dose and continue off-label full dose until platelet count ≤ 25 × 10^9/L
Platelet count ≤ 25 × 10^9/L	Discontinuation of peginterferon

References

1. Manns MP, McHutchison JG, Gordon SC *et al.* Peginterferon alfa-2b plus ribavirin compared with interferon alfa-2b plus ribavirin for initial treatment of chronic hepatitis C: a randomised trial. *Lancet* 2001;358:958–965.
2. Fried MW, Shiffman ML, Reddy KR *et al.* Peginterferon alfa-2a plus ribavirin for chronic hepatitis C virus infection. *New England Journal of Medicine* 2002;347:975–982.
3. McHutchison JG, Manns M, Patel K *et al.* Adherence to combination therapy enhances sustained response in genotype-1-infected patients with chronic hepatitis C. *Gastroenterology* 2002;123:1061–1069.
4. Reddy KR, Shiffman ML, Morgan TR *et al.* Impact of ribavirin dose reductions in hepatitis C virus genotype 1 patients completing peginterferon alfa-2a/ribavirin treatment. *Clinical Gastroenterology and Hepatology* 2007;5:124–129.
5. De Franceschi L, Fattovich G, Turrini F, *et al.* Hemolytic anemia induced by ribavirin therapy in patients with chronic hepatitis C virus infection: role of membrane oxidative damage. *Hepatology* 2000;31:997–1004.
6. Reau N, Hadziyannis SJ, Messinger D, Fried MW, Jensen DM. Early predictors of anemia in patients with hepatitis C genotype 1 treated with peginterferon alfa-2a (40KD) plus ribavirin. *American Journal of Gastroenterology* 2008;103:1981–1988.
7. Roche. Prescribing information. Available at www.rocheusa.com
8. Prescribing information. www.epogen.com, www.procrit.com
9. Afdhal NH, Dieterich DT, Pockros PJ *et al.* Epoetin alfa maintains ribavirin dose in HCV-infected patients: a prospective, double-blind, randomized controlled study. *Gastroenterology* 2004;126:1302–1311. **Highlights role of epoetin alfa in improving anaemia and maintaining ribavirin dose.** ⚷
10. Shiffman ML, Salvatore J, Hubbard S *et al.* Treatment of chronic hepatitis C virus genotype 1 with peginterferon, ribavirin, and epoetin alpha. *Hepatology* 2007;46:371–379.
11. Stravitz RT, Chung H, Sterling RK *et al.* Antibody-mediated pure red cell aplasia due to epoetin alfa during antiviral therapy of chronic hepatitis C. *American Journal of Gastroenterology* 2005;100:1415–1419.
12. Amgen. Prescribing information. Available at www.aranesp.com
13. Younossi ZM, Nader FH, Bai C *et al.* A phase II dose finding study of darbepoetin alpha and filgrastim for the management of anaemia and neutropenia in chronic hepatitis C treatment. *Journal of Viral Hepatitis* 2008;15:370–378.
14. Kugelmas M. Do growth factors improve SVR in chronic HCV-genotype 1 patients treated with peg-interferon and ribavirin? [Abstract]. *Hepatology* 2008;48(Suppl 1):402A.
15. Metwally MA, Zein CO, Zein NN. Clinical significance of hepatic iron deposition and serum iron values in patients with chronic hepatitis C infection. *American Journal of Gastroenterology* 2004;99:286–291.
16. Bonkovsky HL. Iron as a comorbid factor in chronic viral hepatitis. *American Journal of Gastroenterology* 2002;97:1–4.
17. Antonini MG, Babudieri S, Maida I *et al.* Incidence of neutropenia and infections during combination treatment of chronic hepatitis C with pegylated interferon alfa-2a or alfa-2b plus ribavirin. *Infection* 2008;36:250–255.
18. Roche. Prescribing information. Available at www.pegasys.com
19. Schering. Prescribing information. Available at www.pegintron.com
20. Koirala J, Gandotra SD, Rao S *et al.* Granulocyte colony-stimulating factor dosing in pegylated interferon alpha-induced neutropenia and its impact on outcome of anti-HCV therapy. *Journal of Viral Hepatitis* 2007;14:782–787.
21. Koskinas J, Zacharakis G, Sidiropoulos J *et al.* Granulocyte colony stimulating factor in HCV genotype-1 patients who develop Peg-IFN-alpha2b related severe neutropenia: a preliminary report on treatment, safety and efficacy. *Journal of Medical Virology* 2009;81:848–852. **Demonstrates the impact of G-CSF in increasing neutropenia caused by peginterferon.** ⚷
22. Afdhal N, McHutchison J, Brown R *et al.* Thrombocytopenia associated with chronic liver disease. *Journal of Hepatology* 2008;48:1000–1007.
23. Rustgi V. Safety and efficacy of recombinant human IL-11 (oprelvekin) in combination with interferon/ribavirin in hepatitis C patients with thrombocytopenia. *Hepatology* 2002;36(4 Pt 2): 361A [Abstract].
24. McHutchison JG, Dusheiko G, Shiffman ML *et al.* Eltrombopag for thrombocytopenia in patients with cirrhosis associated with hepatitis C. *New England Journal of Medicine* 2007;357:2227–2236. **Proof of concept study demonstrating an improvement in platelet count by the use of thrombopoietin receptor agonist in patients with cirrhosis related thrombocytopenia.** ⚷

16 Management of patients with multiple HCV genotypes

Peter Ferenci

Department of Internal Medicine III, Division of Gastroenterology and Hepatology, Medical University of Vienna, Vienna, Austria

LEARNING POINTS

- Infection with multiple HCV genotypes may occur in up to 10% of infected patients.

- The optimal assay system for identifying multiple genotypes is unclear and current assays may underestimate the prevalence of this disorder.

- The pathological and clinical relevance of infection with multiple genotypes is unclear but there may be compartmentalization of the different strains and a dominant strain may emerge.

- Therapy for patients with multiple genotypes should probably involve a treatment duration dictated by the most treatment-insensitive strain.

Introduction

Hepatitis C virus (HCV) may be divided into at least six major genotypes and more than 30 subtypes according to the phylogenies of available HCV sequences [1]. Moreover, even in patients infected with a single HCV subtype, HCV circulates as a group of variants with up to 10% nucleotide sequence difference, termed quasi-species. Perhaps due to the lack of protective immunity, superinfection by different HCV isolates in patients with chronic HCV is clinically observed, particularly in individuals at very high risk for infection, such as injection drug users, patients on haemodialysis and patients who received multiple blood transfusions in the era before HCV screening of blood

Clinical Dilemmas in Viral Liver Disease, 1st edition. Edited by Graham R. Foster and K. Rajender Reddy. © 2010 Blackwell Publishing.

donors was introduced. Multiple infection by different HCV genotypes may be of great clinicopathological interest.

Extent of the problem

The extent of infection with multiple different subtypes/genotypes of HCV simultaneously in a given individual is controversial. Basically there are two different scenarios that may result in the presence of more than one genotype: superinfection by another genotype of a patient already infected with a single genotype [2] or co-infection with multiple genotypes.

The results of studies about frequency and clinical implications of co-infections are conflicting, possibly due to problems associated with testing for HCV genotype and subtypes. Using serological methods it has been shown that patients infected with a single genotype of HCV may experience transient or occult superinfection with different genotypes of HCV [3]. Today, the most commonly used genotyping test is the line probe assay, which explores changes in the 5′ untranslated region (5′-UTR). Using this testing methodology, multiple HCV genotypes were detected in 10.8% of HCV monoinfected patients [4] and in 5% of HCV/HIV co-infected patients [5]. In the latter group, the presence of multiple HCV genotypes was associated with faster HIV progression. However, it should be noted that the 5′-UTR genotyping approach is not necessarily the most appropriate way to identify infection with multiple genotypes. One consistent error in conventional 5′-UTR-based assays is between subtypes 1a and 1b; about 20% of subtype 1a isolates may be misclassified as subtype 1b due to differences in only a single nucleotide [6,7]. Thus more accurate tests have to be used to ensure that multiple infections with different viral strains are detected.

One attractive explanation for the persistence of multiple different genotypes of HCV is that the different genotypes may persist in different viral reservoirs. Extensive distribution of HCV genomes throughout non-hepatic reservoirs has been described, and some evidence supports the hypothesis that different HCV variants may acquire specific tropism for hepatic versus non-hepatic reservoirs. However, the issue remains controversial, and one of the major limitations in reaching consensus about this aspect of HCV virology is that there are many technical approaches described for assessing HCV genotype [8].

Clinical implications of infection with multiple genotypes

The clinical implications of infection with multiple HCV genotypes are unknown and the clinical trials completed so far have almost invariably excluded such patients, leading to difficulties in assessing the impact of infection with multiple genotypes on treatment response. The setting of liver transplantation where both recipient and donor are infected with different HCV strains provides an interesting scenario for studying host–virus and virus–virus interactions, although the immunosuppression used to prevent rejection of the transplanted liver may modify the nature of the interactions. In six HCV-positive liver donor–recipient pairs, serial serum samples were collected at multiple time points. At each time point, HCV genotype was determined by restriction fragment length polymorphism analysis and phylogenetic analysis. Furthermore, three full-length HCV isolates at the earliest time points after liver transplantation were selectively sequenced, including both 5′ and 3′ ends. Detailed genetic analyses showed that only one strain of HCV could be identified at each time point in all six cases. Recipient HCV strains took over in three cases, whereas donor HCV strains dominated after liver transplantation in the remaining patients. In all six cases studied, no genetic recombination was detected among HCV quasi-species or between donor and recipient HCV strains [9]. Similar observations have been made by others [10] and these suggest that in multiply infected patients one viral sequence will dominate.

A French study [11] investigated 119 patients with previously untreated chronic HCV infection. The internal ribosomal entry site (IRES) of HCV RNA was amplified and compared between plasma and peripheral blood mononuclear cells (PBMCs) by means of single-strand conformational polymorphism (SSCP) analysis, line-probe assay and cloning sequencing. The IRES SSCP patterns differed between plasma and PBMCs in 54 (48%) of 113 assessable patients; 24% of these patients were co-infected by two HCV types or subtypes, only one of which was detectable in PBMCs ($N = 25$) or in plasma ($N = 2$). SSCP-defined compartmentalization was more frequent in former drug users than in others, and less frequent in patients with genotype 1 HCV in plasma. Patients co-infected by two or more HCV variants were more likely to experience a sustained virological response to peginterferon/ribavirin combination therapy. In contrast, a large study in HCV patients from Alaska did not confirm the presence of compartmentalization. A large proportion of mixed-genotype and switching-genotype patterns generated by 5′-UTR analysis were not reproducible using the heteroduplex mobility analysis approach [8].

Summary

Infections with multiple HCV genotypes may occur in some patients, but technical issues regarding optimal test procedures have to be resolved before the clinical implications of this condition can be assessed. Some studies indicate that the presence of multiple genotypes has important implications for choosing therapeutic regimens but this has not been universally accepted. In clinical practice the dominance of one viral genotype will usually ensure that only one viral strain is detected but it is prudent to ensure that a recent genotyping result is used to determine treatment duration as reinfection (or reactivation) of other strains may lead to a change in the dominant genotype over time. In patients who relapse following therapy, many clinicians repeat the viral genotyping assessment to ensure that activation is with the dominant pretreatment strain.

References

1. Robertson B, Myers G, Howard C *et al.* Classification, nomenclature, and database evelopment for hepatitis C virus (HCV) and related viruses: proposals for standardization. *Archives of Virology* 1998;143:2493–2501.

2. Aberle JH, Formann E, Steindl-Munda P *et al.* Prospective study of viral clearance and CD4(+) T-cell response in acute hepatitis C primary infection and reinfection. *Journal of Clinical Virology* 2006;36:24–31.

3. Toyoda H, Fukuda Y, Hayakawa T *et al.* Presence of multiple genotype-specific antibodies in patients with persistent infection with hepatitis C virus (HCV) of a single genotype:

evidence for transient or occult superinfection with HCV of different genotypes. *American Journal of Gastroenterology* 1999;94:2230–2236. **Prevalence of multiple genotypic infections.** 🔑

4. Giannini C, Giannelli F, Monti M *et al.* Prevalence of mixed infection by different hepatitis C virus genotypes in patients with hepatitis C virus-related chronic liver disease. *Journal of Laboratory and Clinical Medicine* 1999;134: 68–73.

5. van Asten L, Prins M. Infection with concurrent multiple hepatitis C virus genotypes is associated with faster HIV disease progression. *AIDS* 2004;18:2319–2324.

6. Cantaloube J-F, Laperche S, Gallian P, Bouchardeau F, de Lamballerie X, de Micco P. Analysis of the 5′ noncoding region versus the NS5b region in genotyping hepatitis C virus isolates from blood donors in France. *Journal of Clinical Microbiology* 2006;44:2051–2056.

7. Chen Z, Weck KE. Hepatitis C virus genotyping: interrogation of the 5′ untranslated region cannot accurately distinguish genotypes 1a and 1b. *Journal of Clinical Microbiology* 2002;40:3127–3134.

8. Li H, Thomassen LV, Majid A *et al.* Investigation of putative multisubtype hepatitis C virus infections in vivo by heteroduplex mobility analysis of core/envelope subgenomes. *Journal of Virology* 2008;82:7524–7532.

9. Fan X, Lang DM, Xu Y *et al.* Liver transplantation with hepatitis C virus-infected graft: interaction between donor and recipient viral strains. *Hepatology* 2003;38:25–33. **Study examining the emergence of different genotyopes during transplantation in patients infected with differing HCV genotypes.** 🔑

10. Vargas HE, Laskus T, Wang L *et al.* Outcome of liver transplantation in hepatitis C virus-infected patients who received hepatitis C virus-infected grafts. *Gastroenterology* 1999;117:149–153.

11. Di Liberto G, Roque-Afonso AM, Kara R *et al.* Clinical and therapeutic implications of hepatitis C virus compartmentalization. *Gastroenterology* 2006;131:76–84.

17 HCV and injecting drug users: how do we approach them?

Olav Dalgard

Medical Department, Oslo University Hospital Rikshospitalet, Oslo, Norway

LEARNING POINTS

- Chronic infection with HCV is common in those who use illicit drugs.

- Illicit drug users may be categorized as regular users, those who are stable on opiate replacement therapy, or as past injectors. Each phase of activity is unstable and many drug users oscillate between the different stages.

- Uptake of antiviral therapy is low in active injectors and in those who are stable on opiate replacement therapy. However, successful therapy has been achieved, particularly in the latter group, and case-by-case assessment is required.

- Treatment in past injectors is common and usually associated with excellent compliance and success rates.

Introduction

Hepatitis C virus (HCV) infection is hyperendemic among injecting drug users. Within a few years of starting drugs, the majority will be exposed to the virus and approximately 50% will develop chronic HCV infection sooner or later [1]. The main route of transmission is obviously sharing of needles but HCV is probably also transmitted within the drug-user community by other routes including sharing of cookers (used to heat the drugs and dissolve them) and cotton filters (used for filtration to remove contaminating material from the drugs) [2].

Chronic HCV infection is a slowly progressive disease and few develop symptoms before they are in their sixth decade [2]. Considering the difficulties in delivering HCV treatment, it seems reasonable to ask whether injecting drug users be

Clinical Dilemmas in Viral Liver Disease, 1st edition. Edited by Graham R. Foster and K. Rajender Reddy. © 2010 Blackwell Publishing.

offered this? In my view the answer is yes. The natural history of injecting drug use frequently manifests as a lifelong history of dependency, with individuals moving between active drug use, maintenance treatment and abstinence of variable duration [3]. In other words, in a great numbers of HCV patients the drug dependency will always be there and HCV infection will have to be dealt with within this frame. It is also important to note that the response to HCV treatment is strongly associated with the age of the patient. In fact for every decade treatment is postponed, the chance of obtaining a sustained virological response (SVR) will decrease by approximately 10% [4]. Therefore, in injecting drug users with an indication for HCV therapy, treatment should be delivered as soon as possible and during any phase of drug addiction.

This chapter reviews some of the experience gathered so far on providing HCV care to injecting drug users.

The problems

There are several challenges that have to be understood and dealt with before effective HCV care can be provided to this patient group.

1 Treatment uptake: even though there are numerous drug users in need of HCV therapy, only a minority are treated. Why this is the case and how we should reach the unreachable is unclear.
2 Adherence: it is still unclear whether drug users who start HCV treatment are less likely to adhere to treatment. If so, we need to develop strategies that allow us to help drug users to adhere to therapy.
3 Side effects of HCV treatment are numerous and sometimes even dangerous. It is unclear how best these can be safely managed within the context of drug dependency.
4 Relapse to drug use: it is unknown whether there is an increased risk of relapse to drug use in patients who are

currently abstinent or on maintenance therapy when HCV treatment is delivered.

5 Reinfection: even though HCV may be successfully treated in drug use, it may be futile due to a high risk of reinfection.

Approaches to therapy during different phases of addiction

Phase 1: active drug use

Active injecting drug users are difficult to reach. In Oslo we performed an epidemiological study among users of the needle exchange programme within the city [5]. Drug users willingly took part in the study and 420 were tested for anti-HCV and HCV RNA in serum. HCV RNA was detectable in 200 and these received a letter with information about the disease they had contracted and an invitation to come to the outpatient clinic at a local hospital for further diagnostics and eventually treatment. Only four of the 200 showed up: two were treated and one achieved SVR. In Amsterdam a stronger effort has been made to reach this patient group [6]. A project has been developed with a committed nurse, a hepatologist and a specialist on maintenance treatment in the team. The cohort of active drug users in this study comprise 466 persons, among whom 125 have been diagnosed with chronic HCV infection. In the last report from this project 13 have started treatment. This study illustrates that even with major efforts only 10% of injectors access HCV treatment in this population. Better results were recently reported from London. In this study a community-based treatment programme was established and antiviral therapy was offered to all drug users who wanted it [7]. Of the 441 patients who were known to be HCV RNA positive and who attended the specialist addiction services in the area, 58 started treatment and 50% achieved SVR. Neither active drug use nor homelessness was associated with low adherence. In Seattle, a cohort of active drug users were followed regularly with HCV testing. Those who became HCV RNA positive were offered HCV treatment in the acute phase. In 21 patients such treatment was started but only four completed therapy. SVR was obtained in three patients. Unfortunately, two of these were soon reinfected (Wang AASLD 2005).

Phase 2: maintenance treatment

HCV treatment uptake among methadone users has not been well documented, but in this phase of drug dependency it also appears to be low. For example, in Oslo all methadone users with an indication for HCV treatment were offered treatment if HCV RNA was detectable and alanine aminotransferase was elevated and no contraindication was evident [8]. An indication for treatment was found in 180 patients but only 18 started treatment. However, when treatment is started, methadone users seem to adhere well to HCV treatment. In a German trial that included 50 patients stable on methadone and 50 controls infected through drug use but abstinent and without maintenance treatment for 5 years, it was found that 75% of methadone users adhered to therapy with peginterferon alfa and ribavirin compared with 85% of controls [9]. In both methadone users and controls, those who did not comply with treatment almost always stopped treatment within the first 4 weeks of treatment. The SVR rates were 21% in cases and 28% in controls ($P = 0.16$).

Side effects are common during treatment with interferon and ribavirin. Psychiatric side effects including psychosis and serious depression may be induced and suicides have occurred. Drug addiction and psychiatric diseases often coexist and it is therefore a concern that pre-existing psychiatric disease may be seriously exacerbated during interferon treatment. In the German trial, 15 of 50 treated methadone users and 10 of 50 controls started treatment with antidepressive drugs during HCV treatment [9]. Thus, the incidence of depression was high and awareness of the problem is mandatory. Patients with ongoing moderate or grave depression should not start interferon treatment and close contact should be maintained during HCV treatment for patients belonging to this vulnerable group. In several centres, directly observed therapy is administered to injecting drug users by weekly injection of peginterferon, enabling the necessary contact between health provider and patient.

It is conceivable that the side effects and perhaps even the exposure to needles increases the risk of patients on maintenance treatment relapsing to injecting drug use. However, in the German trial no case of relapse during treatment or during the 6-month follow-up period was recorded [9]. In another German study at a detox center, HCV treatment was introduced immediately after methadone [10]. Among the 50 enrolled unstable methadone users, 25 soon relapsed to drug use and three later stated that the relapse was connected to the HCV treatment. SVR had been obtained in 18 patients, and at follow-up 33 months later two were most probably reinfected. The incidence of reinfection was 0–4 per 100 person-years of follow-up [11].

Phase 3: abstinence

It is probably during abstinence that most drug dependents seek HCV treatment. Treatment uptake in these patients is difficult to estimate but is probably not very different from that for HCV patients in general. It was recently calculated that treatment uptake in most of Europe ranged from 5 to 15% [11].

In a Scandinavian treatment trial, 432 patients with genotype 2 or 3 infection were included [12]. Previous frequent drug use was reported by half of the patients included in the study. Approximately 80% took more than 80% of both drugs more than 80% of the prescribed time. The rate of adherence was independent of whether the patient was a former regular drug user or not. Relapse to drug use was observed in 15 of 186 former regular users and death due to overdose occurred in two of these. In another study by our group we performed a follow-up 5 years after HCV treatment to abstinent drug users [13]. We found that 9 of 27 sustained responders had relapsed to drug use and that one had been reinfected with HCV.

Conclusion

HCV is endemic among injecting drug users. When HCV treatment is indicated, treatment should be provided as soon as possible. Drug dependency often oscillates between three phases: active drug use, maintenance treatment, and abstinence. Treatment uptake is low among active drug users and reinfection may occur. Active drug users who seek treatment for HCV should be considered for therapy on an individual basis. Treatment uptake is probably also low among those on maintenance treatment. These are patients who may be reached and efforts should be made to increase HCV treatment uptake in this group. HCV treatment should preferably be postponed until the patient is stabilized on maintenance treatment. This phase often provides the opportunity to deliver directly observed therapy. Treatment to abstinent drug users is as effective as in non-drug users. Relapse to drug use may occur, but reinfection is a rare event. Psychatric illnesses are common among the drug dependent and high awareness of psychiatric side effects during HCV treatment is important.

References

1. Roy K, Hay G, Andragetti R, Taylor A, Goldberg D, Wiessing L. Monitoring hepatitis C virus infection among injecting drug users in the European Union: a review of the literature. *Epidemiology and Infection* 2002;129:577–585. **Overview of HCV infection in injecting drug users in Europe.** ⚷

2. Hagan H, Thiede H, Weiss NS, Hopkins SG, Duchin JS, Alexander ER. Sharing of drug preparation equipment as a risk factor for hepatitis C. *American Journal of Public Health* 2001;91:42–46.

3. Hser YI, Hoffman V, Grella CE, Anglin MD. A 33-year follow-up of narcotics addicts. *Archives of General Psychiatry* 2001;58:503–508.

4. Foster GR, Fried MW, Hadziyannis SJ, Messinger D, Freivogel K, Weiland O. Prediction of sustained virological response in chronic hepatitis C patients treated with peg-interferon alfa-2a (40KD) and ribavirin. *Scandinavian Journal of Gastroenterology* 2007;42:247–255.

5. Dalgard O, Egeland A, Ervik R, Vilimas K, Skaug K, Steen TW. [Risk factors for HCV transmission among injecting drug users in Oslo.] *Tidsskrift for den Norske Lægeforening* 2009;129:101–104.

6. Lindenburg KW, Schinkel K, Jansen J *et al.* Hepatitis C screening and treatment among drug users in Amsterdam: interim results of the inclusion procedure in the Dutch C project. *Hepatology* 2006;44:A370.

7. Wilkinson M, Crawford V, Tippet A *et al.* Community based treatment for chronic hepatitis C in drug users: high rates of compliance with therapy despite on-going drug use (HCV in drug users). *Alimentary Pharmacology and Therapeutics* 2008 [Epub ahead of print].

8. Krook AL, Stokka D, Heger B, Nygaard E. Hepatitis C treatment of opioid dependants receiving maintenance treatment: results of a Norwegian pilot study. *European Addiction Research* 2007;13:216–221.

9. Mauss S, Berger F, Goelz J, Jacob B, Schmutz G. A prospective controlled study of interferon-based therapy of chronic hepatitis C in patients on methadone maintenance. *Hepatology* 2004;40:120–124.

10. Backmund M, Meyer K, Von Zielonka M, Eichenlaub D. Treatment of hepatitis C infection in injection drug users. *Hepatology* 2001;34:188–193.

11. Backmund M, Meyer K, Edlin BR. Infrequent reinfection after successful treatment for hepatitis C virus infection in injection drug users. *Clinical Infectious Diseases* 2004;39:1540–1543. **Reinfection rates in successfully treated injecting drug users.** ⚷

12. Dalgard O, Bjoro K, Ring-Larsen H *et al.* Pegylated interferon alfa and ribavirin for 14 versus 24 weeks in patients with hepatitis C virus genotype 2 or 3 and rapid virological response. *Hepatology* 2008;47:35–42.

13. Dalgard O, Bjoro K, Hellum K *et al.* Treatment of chronic hepatitis C in injecting drug users: 5 years' follow-up. *European Addiction Research* 2002;8:45–49.

14. Wang C, Cook L, Krows M *et al.* Randomized trial of pegylated interferon for the treatment of acute HCV in Seattle Injection Drug users. *Hepatology* 2005;42:673A.

18 HCV with and without autoimmune features: how do you sort them out and manage?

M. Shadab Siddiqui, Steven L. Flamm

Northwestern Feinberg School of Medicine

LEARNING POINTS

- Antiviral therapy for HCV comprises peginterferon alfa and ribavirin, which are thought to have immunostimulatory activities.

- Medical therapy of autoimmune hepatitis is with immunosuppressive medications.

- Autoantibody positivity (ANA, SMA, anti-LKM1), which is central to the diagnosis of autoimmune hepatitis, is also common in the setting of chronic HCV.

- In general, ANA or SMA positivity in the setting of HCV does not affect disease progression or response to antiviral therapy.

- Occasionally, chronic HCV with autoimmune features may be present. Since antiviral therapy with immunostimulatory medications can exacerbate underlying immune processes, it is important to identify these patients. High-titre ANA or SMA positivity, unusually highly elevated liver enzymes and liver biopsy suggestive of autoimmune hepatitis should heighten suspicion of chronic HCV with autoimmune features.

- In general, antiviral therapy of HCV should proceed in the usual fashion in the setting of ANA or SMA positivity; however, if HCV with autoimmune features is suspected, antiviral therapy with interferon alfa-based medical regimens should be deferred.

Clinical Dilemmas in Viral Liver Disease, 1st edition. Edited by Graham R. Foster and K. Rajender Reddy. © 2010 Blackwell Publishing.

Introduction

Hepatitis C virus (HCV) is a linear single-stranded RNA virus of the *Flaviviridae* family that was first identified in 1980 as the major causal agent of non-A, non-B hepatitis. It is estimated that there are 170 million people infected worldwide with HCV, with a global prevalence of 3% [1]. Approximately 30% of patients with chronic disease will develop cirrhosis over an estimated 20-year period. Almost all afflicted patients have histological hepatitis, although there are no pathognomonic features for HCV. Findings include focal areas of necrosis, periportal necrosis, chronic inflammation and fibrosis. Steatosis is also common. Peginterferon alfa-2a or alfa-2b in combination with ribavirin comprise the standard treatment regimen for HCV. Although the precise mechanisms of action are unclear, peginterferon is thought to have immunostimulatory activities.

Conversely, autoimmune hepatitis (AIH) is a progressive chronic inflammatory hepatitis of uncertain aetiology. It has been identified throughout the world. The clinical presentation is wide, ranging from asymptomatic disease to chronic non-specific symptoms such as fatigue. Patients may present with complications of cirrhosis. Alternatively, severe acute hepatitis may be observed. There is no single definitive diagnostic test that confirms the diagnosis; however, serological tests are important including antinuclear antibody (ANA), smooth muscle antibody (SMA) and anti-LKM1. Liver biopsy is vital to the diagnosis. Findings may include periportal necrosis, periportal plasma cell infiltration and fibrosis. It is important to accurately diagnose this condition as it is responsive to immunosuppressive therapy.

Chronic HCV infection is associated with several immuno-logical abnormalities, such as production of autoantibodies and cryoglobulins [2]. Although some of the immunological disorders, such as mixed cryoglobulinaemia or membrano-proliferative glomerulonephritis, may affect clinical out-come the presence of non-organ-specific antibodies (i.e. ANA, SMA) is of uncertain clinical relevance [3]. When detection of anti-HCV antibodies and HCV RNA became available, the first autoantibodies to be associated with HCV were those recognized as markers of AIH including SMA, ANA and anti-LKM1 [4]. Since then, other autoantibodies including anti-neutrophil cytoplasmic antibody (ANCA), anti-parietal cell antibody, anti-thyroid antibodies and rheumatoid factor have been associated with chronic HCV, although the clinical significance remains unclear [5].

In this chapter, the roles of ANA, SMA and anti-LKM1 are discussed with regard to chronic HCV infection and its link to autoimmune phenomena. Further, the evaluation and management of patients with HCV and autoimmune features are discussed.

Prevalence

There is wide variability in the reported prevalence of autoantibodies in chronic HCV (Table 18.1). This is likely related to the different laboratory techniques used to detect autoantibodies, the titres at which positive results are reported, and geographical and ethnic variations in the populations examined [6]. Studies show that SMA is the most frequently detected autoantibody in HCV, identified in 10–66% of cases. ANA occurs in 7–63% of chronic HCV patients in comparison with 5% of healthy controls [6]. Treatment of HCV with autoimmune features may exacerbate underlying AIH, so resolving the dilemma of

whether or not autoantibody positivity has clinical rele-vance is important [7].

Prevalence of ANA

ANA is an autoantibody directed against various nuclear antigens including DNA, RNA, histones, acidic nuclear proteins, or complexes of these molecular elements. In a cross-sectional study of adult naive patients with biopsy-proven chronic HCV from South America, the incidence of ANA positivity was 9.4% when an ANA titre of 1 : 80 was considered positive [2]. A similar study from the UK documented an incidence of 5.6% when an ANA titre of either 1 : 32 or 1 : 40 was considered positive [6]. Furthermore, the presence of ANA was associated with increasing age (45 vs. 39 years; $P < 0.001$). In an Italian cohort the incidence of ANA positivity was 7.7% when a titre of 1 : 40 was considered positive [8]. Once again, an association between increasing age and presence of ANA positivity was documented. It is possible that the relationship between age and presence of ANA could represent an ageing immune system that is more prone to developing autoantibodies.

Prevalence of SMA

Much like ANA, the variability of SMA positivity is likely multifactorial. SMA tends to be the most common auto-antibody encountered in chronic HCV infection. In a cohort from the UK, the documented incidence of SMA was 10.8%, whereas it was 12.7–20% in two Italian cohorts [4,6].

Prevalence of ANA and SMA

Whereas the prevalence of autoantibody positivity in the setting of chronic HCV was 23.5% and 17.9% in Italian and British cohorts, respectively, the presence of concomitant

TABLE 18.1 Prevalence of autoantibodies in chronic HCV infection.

Autoantibodies	Prevalence	Comment
ANA	9–38%	Does not alter clinical course or predict response to treatment
Anti-SMA	5–91%	Does not alter clinical course or predict response to treatment
Anti-LKM1	0–10%	Presence of anti-LKM1 may lead to marked elevation in liver function tests in patients with HCV on interferon-based therapy
Rheumatoid factor	8–76%	Significance unclear
Anti-thyroid antibodies	9–20%	May be at increased risk for thyroid dysfunction following interferon-based therapy

antibody positivity was 2.1% in the Italian study and 1.5% in the British study [6,8].

Prevalence of LKM1 antibody

The target of anti-LKM1 is the isoform 2D6 of the cytochrome P450 family, located in the microsomal fraction of the hepatocyte. However, it may also be exposed on the plasma membrane, thus allowing accessibility to immune system effectors [9]. In patients with chronic HCV infection, the overall prevalence of anti-LKM1 in adult populations tends to be low, ranging from 0 to 10% [3,10–12].

Pathophysiology

There is increasing evidence that autoantibody production appears to be due to non-specific activation of the immune system during the course of chronic HCV infection. HCV is capable of infecting lymph nodes, which can then serve as haematopoietic reservoirs [13]. These reservoirs can potentially play a role in viral persistence through mechanisms such as immune escape and viral modulation of the immune system. In fact, the infected phenotypes in lymph nodes are primarily CD20 B cells, which can be responsible for antibody production [13]. It is possible that B cells and other lymphocytes circulating in blood through the liver may become infected. Local infection within the perihepatic lymph nodes may then be established. Alternatively, HCV infection might spread locally through the lymphatics to perihepatic lymph nodes where B cells and other lymphocytes become infected.

It is possible that the interaction between B lymphocytes and HCV leads to B-lymphocyte proliferative disorders, ranging from autoantibody production to lymphoma. In fact, an *in vitro* recombinant form of the major HCV envelope protein E2 binds with high affinity to the CD81 molecule, which is present on not only hepatocytes but also B lymphocytes [14]. On B lymphocytes, CD81 associates with CD21 and CD19, forming a complex that when appropriately engaged can lower the B-cell activation threshold [15]. HCV targets this complex via E2 and perhaps delivers a costimulatory signal to B cells, leading to activation and production of autoantibodies *in vivo*.

Finally, there is an additional hypothesis that molecular mimicry might play an important role in the production of LKM1 autoantibodies. LKM1 autoantibodies specifically target cytochrome P450IID6 (CYP2D6), a protein located on the cytoplasmic side of the endoplasmic reticulum of hepatocytes. It appears that circulating autoantibodies in patients with HCV who are also LKM1 positive are directed against conformational epitopes of CYP2D6, while autoantibodies in type 2 AIH recognize linear epitopes on CYP2D6 [16]. Using immunoprecipitation and absorption with CYP2D6-absorbing resin, molecular mimicry at the B-cell level between CYP2D6 and HCV NS3 and NS5a proteins has been confirmed [16]. This suggests that the antibodies that recognize CYP2D6 also recognize NS3, NS5a, or NS3 and NS5a, leading in some cases to anti-LKM1 positivity. The putative regions of NS3 and NS5a that cross-react with CYP2D6 are highly conserved in HCV genotypes 1a, 1b, 2, 3, 4, 5 and 6, elucidating the possible presence of anti-LKM1 in all genotypes.

Clinical significance of presence of autoantibodies

There is ongoing debate about the clinical significance of autoantibodies in patients with chronic HCV infection. After the identification of HCV as the aetiology of non-A, non-B hepatitis, the first-generation diagnostic antibody tests were insensitive. In fact, the first-generation enzyme immunoassays (EIA-1) were positive in only 80% of patients infected with chronic HCV [17]. This was primarily due to the fact that EIA-1 only used a single target antigen. Not only was EIA-1 insensitive, false-positive results were common. In particular, patients with AIH occasionally had HCV EIA-1 positivity. Unfortunately, some chronic HCV patients with negative EIA-1 but positive autoantibodies were misidentified as having AIH and were erroneously treated with immunosuppressive medications. Alternatively, some AIH patients with false-positive HCV EIA-1 and positive autoantibodies were misidentified and treated with antiviral therapy.

The first-generation HCV EIA-1 test subsequently evolved into a multi-antigen test (EIA-2 and later EIA-3) that not only improved the sensitivity to 97% but also allowed earlier identification of acute infection and fewer false-positive results [18]. This led to the appropriate diagnosis and treatment of chronic HCV and AIH. However, the question of whether the presence of autoantibodies alters disease course or response to treatment of HCV was unresolved.

Multiple epidemiological studies have evaluated this issue, and it appears that the presence of ANA or SMA does not affect disease progression or response to therapy. In a cross-sectional study of 234 patients with biopsy-proven chronic HCV and

ANA positivity, the prevalence of ANA was not associated with fibrosis stage or portal/periportal and lobular necroinflammatory changes [2]. Furthermore, histological features of AIH such as lymphoplasmacytic infiltration and hepatocyte rosettes were not found in ANA-positive patients. The presence of ANA did not influence response to antiviral therapy. The incidence of on-treatment flares in alanine aminotransferase (ALT) was 12%, and the ALT elevations were mild (about two to three times the upper limit of normal). There was no correlation between ALT flares on treatment and ANA positivity [2]. Similarly, in a British cohort of 927 patients, there was no association between total Ishak score, necroinflammatory grade, fibrosis, viral genotype, or liver panel values in patients with chronic HCV infection who were ANA positive, SMA positive, or both [6].

Although the presence of ANA and SMA might reflect epiphenomena, the presence of anti-LKM1 may indicate a propensity towards worsening liver enzyme elevations with interferon-based therapy. In a retrospective study in which 60 patients with chronic HCV infection and anti-LKM1 positivity were compared with age- and sex-matched patients with chronic HCV infection and anti-LKM1 negativity, there was a 7% likelihood of developing severe liver enzyme elevations (10 times the upper limit of normal) on interferon therapy [9]. Interestingly, two patients developed *de novo* anti-LKM1 positivity during a hepatitis flare in the group with anti-LKM1 negativity. Furthermore, of the 22 patients with chronic HCV and anti-LKM1 positivity, anti-LKM1 disappeared in 11 of 12 patients achieving a sustained virological response (SVR) but in only 4 of 10 in non-responders or relapsers. One patient treated with peginterferon did not develop a marked elevation of liver enzymes. It is possible that the pharmacokinetics of different interferon formulations could influence the development of autoimmune phenomena. Continuous stimulation of the immune system with peginterferon could avoid the 'bolus' stimulation of the immune system observed with the non-pegylated formulation, thereby preventing the formation of anti-LKM1. Treatment with proinflammatory interferon may unmask latent type 2 AIH. Of note, none of the patients in these studies had histological, clinical or biochemical features consistent with AIH. Furthermore, treatment of HCV infection led to clinical improvement, and SVR was usually associated with clearance of autoantibodies. This would not be the case if there were an underlying autonomous autoimmune process.

Although ANA or SMA positivity in the setting of confirmed HCV infection usually has no clinical implications, occasionally patients with HCV have high-titre autoantibody positivity. There is little literature regarding this issue and much of the experience is anecdotal. In some of these cases, ANA is elevated for unclear reasons. In other patients, ANA is elevated for other reasons such as lupus erythematosus. Finally, a small number of patients have HCV with an autoimmune component. Such patients tend to have higher liver enzyme elevations than normally encountered with chronic HCV infection. Biopsy may reveal an aggressive histological picture with periportal and lobular inflammation and increased plasma cells. If antiviral therapy is instituted, liver enzymes should be followed closely early in therapy. If liver enzymes rise markedly, it would suggest a possible exacerbation of an autoimmune component of chronic liver disease, and antiviral therapy should be discontinued.

Summary and recommendations

Autoantibody positivity in the setting of chronic HCV infection is common. Alternatively, HCV EIA positivity may be observed as a false-positive result in the setting of AIH. ANA and SMA positivity does not impact on the natural history of HCV, nor does it affect response to antiviral therapy. However, in the setting of high-titre ANA or SMA positivity, an autoimmune component of chronic liver disease must be contemplated. It is important to distinguish these issues prior to commencing medical therapy. Treatment of confirmed HCV with an autoimmune component or AIH with false-positive HCV EIA testing with immunomodulatory interferon alfa-based medical regimens exacerbates the underlying autoimmune process.

In all patients with presumed chronic HCV infection as identified by EIA positivity, HCV must be confirmed by HCV RNA testing prior to commencing antiviral therapy. For patients with confirmed HCV and autoantibody positivity, an autoimmune component must be considered. Since there is little literature on this issue, recommendations are based on experience (Figure 18.1). If autoantibody titre is high (ANA > 1 : 160 or SMA > 1 : 80), especially if liver enzyme elevations are higher than usual (ALT more than eight times upper limit of normal), suspicion of an autoimmune component should be heightened. Liver biopsy should be performed prior to commencing antiviral therapy of HCV. If the biopsy is not suggestive of HCV with autoimmune features, plans for antiviral therapy of HCV should

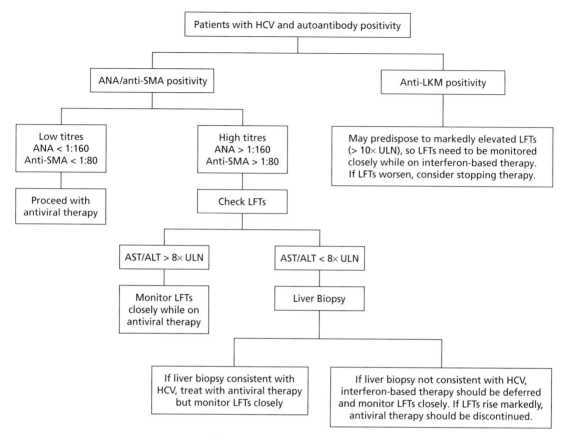

FIG. 18.1 Algorithm for patients with HCV infection and autoantibody positivity. AST/ALT, aspartate aminotransferase/alanine aminotransferase; LFTs, liver function tests; ULN, upper limit of normal.

proceed. However, if the biopsy is suggestive of HCV with autoimmune features, interferon alfa-based medical regimens should be deferred. If HCV therapy is administered, liver enzymes should be followed closely throughout the early weeks of therapy, and if liver enzymes rise markedly antiviral therapy should be discontinued.

References

1. Bandy U. Hepatitis C virus (HCV): a silent epidemic. *Medicine and Health Rhode Island* 1999;82:223–224.

2. Narciso-Schiavon JL, Freire FC, Suarez MM *et al*. Antinuclear antibody positivity in patients with chronic hepatitis C: clinically relevant or an epiphenomenon? *European Journal of Gastroenterology and Hepatology* 2009;21:440–446.

3. Obermarmayer-Straub P, Manns MP. Hepatitis C and D, retroviruses and autoimmune manifestations. *Journal of Autoimmunity* 2001;16:275–285.

4. Zauli D, Cassani F, Bianchi FB. Auto-antibodies in hepatitis C. *Biomedicine and Pharmocotherapy* 1999;53:234–241.

5. Vergani D. Non-organ specific autoantibodies in HCV infection: markers or makers of disease? *Gut* 1999;45:328–329.

6. Williams MJ, Lawson K, Neal R *et al*. Autoantibodies in chronic hepatitis C virus infection and their association with disease profile. *Journal of Viral Hepatitis* 2009;16:325–331. **This is an important trial evaluating the prevalence as well as significance of ANA and anti-SMA in patients with chronic HCV infection. The paper reinforces the view that the prevalence of ANA and anti-SMA is not low and that the presence of these autoantibodies does not alter the natural history of chronic HCV infection or predict outcome to therapy.**

7. Manns MP, Wedemeyer H, Cornberg M. Treating viral hepatitis C: efficacy, side effects, and complications. *Gut* 2006;55:150–159.

8. Squadrito G, Previti M, Lenzi M *et al*. High prevalence of non-organ specific auto-antibodies in hepatitis C virus-infected

cirrhotic patients from southern Italy. *Digestive Diseases and Sciences* 2004;48:349–353.

9. Ferri S, Muratori L, Quarneti C *et al*. Clinical features and effect of antiviral therapy on anti-liver/kidney microsomal antibody type 1 positive chronic hepatitis C. *Journal of Hepatology* 2009;50:1093–1101. **This an important paper that evaluates the prevalence of anti-LKM1 in patients with chronic HCV infection. Furthermore, it shows a possible correlation between high titres of anti-LKM1 in patients with biopsy-proven chronic HCV infection and marked liver enzyme elevation while on interferon therapy.** ☞

10. Cassani F, Cataleta M, Valentini P *et al*. Serum autoantibodies in chronic hepatitis C: comparison with autoimmune hepatitis and impact on the disease profile. *Hepatology* 1997;26:561–566.

11. Reddy KR, Krawitt EL, Homberg JC *et al*. Absence of LKM-1 antibody in hepatitis C viral infection in the United States of America. *Journal of Viral Hepatitis* 1995;2:175–179.

12. Muratori P, Muratori L, Verucchi G *et al*. NOSA in children with chronic hepatitis C: clinical significance and impact on interferon treatment. *Clinical Infectious Diseases* 2003;37:1320–1326.

13. Pal S, Sullivan D, Kim S *et al*. Productive replication of hepatitis C virus in perihepatic lymph nodes in vivo: implications of HCV lymphotrophism. *Gastroenterology* 2006;130:1107–1116.

14. Pileri P, Yasushi Y, Campagnoli S *et al*. Binding of hepatitis C virus to CD81. *Science* 1998;282:938–942. **An important article which showed that the HCV envelope protein E2 is able to bind to CD81 and suggests a possible explanation for how HCV can lead to activation of the immune system and lead to such clinically relevant phenomena as production of autoantibodies and malignancies.** ☞

15. Fearon DT, Carter RH. The CD19/CR2/TAPA-1 complex of B lymphocytes: linking natural to acquired immunity. *Annual Review of Immunology* 1995;13:127–149.

16. Marceau G, Lapierre P, Beland K, Soudeyns H, Alvarez F. LKM1 autoantibodies in chronic hepatitis C infection: a case of molecular mimicry? *Hepatology* 2005;42:675–682.

17. Gretch DR, Lee W, Corey L. Use of aminotransferase, hepatitis C antibody, and hepatitis C polymerase chain reaction RNA assays to establish the diagnosis of hepatitis C virus infection in a diagnostic virology laboratory. *Journal of Clinical Microbiology* 1992;30:2145–2149.

18. Barrera J, Prancis B, Ercilla G *et al*. Improved detection of anti-HCV in post-transfusion hepatitis by a third-generation ELISA. *Vox Sanguinis* 1995;68:15–18.

19 HCV and iron excess: the interaction and how to handle it

Bryan D. Maliken, Kris V. Kowdley

Benaroya Research Institute and Center for Liver Disease, Digestive Disease Institute, Virginia Mason Medical Center, Seattle, Washington, USA

LEARNING POINTS

- On the first visit, measure iron parameters in all patients (serum iron, ferritin, and transferrin-iron saturation) to establish a baseline and determine if iron overload is present.

- Perform *HFE* genotyping in all patients who have transferrin-iron saturation above 45% and/or ferritin greater than 500 ng/mL.

- Iron depletion via phlebotomy is appropriate if hepatic iron stores are increased (> 2+) and if the patient is not a candidate for interferon/ribavirin combination therapy.

- Consider phlebotomy in cirrhotics with increased iron stores to reduce progression and to possibly reduce the risk of hepatocellular carcinoma.

- Iron depletion before the initial round of treatment with interferon/ribavirin combination therapy is not indicated unless the patient has concomitant hereditary haemochromatosis.

Since the initial description in 1992 by Di Bisceglie *et al.* [1], many studies have confirmed that hepatitis C virus (HCV) infection is associated with elevation in serum iron parameters (iron, ferritin, transferrin-iron saturation) compared with non-HCV-infected control subjects. Di Bisceglie *et al.* reported that 36% of patients with chronic HCV infection had elevated serum iron values and increased stainable iron in Kupffer cells and hepatocytes [1]. Similar staining patterns have been noted in subsequent studies and further

Clinical Dilemmas in Viral Liver Disease, 1st edition. Edited by Graham R. Foster and K. Rajender Reddy. © 2010 Blackwell Publishing.

support the assertion that HCV is associated with hepatic iron accumulation in a mixed pattern of deposition [2,3]. Furthermore, patients with chronic HCV infection have markedly raised levels of iron compared to those with cholestatic or autoimmune liver disease [4]. Ferrara *et al.* [5] recently suggested that serum ferritin, an easily measured parameter, might predict therapeutic response at different points during antiviral treatment and may be a marker for disease progression.

Although there are data supporting the premise that hepatic iron deposition may be caused by HCV, it is also possible that increased iron deposition in these patients may be due to coexisting factors such as age, race, gender, body mass index (BMI), HCV genotype, viral load, insulin resistance and alcohol use [6,7]. In particular, African-American race has been found to be a unique contributor to elevated iron indices in the context of HCV infection. A standardized analysis showed that HCV-infected African-Americans with elevated liver enzymes were much more prone to have increased iron stores (odds ratio 17.8) [8]. Although some have proposed that hepatic iron deposition may result from damaged hepatocytes, the overall mechanism of iron accumulation remains uncertain [9]. Regardless of the cause of increased hepatic iron, once present this metal may exacerbate liver injury and hepatic fibrosis via the Fenton reaction, leading to generation of hydroxyl radicals that act on structural macromolecules and DNA [10]. In one study, 8-hydroxy-2′-deoxyguanosine, a marker for DNA damage in the liver, was shown to increase in parallel with hepatic iron stores in HCV-infected patients, suggesting that iron may be implicated in oxidative stress and progression of fibrosis [11].

There are conflicting data regarding the relationship between *HFE* mutations, hepatic iron accumulation and disease severity in chronic HCV infection. Several studies have found a positive relationship between *HFE* mutations and increased liver iron storage [12–17]. However, the relationship between increased hepatic iron and advanced fibrosis has been less clear, with a direct relationship in some studies [13,14,18–20] but not in others [2,21–25]. Some studies have found that both the C282Y and H63D mutations are associated with increased inflammation and fibrosis, whereas others have found a much weaker association with the H63D mutation than the C282Y mutation [13,14,18–20]. We previously found both H63D and C282Y mutations to be associated with more rapid progression of chronic HCV infection after adjustment for duration of disease [13]. Both the H63D and C282Y mutations were strongly associated with advanced fibrosis, with odds ratios of 22 and 30, respectively [13].

It has been well established that iron overload is associated with lower rates of sustained virological response (SVR) to interferon monotherapy [3,26,27]. Following this discovery, studies were conducted to test the effect of pretreatment phlebotomy on SVR in treatment-naive patients [28–32]. Most have shown a trend towards increased SVR [28–31] and improved iron indices and aminotransferase levels [28–32]. A recent meta-analysis of six randomized controlled studies showed a significant difference between the phlebotomy and control groups, with SVR of 27% and 12%, respectively ($P < 0.0001$) [33].

Similar phlebotomy studies were performed in groups of patients who had previously not responded to interferon monotherapy [34–38]. The largest trial, performed by Di Bisceglie *et al.* [34], did not show increased SVR in iron-depleted patients but did show decreased levels of liver injury and improved aminotransferase levels. Many other studies have shown improved aminotransferase levels as well [35–38], but only two studies showed significance for improved SVR [37,38]. Overall, iron depletion prior to interferon monotherapy has been shown to be effective in lowering aminotransferase levels and iron indices, but is inconclusive with regard to change in SVR. Furthermore, the results of these studies is becoming less relevant in current practice as monotherapy has been replaced with interferon/ribavirin combination therapy, which has been shown to have much higher response rates [39].

While pretreatment liver iron concentration can be a predictor of non-response in monotherapy, SVR is generally found to be independent of iron parameters with combination interferon and ribavirin therapy [40–42]. The exception is a study by Fujita *et al.* [43]. These authors measured total iron liver score in 103 HCV-infected patients before and after 24 weeks of combination therapy and found that this variable was the only factor independently associated with non-response to combination therapy ($P = 0.0277$). Most other studies have shown no association between hepatic iron concentration and response to combination therapy [40–42]; two studies suggested that high serum ferritin levels at baseline were associated with non-response [40,44]. In summary, the bulk of the evidence suggests that iron studies and hepatic iron concentration are not likely to predict response to combination therapy; the role of serum ferritin as a predictor of response remains unclear.

Recent work has also examined the relationship between *HFE* mutations and response to combination therapy. Bonkovsky *et al.* [12] recently found in a study of 363 patients that H63D mutations actually predicted a higher rate of SVR ($P = 0.009$). There was an inverse relationship between SVR and stainable iron in portal triads and endothelial cells, suggesting that location of hepatic iron may be more important than concentration [12]. In contrast, a smaller study with 34 patients showed that patients with any *HFE* mutations were much less likely to achieve SVR [45]. Based on the data discussed previously on *HFE* mutations, it is clear that combination therapy is still the best choice for antiviral treatment as its effectiveness is widely considered independent of iron status.

Combination therapy is clearly proven to be the most effective therapy in most HCV-infected patients; however, there are situations where alternative therapies may be recommended, such as for non-responders and patients who cannot tolerate antiviral therapy. In these situations, it is reasonable to recommend iron reduction with phlebotomy because has been shown to significantly reduce alanine aminotransferase (ALT) levels in both treatment-naive and non-responder patients [28–32,34–38,46–48]. This significant improvement in biochemical response highlights the possibility that if iron depletion is maintained, it may help to reduce hepatic necroinflammation and fibrosis in HCV-infected patients. It may also be worthwhile for patients to consider an iron-restricted diet as Tandon *et al.* [49] have shown that treatment with a 50% reduced iron rice/casein-based diet was associated with significant improvement serum iron, transferrin-iron saturation, and serum ALT levels.

It is possible that iron depletion via phlebotomy has the potential to prevent DNA damage and development of hepatocellular carcinoma (HCC). Several studies have demonstrated that hepatic iron concentration is a relevant factor in the development of HCC [50]. Cirrhosis associated with HCV infection is accompanied by increased hepatic iron concentration [51]. Markers of iron-related damage such as 8-hydroxy-2'-deoxyguanosine are commonly found to be elevated in patients with HCC, especially those with increased hepatic iron, and are thought to indicate a hepatic microenvironment prone to cancerous mutations [52].

Chapoutot *et al.* [50] compared patients with chronic HCV infection, cirrhosis and HCC with non-cancer patients and found that iron deposits were much more common in the HCC group than in controls ($P = 0.0056$). *HFE* mutations have been examined in patients with chronic HCV infection and HCC, with some studies showing positive correlations [53,54] and others negative correlations [55,56]. It is possible that iron may be the more pertinent risk factor for HCC in chronic HCV infection rather than *HFE* mutations.

TABLE 19.1 Summary of studies examining iron depletion therapy for treatment-naive patients and prior non-responders.

Reference	No. of patients		IFN treatment	SVR		End biochemical response/sustained biochemical response	
	IFN	Iron reduction + IFN		IFN	Iron reduction + IFN	IFN	Iron reduction + IFN
Treatment-naive patients							
Carlo *et al.* [31]	40	43	6 MU IFN alfa-2b or alfa-2a q.o.d. for 6 months; then 3 MU q.o.d. for 6 months	6 (15%)	12 (28%)	18 (45%)/ 8 (20%)	24 (56%)/ 16 (37%)
Fargion *et al.* [29]	57	57	6 MU IFN alfa-2b t.i.w. for 4 months; then 3 MU t.i.w. for 8 months	9 (15.8%)	16 (28.1%)	18 (32%)/ 15 (26%)	24 (42%)/ 19 (33%)
Fong *et al.* [30]	21	17	3 MU IFN alfa-2b t.i.w. for 6 months	1 (4.8%)	5 (29.4%)	6 (29%)/ 1 (4.8%)	9 (53%)/ 6 (35%)
Fontana *et al.* [28]	42	40	3 MU IFN alfa-2b t.i.w. for 6 months	3 (7%)	7 (17%)	20 (48%)/ 6 (14%)	25 (63%)/ 11 (28%)
Piperno *et al.* [32]	61	20	3 MU IFN alfa-2b t.i.w. for 12 months	NR	0 (0%)	21 (34%)/ 13 (21%)	1 (5%)/ 1 (5%)
Non-responders							
Alexander *et al.* [36]	18	N/A	NR	NR	N/A	4 (22%)	N/A
Di Bisceglie *et al.* [34]	32*	32	Not known	0 (0%)	0 (0%)	ALT (×ULN) 2.9 to 1.9†	ALT (×ULN) 3.2 to 1.6†
Guyader *et al.* [35]	No control	Pilot study $N = 15$	Min. 3 MU IFN t.i.w. for 3 months	N/A	0 (0%)	N/A	2 (13%)/0
Tsai *et al.* [37]	No control	20	3 MU IFN alfa-2b t.i.w. for 6 months	N/A	3/20 (15%)	N/A	11 (55%)/ 10 (50%)
Van Thiel	15	15	5 MU IFN daily for 6 months	2 (13%)	9 (60%)	2 (13%)	7 (47%)

* Iron reduction only (not IFN alone).
† 24 weeks after treatment.
ALT, alanine aminotransferase; IFN, interferon; NR, not reported; t.i.w., three times weekly; ULN upper limit of normal.

Studies investigating iron depletion therapy to prevent HCC have shown some promising results. Kato *et al.* [57] performed iron depletion therapy in 35 patients with moderate to severe liver fibrosis who were likely to progress to HCC and who could not tolerate, or previously failed to respond to, antiviral therapy. Treatment was associated with significantly decreased ALT levels and was independently associated with a lowered risk of HCC ($P = 0.0337$) compared with controls. Additional studies are needed to further explore the effect of iron depletion for this indication.

In summary, increased serum and hepatic iron levels are relatively common in patients with chronic HCV infection. We postulate that the combined action of HCV and the generation of free radicals by iron may increase the rate at which liver damage occurs, especially in patients with cirrhosis when iron accumulation may occur at a faster rate. *HFE* mutations are associated with increased hepatic iron concentration. Although hepatic iron content predicts a negative response to interferon monotherapy, the SVR with interferon/ribavirin combination therapy is independent of iron markers. Treatment with iron depletion is associated with the prevention of hepatic complications in patients with hereditary haemochromatosis but has not been shown to clearly improve prognosis in chronic HCV infection except in pilot studies (Table 19.1). Phlebotomy may be considered for patients with advanced fibrosis and increased iron stores (> 2+ stainable iron on biopsy with or without serum ferritin > 500 ng/mL) who are either not candidates for combination therapy or have been previously treated without success; in such patients, iron depletion is associated with improved serum liver biochemical tests and may slow progression of liver disease and reduce the risk of HCC.

References

1. Di Bisceglie AM, Axiotis CA, Hoofnagle JH, Bacon BR. Measurements of iron status in patients with chronic hepatitis. *Gastroenterology* 1992;102:2108–2113.
2. Hezode C, Cazeneuve C, Coue O *et al.* Liver iron accumulation in patients with chronic active hepatitis C: prevalence and role of hemochromatosis gene mutations and relationship with hepatic histological lesions. *Journal of Hepatology* 1999;31:979–984.
3. Olynyk JK, Reddy KR, Di Bisceglie AM *et al.* Hepatic iron concentration as a predictor of response to interferon alfa therapy in chronic hepatitis C. *Gastroenterology* 1995;108:1104–1109. **One of many papers assessing the impact of hepatic iron on treatment response.** 🔑🔒
4. Cotler SJ, Bronner MP, Press RD *et al.* End-stage liver disease without hemochromatosis associated with elevated hepatic iron index. *Journal of Hepatology* 1998;29:257–262.
5. Ferrara F, Ventura P, Guido M *et al.* Serum ferritin as a predictor of treatment outcome in patients with chronic hepatitis C. *American Journal of Gastroenterology* 2009;104:605–616.
6. Alter MJ, Kruszon-Moran D, Nainan OV *et al.* The prevalence of hepatitis C virus infection in the United States, 1988 through 1994. *New England Journal of Medicine* 1999;341:556–562.
7. Ioannou GN, Dominitz JA, Weiss NS, Heagerty PJ, Kowdley KV. Racial differences in the relationship between hepatitis C infection and iron stores. *Hepatology* 2003;37:795–801.
8. Nelson JE, Kowdley KV. Iron and hepatitis C. *Current Hepatitis Reports* 2004;3:140–147.
9. Bonkovsky HL, Banner BF, Rothman AL. Iron and chronic viral hepatitis. *Hepatology* 1997;25:759–768.
10. Thursz M. Iron, haemochromatosis and thalassaemia as risk factors for fibrosis in hepatitis C virus infection. *Gut* 2007;56:613–614.
11. Fujita N, Sugimoto R, Ma N *et al.* Comparison of hepatic oxidative DNA damage in patients with chronic hepatitis B and C. *Journal of Viral Hepatitis* 2008;15:498–507.
12. Bonkovsky HL, Naishadham D, Lambreacht RW *et al.* Roles of iron and HFE mutations on severity and response to therapy during retreatment of advanced chronic hepatitis C. *Gastroenterology* 2006;131:1440–1451.
13. Tung BY, Emond MJ, Bronner MP, Raaka SD, Cotler SJ, Kowdley KV. Hepatitis C, iron status, and disease severity: relationship with HFE mutations. *Gastroenterology* 2003;124:318–326. **Importance of *HFE* mutations in iron overload.** 🔑🔒
14. Smith BC, Grove J, Guzail MA *et al.* Heterozygosity for hereditary hemochromatosis is associated with more fibrosis in chronic hepatitis C. *Hepatology* 1998;27:1695–1699.
15. Piperno A, Vergani A, Malosio D *et al.* Hepatic iron overload in patients with chronic viral hepatitis: role of HFE gene mutations. *Hepatology* 1998;28:1105–1109.
16. Bonkovsky HL, Troy N, McNeal K *et al.* Iron and HFE or TfR1 mutations as comorbid factors for development and progression of chronic hepatitis C. *Journal of Hepatology* 2002;37:848–854.
17. Kazemi-Shirazi L, Datz C, Maier-Dobersberger T *et al.* The relation of iron status and hemochromatosis gene mutations in patients with chronic hepatitis C. *Gastroenterology* 1999;116:127–134.
18. Erhardt A, Maschner-Olberg A, Mellenthin C *et al.* HFE mutations and chronic hepatitis C: H63D and C282Y heterozygosity are independent risk factors for liver fibrosis and cirrhosis. *Journal of Hepatology* 2003;38:335–342.

19. Gehrke S, Stremmel W, Mathes I, Riedel H, Bents K, Kallinowski B. Hemochromatosis and transferrin receptor gene polymorphisms in chronic hepatitis C: impact on iron status, liver injury, and HCV genotype. *Journal of Molecular Medicine* 2003;81:780–787.

20. Geier A, Reugels M, Weiskirchen R *et al.* Common heterozygous hemochromatosis gene mutations are risk factors for inflammation and fibrosis in chronic hepatitis C. *Liver International* 2004;24:285–294.

21. Thorburn D, Curry G, Spooner R *et al.* The role of iron and haemochromatosis gene mutations in the progression of liver disease in chronic hepatitis C. *Gut* 2002;50:248–252.

22. Lal P, Fernandes H, Koneru B, Albanese E, Hameed M. C282Y mutation and hepatic iron status in hepatitis C and cryptogenic cirrhosis. *Archives of Pathology and Laboratory Medicine* 2000;124:1632–1635.

23. Pirisi M, Scott CA, Avellini C *et al.* Iron deposition and progression of disease in chronic hepatitis C. *American Journal of Clinical Pathology* 2000;113:546–554.

24. Negro F, Samii K, Rubbia-Brandt L *et al.* Hemochromatosis gene mutations in chronic hepatitis C patients with and without liver siderosis. *Journal of Medical Virology* 2000;60:21–27.

25. Hohler T, Leininger S, Kohler HH, Schirmacher P, Galle PR. Heterozygosity for the hemochromatosis gene in liver diseases: prevalence and effects on liver histology. *Liver* 2000;20:482–486.

26. Van Thiel DH, Friedlander L, Fagiuoli S, Wright HI, Irish W, Gavaler JS. Response to interferon α therapy is influenced by the iron content of the liver. *Journal of Hepatology* 1994;20:410–415.

27. Ikura Y, Morimoto H, Johmura H, Fukui M, Sakurai M. Relationship between hepatic iron deposits and response to interferon in chronic hepatitis C. *American Journal of Gastroenterology* 1996;91:1367–1373.

28. Fontana RJ, Israel J, LeClair P *et al.* Iron reduction before and during interferon therapy of chronic hepatitis C: results of a multicenter, randomized, controlled trial. *Hepatology* 2000;31:730–736.

29. Fargion S, Fracanzani AL, Rossini A *et al.* Iron reduction and sustained response to interferon-α therapy in patients with chronic hepatitis C: results of an Italian multicenter randomized study. *American Journal of Gastroenterology* 2002;97:1204–1210.

30. Fong TL, Han SH, Tsai NC *et al.* A pilot randomized, controlled trial of the effect of iron depletion on long-term response to alpha-interferon in patients with chronic hepatitis C. *Journal of Hepatology* 1998;28:369–374.

31. Carlo C, Daniela P, Giancarlo C. Iron depletion and response to interferon in chronic hepatitis C. *Hepato-Gastroenterology* 2003;50:1467–1471.

32. Piperno A, Sampietro M, D'Alba R *et al.* Iron stores, response to α-interferon therapy, and effects of iron depletion in chronic hepatitis C. *Liver* 1996;16:248–254.

33. Desai TK, Jamil LH, Balasubramaniam M, Koff R, Bonkovsky HL. Phlebotomy improves therapeutic response to interferon in patients with chronic hepatitis C: a meta-analysis of six prospective randomized controlled trials. *Digestive Diseases and Sciences* 2008;53:815–822.

34. Di Bisceglie AM, Bonkovsky HL, Chopra S *et al.* Iron reduction as an adjuvant to interferon therapy in patients with chronic hepatitis C who have previously not responded to interferon: a multicenter, prospective, randomized, controlled trial. *Hepatology* 2000;32:135–138.

35. Guyader D, Boucher E, Andre P *et al.* A pilot study of iron depletion as adjuvant therapy in chronic hepatitis C patients not responding to interferon. *American Journal of Gastroenterology* 1999;94:1696–1698.

36. Alexander J, Tung BY, Croghan A, Kowdley KV. Effect of iron depletion on serum markers of fibrogenesis, oxidative stress and serum liver enzymes in chronic hepatitis C: results of a pilot study. *Liver International* 2007;27:268–273.

37. Tsai N, Zuckerman E, Han SH, Goad K, Redeker AG, Fong TL. Effect of iron depletion on long-term response to interferon-alpha in patients with chronic hepatitis C who previously did not respond to interferon therapy. *American Journal of Gastroenterology* 1997;92:1831–1834.

38. Van Thiel DH, Friedlander L, Molloy PJ *et al.* Retreatment of hepatitis C interferon non-responders with larger doses of interferon with and without phlebotomy. *Hepato-Gastroenterology* 1996;43:1557–1561.

39. McHutchinson JG, Gordon SC, Schiff ER *et al.* Interferon alfa-2b alone or in combination with ribavirin as initial treatment for chronic hepatitis C. *New England Journal of Medicine* 1998;339:1485–1492.

40. Hofer H, Osterreicher C, Jessner W *et al.* Hepatic iron concentration does not predict response to standard and pegylated-IFN/ribavirin therapy in patients with chronic hepatitis C. *Journal of Hepatology* 2004;40:1018–1022.

41. Rulyak SJ, Eng SC, Patel K, McHutchinson JG, Gordon SC, Kowdley K. Relationships between hepatic iron content and virologic response in chronic hepatitis C patients treated with interferon and ribavirin. *American Journal of Gastroenterology* 2005;100:332–337.

42. Pianko S, McHutchison JG, Gordon SC *et al.* Hepatic iron concentration does not influence response to therapy with interferon plus ribavirin in chronic HCV infection. *Journal of Interferon and Cytokine Research* 2002;22:483–489.

43. Fujita N, Sugimotot R, Urawa N *et al.* Hepatic iron accumulation is associated with disease progression and resistance to interferon/ribavirin combination therapy in chronic

hepatitis C. *Journal of Gastroenterology and Hepatology* 2007;22:1886–1893.

44. Distante S, Bjoro K, Hellum KB *et al.* Raised serum ferritin predicts non-response to interferon and ribavirin treatment in patients with chronic hepatitis C infection. *Liver* 2002;22:269–275.

45. Coelho-Borges S, Cheinquer H, Cheinquer N, Krug L, Ashton-Prollo P. HFE gene mutations prevent sustained virological response to interferon plus ribavirin in chronic hepatitis C patients with serum markers of iron overload. *American Journal of Gastroenterology* 2002;97:1570–1572.

46. Yano M, Hayashi H, Yoshioka K *et al.* A significant reduction in serum alanine aminotransferase levels after 3-month iron reduction therapy for chronic hepatitis C: a multicenter, prospective, randomized, controlled trial in Japan. *Journal of Gastroenterology* 2004;39:570–574.

47. Yano M, Hayashi H, Wakusawa S *et al.* Long term effects of phlebotomy on biochemical and histological parameters of chronic hepatitis C. *American Journal of Gastroenterology* 2002;97:133–137.

48. Kawamura Y, Akuta N, Sezaki H *et al.* Determinants of serum ALT normalization after phlebotomy in patients with chronic hepatitis C infection. *Journal of Gastroenterology* 2005;40:901–906.

49. Tandon N, Thaker V, Kumkar R, Guptan C, Sarin SK. Beneficial influence of an indigenous low-iron diet on serum indicators of iron status in patients with chronic liver disease. *British Journal of Nutrition* 2000;83:235–239.

50. Chapoutot C, Esslimani M, Joomaye Z *et al.* Liver iron excess in patients with hepatocellular carcinoma developed on viral C cirrhosis. *Gut* 2000;46:711–714.

51. Casaril M, Stanzial AM, Tognella P *et al.* Role of iron load on fibrogenesis in chronic hepatitis C. *Hepato-Gastroenterology* 2000;47:220–225.

52. Kato J, Kobune M, Nakamura T *et al.* Normalization of elevated hepatic 8-hydroxy-2′-deoxyguanosine levels in chronic hepatitis C patients by phlebotomy and low iron diet. *Cancer Research* 2001;61:8697–8702.

53. Cauza E, Peck-Radosavljevic M, Ulrich-Pur H *et al.* Mutations of the HFE gene in patients with hepatocellular carcinoma. *American Journal of Gastroenterology* 2003;98:442–447.

54. Hellerbrand C, Poppl A, Hartmann A, Scholmerich J, Lock G. HFE C282Y heterozygosity in hepatocellular carcinoma: evidence for an increased prevalence. *Clinical Gastroenterology and Hepatology* 2003;1:279–284.

55. Lauret E, Rodriguez M, Gonzalez S *et al.* HFE gene mutations in alcoholic and virus-related cirrhotic patients with hepatocellular carcinoma. *American Journal of Gastroenterology* 2002;97:1016–1021.

56. Boige V, Castera L, de Roux N *et al.* Lack of association between HFE gene mutations and hepatocellular carcinoma in patients with cirrhosis. *Gut* 2003;52:1178–1181.

57. Kato J, Miyanishi K, Kobune M *et al.* Long-term phlebotomy with low-iron diet therapy lowers risk of development of hepatocellular carcinoma from chronic hepatitis C. *Journal of Gastroenterology* 2007;42:830–836.

20 Management of patients with genotype 3 chronic hepatitis C: can we change the duration of therapy?

Alessandra Mangia, Valeria Piazzolla, Angelo Andriulli

Division of Gastroenterology, Hospital Casa Sollievo della Sofferenza, IRCCS, San Giovanni Rotondo, Foggia, Italy

LEARNING POINTS

- Patients infected with genotype 2 and 3 HCV have traditionally been regarded as easy to treat. However, patients with genotype 3 HCV have significantly lower response rates than those with genotype 2 infection.

- The on-treatment virological response is increasingly being used to determine the duration of therapy in patients with chronic HCV infection and a rapid virological response (i.e. undetectable HCV RNA after 4 weeks of therapy) is increasingly used as an indication that a shortened duration of therapy may be effective.

- In the absence of a rapid virological response, patients with genotype 3 HCV respond less well than genotype 2 HCV patients, even after 24 weeks of treatment.

- In patients with genotype 3 HCV, advanced liver damage is the most important adverse factor associated with the absence of a rapid virological response and/or of a poor response after an early response and the reduced response occurs in patients treated with either a short or a standard courses of antiviral therapy.

Introduction

Hepatitis C virus (HCV) is an RNA virus that belongs to the family *Flaviviridae*. Six HCV genotypes exist, of which genotypes 1, 2, 3 and 4 are most prevalent worldwide. While the evaluation of HCV genotypes bears no relevance

Clinical Dilemmas in Viral Liver Disease, 1st edition. Edited by Graham R. Foster and K. Rajender Reddy. © 2010 Blackwell Publishing.

to the natural history of the liver disease, they impact substantially on both duration and outcome of antiviral therapy. Compared with genotype 1, genotype 2 and 3 infections are consistently associated with significantly higher rates of sustained virological response (SVR) [1]. When genotypes 2 and 3 are considered as a homogeneous group, combination therapy with peginterferon and ribavirin for 24 weeks achieves SVR in over 70–80% of individuals, whereas no more than 40% of patients harbouring genotype 1 infection will clear the virus after a 48 week-course of treatment [1–3]. It has become common to label the former patients 'easy to treat' and the latter 'difficult to treat'. The difference in SVR rates between these two categories of patients is most likely a reflection of viral kinetics in response to interferon therapy, as viral decline among genotype 2 and 3 infections is up to eight times faster than that of genotype 1 [4].

In this chapter we discuss the emerging data on virological response in patients with genotype 3 HCV infection as reported in different studies of either standard or abbreviated courses of treatment, and discuss the most appropriate course of therapy and investigate whether host-related factors play a role in the response rate to antiviral therapy in patients with this viral genotype.

Genotype 3 infections are not easy to treat

It has been ascertained only recently that even among easy-to-treat patients, there are differences in SVR rates that can be achieved after the standard course of 24 weeks of combination therapy (Table 20.1). The original observation of a lower rate of SVR in patients harbouring genotype 3

TABLE 20.1 Sustained virological response rates in patients infected with HCV genotype 3 and genotype 2 after 24 weeks of therapy with peginterferon and ribavirin.

Reference	Year	HCV-3		HCV-2	
		No. of patients	SVR (%)	No. of patients	SVR (%)
Zeuzem et al. [5]	2004	183	79	42	93
Mangia et al. [23]	2005	17	76	53	76
Shiffman et al. [13]	2007	369	66	356	75
Powis et al. [21]	2008	81	75	276	85
Jacobson et al. [18]	2006	251	60	298	71
Bailey et al. [19]	2007	389	72	276	79
Aghemo et al. [20]	2008	71	75	136	78
Lagging et al. [29]	2008	139	78	49	82

HCV in comparison with those with genotype 2 infection [5] has been substantially corroborated by the finding of a recent meta-analysis: after pooling the results from eight studies that enrolled 2275 patients treated for 24 weeks with peginterferon and ribavirin, the SVR rate among genotype 3 infections was 74% (95% CI 71.8–77.1) compared with 68% (95% CI 66.0–71.2) among those patients with genotype 2, and the pooled estimate of the difference was 8.7% (95% CI 5.1–12.3) [6].

Unfavourable predictors of SVR in genotype 3 infection

A clear biological explanation for the difference in SVR rates between genotype 2 and genotype 3 infection is not obvious. There are several conceivable claims for the reduced response in genotype 3 infection, including higher amount of liver steatosis, insulin resistance, advanced fibrosis and cirrhosis, and high viral load.

Liver steatosis

The 2.5-fold increased prevalence of steatosis in patients with HCV infection suggests that the virus *per se* promotes the accumulation of fat into the hepatocyte [7]. The association seems to prevail in patients infected with genotype 3. Studies *in vitro* and in experimental animals indicate the existence of 'steatogenic' sequences in the core region of the HCV genome. Of note, the core protein from HCV genotype 3 isolates is about threefold more efficient than the corresponding protein from genotype 1 isolates in reducing lipid export from the hepatocyte and inducing lipid accumulation in the liver [8]. The degree of hepatic fat accumulation correlates with levels of HCV replication and the condition may be reversed by inducing a sustained viral clearance with a course of antiviral therapy [9]. Given the documented impact of steatosis on the development of liver fibrosis [10], it may be hypothesized that the poorer outcome of antiviral therapy in genotype 3-infected patients may, at least in part, be explained by a higher frequency of patients with steatosis [10,11]. A complementary explanation would refer to experimental data showing that liver steatosis increases hepatic expression of factors that inhibit interferon signalling, such as SOCS-3, a mechanism that, at least in patients with genotype 1 infection, would reduce the likelihood of achieving SVR with appropriate therapy [12]. However, the association between liver steatosis and poor outcome of therapy among genotype 3-infected patients has not been uniformly reported [13].

Insulin resistance and obesity

Liver steatosis has been recently outlined as a further component of the metabolic syndrome [14]. As it may aggravate liver disease in patients with genotype 3 and those with other genotypes, it is still uncertain whether hepatic fibrosis is a secondary effect of steatosis or a direct consequence of insulin resistance. Recent investigation would indicate that virus-induced steatosis as seen in genotype 3-infected patients did not appear to directly promote hepatic fibrogenesis, a condition that was primarily correlated with insulin resistance [15].

Insulin resistance may also explain the lower rates of SVR observed in obese patients. Patients with a body mass index (BMI) above 30 kg/m^2 constitute one of the most difficult-to-treat groups, independently of the infecting genotype, as shown in several studies [16]. In African-Americans, BMI, diabetes and hypertension are all associated with the lower response rate to antiviral therapy [17]. In HCV genotype 3 patients, SVR rates were lower and declined with increasing weight when a flat dose of 800 mg ribavirin daily was used in combination with peginterferon [18].

Advanced fibrosis/cirrhosis

One of the most consistently reported observations when treating patients with chronic HCV infection is the hypo-responsiveness that characterizes patients with cirrhosis compared with those who do not have cirrhosis after completion of the standard 24 weeks of treatment.

Among 241 HCV genotype 3 patients enrolled in the 24-week treatment arm of the Accelerate study, SVR was observed in 49% of cirrhotic patients and in 70% of those without cirrhosis [13]. An inverse correlation between stage of fibrosis and SVR in genotype 3 infection was also reported in the observational POWeR study, where SVR rates were 47% and 68% in patients with or without liver cirrhosis, respectively [19]. In an Italian retrospective observational study including patients treated with peginterferon and ribavirin combination, only 6 of 17 (35%) patients with genotype 3 and cirrhosis were responders after 24 weeks of therapy compared with 62 of 74 (84%) non-cirrhotic patients. These disappointing results were attributed to the high rate of relapse in cirrhotic patients (57% vs. only 9% in non-cirrhotic patients) [20]. Similar results were reported in a Canadian study, where only 2 of 12 (37%) genotype 3-infected patients with advanced fibrosis were responders, as opposed to 7 of 9 (79%) equally staged patients with genotype 2 [21]. Although the validity of the conclusions reached in some of these studies is limited by the small number of patients with cirrhosis enrolled, overall these results confirm that in patients with genotype 3 treated with the standard 24-week course the presence of cirrhosis reduces the likelihood of attaining SVR.

Viral load

The other factor associated with a lower SVR rate in patients with genotype 3 in comparison with genotype 2 is viral load at baseline evaluation. In 185 patients infected with genotype 3, after a standard course of peginterferon alfa-2b and ribavirin, the occurrence of relapse was associated with both HCV RNA levels at baseline and amount of steatosis [5]. In patients with HCV RNA levels above 600 000 IU/mL enrolled in the large community-based Win-R study, the relapse rate was up to 16%, whereas it was only 6% in patients with HCV RNA levels below this cut-off [18]. However, discordant data were provided in subsequent studies [20,22]. In particular, in 374 patients enrolled in the registration studies of peginterferon alfa-2a and ribavirin, high baseline levels were not associated with lower SVR [22]. After reviewing this issue with a meta-analytical approach, we have found that among high-viraemic patients SVR rate in genotype 2-infected patients was 24.9% higher than the rate in genotype 3-infected patients, while among low-viraemic patients the difference amounted to 7.1%.

Variations on the standard schedule of antiviral therapy: the role of rapid virological response

Treatment guidelines for chronic HCV infection recommend treating patients with genotype 2 and 3 with either of the two peginterferons commercially available in combination with low-dose ribavirin (800 mg daily) for a duration of 24 weeks. Several attempts to further simplify treatment have focused on decreasing the recommended dosages of either peginterferon or ribavirin, and on shortening the duration to 12 or 16 weeks [23–26].

As reported in recent studies, in patients with genotype 2 and 3 who clear the virus by 4 weeks, i.e. who achieve a rapid virological response (RVR), length of treatment might be safely reduced to 16, 14 or even 12 weeks of therapy without compromising SVR rates [23–26]. RVR is now considered as the most valuable tool predicting ultimate SVR in all HCV-infected patients, not only among those with the easy-to-treat genotype. The question whether patients with genotype 3 and RVR respond equally well as those with genotype 2 to an abbreviated course of therapy remains unanswered.

Only a few studies on short courses of antiviral therapy have separately evaluated RVR in patients with genotype 2 and 3; the respective data are reported in Table 20.2. It is of note that after RVR, SVR rates in genotype 2- and 3-infected patients were not different. Of 632 genotype 3 patients, globally evaluated in five studies [13,25–27,29], SVR was observed in 480 (76%) individuals; of 490 genotype 2 patients, SVR was reported in 402 (82%).

TABLE 20.2 Sustained virological response rates in patients with viral clearance at week 4 after starting antiviral therapy: comparison of outcome after a short (12–16 week) course of therapy in HCV genotype 3 and 2.

Reference	Year	HCV-3		HCV-2	
		No. of patients	SVR (%)	No. of patients	SVR (%)
Andriulli et al. [26]	2005	104	91	157	88
von Wagner et al. [25]	2005	51	76	19	79
Shiffman et al. [13]	2007	230	80	230	86
Dalgard et al. [27]	2008	110	75	29	93
Lagging et al. [29]	2008	137	58	55	56

In contrast, in patients without RVR the difference in SVR rates between the two genotypes is much more pronounced. In the combined analysis of Norwegian and Italian patients, only 46% of 50 genotype 3 patients without RVR attained SVR after the standard 24 weeks of therapy, while 73% of 79 genotype 2 patients were long-term responders [26]. Similar figures were also reported in the Accelerate study where only 30 of 109 genotype 3 patients without RVR eventually cleared the virus after 24 weeks (27%) [13]. Together these results suggest that treatment longer than the recommended 24 weeks may be needed in genotype 3 patients in the absence of RVR.

Cirrhosis and RVR in patients treated with a short course of antiviral therapy

In genotype 3 patients with cirrhosis, the results of the clinical trials are concordant in showing reduced rates after an abbreviated course of therapy. This low response rate may be due to a reduced number of patients achieving RVR due to the advanced liver fibrosis. In our studies, only 48% (13 of 27) of patients with severe fibrosis achieved an RVR as compared with 76% (71 of 94) of those with a lower fibrotic score [26]. Our data are in keeping with those attained by von Wagner et al. [25] in a limited number of HCV genotype 3 patients. In contrast, in the recently published North C Trial, high aspartate aminotransferase to platelet ratio index (APRI) score was used as an non-invasive tool to estimate the severity of liver damage; a high APRI score did not predict RVR, as 21% of patients with RVR and 20% of those without had APRI scores above 2 [27]. Therefore, whether genotype 3 patients with advanced liver damage experience

RVR less often than patients with lesser degrees of liver damage requires further clarification in future studies.

A related question in patients with advanced liver fibrosis receiving shortened courses of antiviral therapy is whether, once they achieve RVR, genotype 3-infected patients maintain this response. Of 718 patients treated for 12 weeks on the basis of achievement of RVR in a large Italian cohort, 108 were infected with genotype 3 and 19% had advanced liver damage. A platelet count lower than 140×10^9/L, considered a surrogate marker of advanced liver damage, was an independent predictor of relapse [28], suggesting that in patients with genotype 3 chronic HCV relapse is common in those with advanced fibrosis who achieve RVR.

Conclusions

In conclusion, not all patients with genotype 3 are easy to treat. In patients receiving the recommended 24 weeks of therapy with peginterferon and ribavirin, non-responder patients had significantly more fibrosis and higher BMI. Both these conditions might be consequent on insulin resistance that may be higher in non-responders than in responders, and insulin resistance may be responsible for the reduced SVR rates seen in these patients. Still a matter of debate is the impact of baseline viraemia on the therapeutic outcome. Studies evaluating the early (week 4) RVR have consistently shown that patients failing to achieve RVR status are poor responders to therapy and might need longer than the currently recommended 24 weeks of antiviral treatment. Patients with genotype 3 and rapid viral clearance may be easily treated with shorter courses of treatment, especially those with less advanced fibrosis and normal BMI. It is unknown whether patients with advanced fibrosis and abnormal BMI can respond to a shortened course of therapy and further studies are needed to determine which patients with genotype 3 can safely be treated with shortened courses of antiviral medication.

References

1. Strader DB, Wright T, Thomas DL, Seeff LB. Diagnosis, management and treatment of hepatitis C. *Hepatology* 2004;39:1147–1171.

2. Fried MW, Schiffman ML, Reddy KR et al. Peginterferon alfa2a plus ribavirin for chronic hepatitis C virus infection. *New England Journal of Medicine* 2002;347:975–982.

3. Manns MP, McHutchinson JG, Gordon SC et al. Peginterferon alfa-2b plus ribavirin compared with interferon alfa-2b plus ribavirin for initial treatment of chronic hepatitis C: a randomized trial. *Lancet* 2001;358:958–956.

4. Zeuzem S, Hermann E, Lee JH et al. Viral kinetics in patients with chronic hepatitis C treated with standard or peginterferon alpha 2a. *Gastroenterology* 2001;120:1438–1447.

5. Zeuzem S, Hultcrantz R, Bourliere M et al. Peginterferon alfa-2b plus ribavirin for treatment of chronic hepatitis C in previously untreated patients infected with HCV genotype 2 or 3. *Journal of Hepatology* 2004;40:993–999.

6. Andriulli A, Leandro G, Mangia A, Iacobellis A, Ippolito A, Zeuzem S. Pooled analysis of outcome of antiviral therapy in HCV genotype 2 and 3 patients. *Alimentary Pharmacology and Therapeutics* 2008;28:397–404. **Summary of responses in patients with genotype 2 and 3 HCV. Comprehensive study of factors affecting response in these easy-to-treat genotypes.** 🔑🔖

7. Hourioux C, Patent R, Morin A et al. The genotype 3-specific hepatitis C virus core protein residue phenylalanine 164 increases steatosis in an in vitro cellular model. *Gut* 2007;56:1302–1308.

8. Abid K, Pazienza V, de Gottardi A et al. An in vitro model of hepatitis C virus genotype 3a-associated tryglicerides accumulation. *Journal of Hepatology* 2005;42:744–751.

9. Kumar D, Farrell GC, Fung C, George J. Hepatitis C virus genotype 3 is cytopathic to hepatocytes: reversal of hepatic steatosis after sustained therapeutic response. *Hepatology* 2002;36:1266–1272.

10. Leandro G, Mangia A, Hui J et al. Relationship between steatosis, inflammation, and fibrosis in chronic hepatitis C: a meta-analysis of individual patient data. *Gastroenterology* 2006;130:1346–1362.

11. Westin J, Lagging M, Dhillon AP et al. Impact of hepatic steatosis on viral kinetics and treatment outcome during antiviral treatment of chronic HCV infection. *Hepatology* 2007;45:1333–1334.

12. Walsh MJ, Jonsson JR, Richardson MM et al. Non-response to antiviral therapy is associated with obesity and increased hepatic expression of suppressor of cytokine signalling 3 (SOCS-3) in patients with chronic hepatitis C, viral genotype 1. *Gut* 2006;55:529–535.

13. Shiffman ML, Suter F, Bacon BR et al. Peginterferon alfa-2a and ribavirin for 16 or 24 weeks in HCV genotype 2 or 3. *New England Journal of Medicine* 2007;357:124–134.

14. Kahn R, Buse J, Ferrannini E, Stern M. The metabolic syndrome: time for a critical apprisal. *Diabetologia* 2005;48: 1684–1699.

15. Bugianesi E, Marchesini G, Gentilcore E et al. Fibrosis in genotype 3 hepatitis C and nonalcholic fatty liver disease: role of insulin resistance and steatosis. *Hepatology* 2006;44:953–955.

16. Sharma P, Balan V, Fernandez J et al. Hepatic steatosis in hepatitis C virus genotype 3 infection: does it correlate with body mass index, fibrosis and HCV risk factors? *Digestive Diseases and Sciences* 2004;49:25–29.

17. Conjevaraiam H, Kleiner DE, Everhart JE et al. Race, insulin resistance and hepatic steatosis in chronic hepatitis C. *Hepatology* 2007;45:80–87.

18. Jacobson IM, Brown RS, Ferlich B et al. Peginterferon alfa-2b and weight-based or flat-dose ribavirin in chronic hepatitis C patients: a randomized trial. *Hepatology* 2007;46:971–981.

19. Bailey RJ, Wong DK, Cooper C et al. Response to peginterferon alfa 2b plus ribavirin combination therapy in genotype 2 and 3 patients with poor baseline prognostic factors: results of the Canadian POWeR program. *Hepatology* 2007;46:A246.

20. Aghemo A, Rumi MG, Soffredini R et al. Impaired response to interferon-alpha2b plus ribavirin in cirrhotic patients with genotype 3a hepatitis C virus infection. *Antiviral Therapy* 2006;11:797–802.

21. Powis J, Peltekian M, Lee SS et al. Exploring differences in response to treatment with peginterferon alpha 2a and ribavirin in chronic hepatitis C between genotypes 2 and 3. *Journal of Viral Hepatitis* 2008;18:52–57.

22. Rizzetto M. Treatment of hepatitis C virus genotype 2 and 3 with pegylated interferon plus ribavirin. *Journal of Hepatology* 2005;42:275–276.

23. Mangia A, Santoro R, Minerva N et al. Peginterferon alfa-2b and ribavirin for 12 vs 24 weeks in HCV genotype 2 or 3. *New England Journal of Medicine* 2005;352:2609–2617.

24. Dalgard O, Bjoro K, Hellum K et al. Short (14 wks) treatment with pegylated interferon alpha-2b and ribavirin in patients with hepatitis C genotype 2/3 virus infection and early virological response. *Hepatology* 2004;40:1260–1265.

25. Von Wagner H, Huber H, Berg T et al. Peginterferon alpha 2a (Pegasys) plus ribavirin (Copegus) for 16 or 24 weeks in

patients with HCV genotype 2 and 3 chronic hepatitis C. *Hepatology* 2001;34:395–403.

26. Andriulli A, Dalgard O, Bjoro K, Mangia A. Short-term treatment duration for HCV-2 and HCV-3 infected patients. *Digestive and Liver Disease* 2006;38:741–748.

27. Dalgard O, Bjoro K, Ring-Larsen H *et al.* Pegylated interferon alfa and ribavirin for 14 versus 24 weeks in patients with hepatitis C virus genotype 2 or 3 and rapid virological response. *Hepatology* 2008;47:35–42.

28. Mangia A, Minerva N, Bacca D *et al.* Determinants of relapse after a short (12 weeks) course of antiviral therapy and re-treatment efficacy of a prolonged course in patients with chronic HCV genotype 2 or 3 infection. *Hepatology* 2009;49:358–363. **Predictive factors influencing treatment outcomes. An important study showing that relapsers after a shortened course of therapy can be successfully retreated with extended duration therapy.** ⚷

29. Lagging M, Langeland N, Pedersen C *et al.* Randomized comparison of 12 or 24 weeks of peginterferon alpha-2a and ribavirin in chronic hepatitis C virus genotype 2/3 infection. *Hepatology* 2008;47:1837–1845.

Management of hepatitis C in children

Maureen M. Jonas

Children's Hospital Boston, Division of Gastroenterology, Boston, Massachusetts, USA

LEARNING POINTS

- Only a minority of individuals with chronic HCV are children, and liver disease is generally mild and slowly progressive in this population. However, some children have advanced liver disease, and others are at risk for future complications such as cirrhosis and hepatocellular carcinoma.

- The majority of new cases of HCV infection in children are due to perinatal transmission. The likelihood of perinatal transmission is about 5% with each pregnancy.

- Children as young as 3 years of age with chronic HCV may be candidates for treatment. The recommended therapy is the combination of peginterferon and ribavirin.

- The success of treatment for chronic HCV in children and adolescents depends on multiple factors such as genotype, viral level, side effects, adherence, close monitoring, and the availability of a supportive and involved family.

Acute hepatitis C virus (HCV) infection is rarely detected in children, and fulminant HCV is rare. Accordingly, there are few data regarding treatment of acute HCV in the paediatric age group. Also, children are only a small proportion of the HCV-infected population, but there are a significant number of children with chronic HCV. Chronic infection is generally asymptomatic during childhood, but long-term infection can lead to significant morbidity and mortality, such as cirrhosis and hepatocellular carcinoma, later in life. The proportion of HCV-infected children who will suffer these serious consequences in unknown, but several paediatric studies have demonstrated that the degree of hepatic fibrosis generally correlates with age and duration of infection, although progression seems to be slower than observed in those infected later in life. Understanding that HCV in children has different modes of acquisition, complications and natural history will influence management and treatment decisions.

The groups of children at risk for HCV infection are listed in Table 21.1. After 1992 and universal testing of blood products, vertical transmission has become the leading source of infection for children. The rate of vertical transmission averages about 5% from most studies. Universal screening of pregnant women is not cost-effective or useful at the present time. The American Academy of Pediatrics (AAP) Committee on Infectious Disease does not recommend testing of pregnant women for HCV unless they have an identifiable risk factor. Vertical transmission is associated with a high incidence of viraemia and abnormal aminotransferases during the first 12 months. Of 70 prospectively followed infants in five European centres during 1990–1999, 93% had abnormal alanine aminotransferase (ALT) during the first 12 months, and only 19% cleared HCV RNA with normal ALT by 30 months of age [1]. Clearance

TABLE 21.1 Children who should be tested for HCV infection.

Children born to mothers with HCV*
International adoptees
Children who received blood or blood products prior to 1992
Adolescents with parenteral exposures
   Intravenous drug use
   Non-professional tattoos or body piercings

---

* Testing for anti-HCV should be done after 15 months of age, since younger infants may be seropositive from passively transferred maternal antibody.

Clinical Dilemmas in Viral Liver Disease, 1st edition. Edited by Graham R. Foster and K. Rajender Reddy. © 2010 Blackwell Publishing.

of viraemia was independent of sex and maternal HIV co-infection. Peak ALT greater than five times normal during the first 18 months and genotype 3 were more common in the patients in whom viraemia resolved spontaneously.

The largest paediatric natural history study to date describes a cohort of 200 HCV-infected children in Europe [2]. The majority had genotype 1b, 45% from vertical transmission and 39% from transfusion. Of these patients 15% had normal ALT and none had jaundice or extrahepatic manifestations. After follow-up of 1–17.5 years (mean 6.2), only 6% achieved sustained virological clearance and normalization of ALT. Liver biopsies were performed in 118 of these patients at various times during follow-up; the majority (76%) had mild hepatitis and low fibrosis scores. One patient (1%) had cirrhosis and one (1%) had severe hepatitis. Greater degrees of fibrosis were seen in children older than 15 years, suggesting long-term effects of chronic HCV infection.

There have been only a few case reports of hepatocellular carcinoma associated with HCV during childhood [3–5]. Liver transplantation for complications of chronic HCV infection during childhood is uncommon. According to the Study of Pediatric Liver Transplantation (SPLIT) Registry that collects data from 37 North American paediatric liver transplant centres, chronic HCV with cirrhosis or 'subacute hepatitis C' was the reason for transplant in 13 of 1378 children (1%) from 1995 through June 2003. For these reasons, the primary indications for treatment of paediatric patients with HCV infection are prevention of future complications and the psychosocial benefits of eradication in this young and vulnerable population.

In 2003 the Food and Drug Administration (FDA) in the USA approved the combination of interferon and ribavirin for the treatment of chronic HCV infection in children aged 3–17 years. Until very recently, this was the only licensed treatment for children with HCV. Studies had demonstrated that response rates depended on genotype and viral load, as in adults. This was illustrated in a study of 118 children [6] who had a 46% overall sustained virological response (SVR) rate. Among children with genotype 1, the SVR rate was 48% in children who had viral levels of 2 million copies/mL or less compared with 26% in those with more than 2 million copies/mL. Children with genotype 2 or 3 HCV had 84% SVR, and younger children had higher SVR rates than adolescents (57% vs. 26 %). Similar findings had been described in an earlier smaller study [7].

There are limited data regarding the use of peginterferon monotherapy or in combination with ribavirin in children.

In an open-label uncontrolled pilot study, 62 children and adolescents, aged 2–17 years (mean 10.6 years), were treated with peginterferon alfa-2b and ribavirin for 48 weeks [3]. The SVR rate was 59%. In 2008, the FDA approved combination therapy with peginterferon alfa-2b and ribavirin for use in children with HCV 3 years and older with compensated liver disease. This decision was supported by the results of a trial [8]. In this study, children with genotype 1 or 4, or genotype 3 with greater than 600 000 IU/mL, were treated for 48 weeks, while those with genotype 2, or genotype 3 with less than 600 000 IU/mL, were treated for 24 weeks. The SVR rate was 55% in the first group and 96% in the second.

A randomized trial of peginterferon alfa-2a with or without ribavirin in children aged 5–17 years was recently reported in abstract form [9]. This study demonstrated the superiority of combination therapy in children, with SVR of 53% in children who received combination therapy compared with 21% in those who received monotherapy. The difference was significant for both genotype 1 and non-genotype 1 infections. Analysis of the pretreatment liver biopsies in this cohort had reaffirmed the generally mild histological disease during childhood, but cases of marked fibrosis and even cirrhosis were observed [10].

In both of these trials, peginterferon and ribavirin were generally well tolerated in these young subjects. Side effects were generally those observed in adults, although weight loss and changes in linear growth velocity are of particular importance in paediatrics (Table 21.2). In the peginterferon alfa-2b trial, weight loss and growth inhibition were common. In addition, 3% were treated for clinical hypothyroidism. In the peginterferon alfa-2a trial, dose reductions and early discontinuation were needed in 51% and 4%, respectively, of those receiving combination therapy, primarily for neutropenia.

Given these considerations and the superior results in adults with peginterferon versus standard interferon, it

TABLE 21.2 Interferon side effects in children and adolescents.

Flu-like symptoms, especially in first few weeks
Weight loss (reversible)
Decreased growth velocity
Neutropenia
Thyroid dysfunction
Depression, behavioural changes (uncommon)

is reasonable to infer that peginterferon, in combination with ribavirin, is the treatment of choice for children with chronic HCV infection who are considered to be appropriate candidates for therapy. There are no published consensus statements or guidelines for treatment of HCV-infected children, and treatment decisions may vary with the child's age and individual disease characteristics. Examination of a liver biopsy may not be a prerequisite for treatment; it is rare to find advanced histology in young children, and the response rates of children with genotype 2 or 3 HCV are so high that baseline biopsies may provide little information regarding either likelihood of response or long-term prognosis. Exceptions are children whose parents want to know the stage of disease in considering treatment, and

those with comorbid diseases in whom the results of a biopsy might influence the decision to treat. In genotype 1 infections, especially in older children, biopsy information might be useful, since the SVR rate is not as high, and those with mild histological changes may choose to wait for the availability of newer more effective therapies (Figure 21.1).

Children as young as 3 years may be considered candidates for combination therapy. Decisions regarding timing of therapy are influenced by disease factors, such as degree of hepatic inflammation and fibrosis, the presence of comorbid diseases, and psychosocial factors such as school and athletic activities, family stability and availability for support, and participation in high-risk behaviours such as intravenous drug use. Treatment might be more strongly

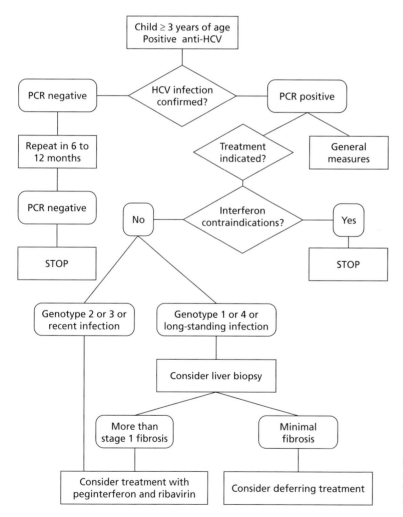

FIG. 21.1 Selection of paediatric patients with chronic HCV for treatment. PCR, polymerase chain reaction.

advocated for children with perinatally acquired HCV who are older than 10 years, those with at least moderate hepatic fibrosis, and in those with a comorbid disease or other features that raise concern for rapid progression. Just as in adults, obesity and insulin resistance might need to be addressed prior to HCV treatment in children, since these factors are likely to decrease the likelihood of SVR in children.

Peginterferon alfa-2b ($60\ \mu g/m^2$ once weekly) has been approved by the FDA for use in children 3 years and older, in combination with ribavirin (15 mg/kg daily in two divided doses). Although peginterferon alfa-2b is most commonly available in standardized doses in a multidose injection device (PegIntron RediPen, Schering Plough), this approach may not be feasible in the smallest children; doses may be individualized using more typical vials of the drug. Ribavirin is available as an oral suspension at a concentration of 40 mg/mL (Rebetol, Schering Plough) to allow accurate dosing and adjustments. Peginterferon alfa-2a ($180\ \mu g/1.73\ m^2$ weekly) can also be used in combination with ribavirin, although this type of interferon is not yet approved for use in this age group, and pharmacokinetic data are only available for children aged 5 years and older. Peginterferon and ribavirin should be given for 24 weeks for genotype 2 and 3, and for 48 weeks for genotype 1 infections. There are insufficient data regarding other genotypes, although the longer course of therapy could be considered for genotype 4 infections, extrapolating from adult data. There are no data using slow early virological response (reduction of at least 2 log IU/mL from baseline but not to undetectable at week 12) to substantiate the provision of 72 weeks of treatment in children with genotype 1 HCV but, once again, a case could be made for extrapolating from these recommendations in adults.

It has been well demonstrated in adults that medication dose reductions and interruptions resulting in less than 80% of recommended doses are clearly associated with suboptimal responses. The success of treatment for chronic HCV infection in children and adolescents depends not only on viral factors such as genotype and viral level, host factors such as age and histological stage, but also on careful medical and psychosocial monitoring by the provider and medical support staff, and the availability of a supportive engaged family. Anticipation and early intervention for side effects such as weight loss, fatigue and behavioural changes can help to promote completion of recommended doses of these medications and ensure the highest likelihood of achieving SVR. There are no data regarding the use of haematopoietic growth factors in children receiving HCV treatment, but most children tolerate some degree of anaemia quite well; although neutropenia was common in the clinical trials, significant infections were not observed. Interferon-associated thyroid dysfunction has been demonstrated in children, just as in adults. In one recent retrospective review, thyroid dysfunction was detected in 17% of children with HCV treated with either standard or pegylated interferon [11]. It would be prudent to monitor thyroid-stimulating hormone and promptly refer children who develop abnormalities for consideration of treatment, although it is transient in most instances.

The general management of children and adolescents with HCV infection includes more than just antiviral therapy. Education about the infection, its natural history and modes of transmission, and risk factors for progression such as alcohol use, obesity and other infections is critical to ensure optimal outcomes. In addition, the clinician can be of importance in dissipation of parental guilt regarding vertical transmission, and destigmatization in school and other social settings, as well as provision of other health measures such as hepatitis A and B immunization, and pregnancy prevention counselling and measures. It is also important to emphasize that children and adolescents with HCV can participate fully in school and extracurricular activities including sports without any more than the standard universal precautions already advocated for these settings.

In summary, the minority of individuals with chronic HCV infection are children, and most children and adolescents with this infection have clinically unapparent and histologically mild liver disease. However, some children have more advanced liver fibrosis, and it has been demonstrated that this is a progressive, albeit slow, disease. Children as young as 3 years of age with chronic HCV infection are candidates for treatment. The recommended treatment is the combination of peginterferon alfa and ribavirin for 24–48 weeks, depending on genotype. In general, children tolerate this therapy well. Consideration of age, family and social factors, and anticipatory management of side effects are important in achieving optimal therapeutic responses.

References

1. Resti M, Jara P, Hierro L *et al.* Clinical features and progression of perinatally acquired hepatitis C virus infection. *Journal of Medical Virology* 2003;70:373–377.

2. Jara P, Resti M, Hierro L *et al.* Chronic hepatitis C virus infection in childhood: clinical patterns and evolution in 224 white children. *Clinical Infectious Diseases* 2003;36:275–280.

3. Schaffner F, Thung SN. Clinicopathology Conferences. End-stage liver disease in a young woman. *Hepatology* 1994;19:534–537.

4. Strickland DK, Hudson MM. Hepatitis C infection and hepatocellular carcinoma after treatment of childhood cancer. *Journal of Pediatric Hematology and Oncology* 2001;23:527–529.

5. González-Peralta R, Langham MR Jr, Andres JM *et al.* Hepatocellular carcinoma in 2 young adolescents with chronic hepatitis C. *Journal of Pediatric Gastroenterology and Nutrition* 2009;48:630–635.

6. González-Peralta R, Kelly DA, Haber B *et al.* Interferon alfa-2b in combination with ribavirin for the treatment of chronic hepatitis C in children: efficacy, safety, and pharmacokinetics. *Hepatology* 2005;42:1010–1018. **This open-label study provided the basis for the approval of combination therapy with interferon and ribavirin in children with chronic HCV.** 🔑

7. Wirth S, Lang T, Gehring S, Gerner P. Recombinant alfa-interferon plus ribavirin therapy in children and adolescents with chronic hepatitis C. *Hepatology* 2002;36:1280–1284.

8. PegIntron package insert. Available at Drugs@FDA.gov (accessed 6/2/09; access approved 3/10/09).

9. Schwarz KB, Gonzalez-Peralta RP, Murray KF *et al.* Peginterferon with or without ribavirin for chronic hepatitis C in children and adolescents: final results of the PEDS-C trial. *Hepatology* 2008;48(4 Suppl):418A. **This recent abstract reports the results of a large randomized trial of peginterferon monotherapy versus combination therapy in children with chronic HCV.** 🔑

10. Goodman ZD, Makhlouf HR, Liu L *et al.* Pathology of chronic hepatitis C in children: liver biopsy findings in the Peds-C trial. *Hepatology* 2008;47:836–883.

11. Raghunaathan KDR, Galacki DM, Quan J, Mitchell PD, Jonas MM. Prevalence and characterization of thyroid abnormalities in children and young adults treated with combination therapy for chronic hepatitis C at a single center. *Gastroenterology* 2009;136(5 Suppl. 1):A-808.

22 Controlling symptoms in chronic HCV on and off treatment: does anything work?

Brenda A. Appolo

Hospital of the University of Pennsylvania, Division of Gastroenterology, Philadelphia, Pennsylvania, USA

LEARNING POINTS

- Individuals chronically infected with HCV demonstrate decreased quality-of-life scores in comparison with healthy controls.

- Patients may have physical, psychosomatic or emotional complaints as a result of their viral hepatitis or as a direct result of side effects related to HCV therapy.

- Almost all patients on HCV therapy experience one or more symptoms. The most common symptoms related to chronic HCV infection include constitutional complaints such as fatigue and malaise, neuropsychiatric symptoms, and associated complaints related to anaemia and dermopathies that may evolve or be exacerbated by HCV treatment.

- The control of symptoms in chronic HCV infection both on and off therapy is clinically challenging and largely supportive in nature.

Introduction

Systematic clinical research describing the signs and symptoms of chronic hepatitis C virus (HCV) infection are limited and therefore begets controversy regarding effective symptom control. The majority of chronically infected individuals are asymptomatic and progression to cirrhosis is typically silent. However, once cirrhosis is established, the rate at which decompensated liver disease develops is about 4% per year in the HCV-infected patient. The diagnosis of

chronic HCV infection is often an incidental finding during the comprehensive evaluation of patients with abnormal transaminases or of at-risk populations such as intravenous drug users or those who received blood products prior to 1992.

While clinically there is a perception that chronic HCV infection is asymptomatic, there is a significant amount of information reflecting a negative impact on patient quality of life. Thus, health-related quality of life (HRQL) assessments are widely adopted in the approach to the chronic HCV-infected individual in conjunction with routine objective laboratory, radiographic and histological assessments. HRQL assessments aim to assess the effects of health on well-being and incorporate extrinsic factors as well, including economic and environmental variables. A number of HCV-specific quality-of-life assessments have been developed, such as SF-36, a self-assessment that incorporates both a physical and mental component (Figure 22.1) [1]. Lower quality-of-life scores have been appreciated in patients who are aware of their diagnosis compared with those who are infected yet unaware of their chronic HCV infection status. Moreover, compensated HCV patients demonstrated diminished quality of life in comparison with healthy controls as a whole. Most notably, chronic HCV-infected patients scored categorically worse in the physical and emotional roles and attributed poor quality of life to extrahepatic complaints of fatigue, malaise, athralgias, depression and poor cognition [1,2].

Symptom control in chronic HCV infection is a clinical challenge, partly due to the subjective symptoms believed to be associated with the disease at baseline, compounded by the well-described adverse effects associated with therapy and psychosocial factors such as drug and alcohol use. The mainstay of chronic HCV therapy comprises once-weekly injections of peginterferon alfa in combination with ribavirin

Clinical Dilemmas in Viral Liver Disease, 1st edition. Edited by Graham R. Foster and K. Rajender Reddy. © 2010 Blackwell Publishing.

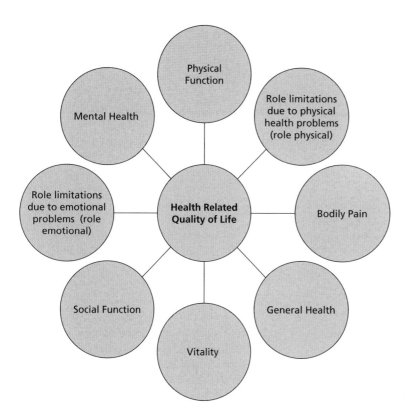

FIG. 22.1 Quality-of-life assessment tools may be generic or specific instruments: the SF-36 (short form questionnaire) is a health survey consisting of 36 questions which target eight domains.

orally. Treatment side effects are often predictable, yet there is some heterogeneity in how best to treat side effects given the lack of double-blind placebo-controlled studies in this area and increasing healthcare costs.

Baseline patient education from the physician and nurse specialist prior to treatment initiation cannot be overestimated and plays a major role in setting a patient's perception about the potential for HCV treatment-induced side effects and the subsequent ability to cope with them. Moreover, it fosters necessary patient–provider trust and continued communication that in turn enables the treating provider to establish individual thresholds for applying side-effect management techniques. Finally, prior to treatment initiation and as part of the initial assessment of a patient pursuing HCV therapy, identification of a social support network (e.g. family, friends, church) will help to improve patient motivation and adherence to therapy and perhaps even to avoid drug and alcohol relapse. It is highly recommended that a patient support person be identified beforehand and be present for patient counselling at baseline.

Flu-like syndrome

Flu-like syndrome is common and often one of the first side effects induced by HCV therapy a patient may experience. Often the symptoms noted include general malaise, fever, anorexia, nausea, vomiting, diarrhoea and body aches. This constellation of symptoms is related to cytokine reactions induced by interferon products as a whole. However, with the advent of once-weekly injections, patients and providers have noted a decrease in frequency of symptoms compared with traditional thrice-weekly preparations. Patients should be educated about these potential side effects, particularly within the first 12 weeks of interferon exposure. Pre-emptive supportive therapy is helpful and includes premedication with paracetamol prior to the interferon injection and continuation of paracetamol dosing as needed over the subsequent 24–48 hours after the interferon injection. Paracetamol doses up to 2 g per 24 hours is acceptable. Additionally, antiemetic and antidiarrhoeal drugs may be employed (Table 22.1).

TABLE 22.1 Commonly encountered side effects related to HCV therapy and suggested adjunctive therapy.

HCV therapy-induced side effects	Suggested adjunctive therapy

Flu-like syndrome
   Malaise
   Fever
   Gastrointestinal upset
   Anorexia
   Body aches
	Paracetamol (2 g/day maximum)
	NSAIDs (limit use in cirrhotics, previous gastrointestinal bleed)
	Proton pump inhibitors/antiemetics (e.g. ondansetron)
	Antidiarrhoeals (loperamide, Lomotil)
	Drobinal, megestrol
	Tramadol, oxycodone (consider APAP max)
	Increased hydration, exercise

Fatigue	Modafinil (non-sleep-deprived patients) Bupropion
Insomnia	Zolpidem, mirtazapine, trazodone
Mood changes, depression, anxiety	Citalopram, escitalopram, bupropion Benzodiazepines (limit use of alprazolam) Presence of mania: low threshold for psychiatry consultation
Cough	Antitussives (guaifenesin, hydrocodone bitartrate) Survey for pulmonary infiltrates (ribavirin related)
Rash	Topical steroids, Benadryl, hydroxyzine
Neutropenia	Filgrastim 300 μg weekly versus as-needed Start: ANC < 500×10^6/L (non-cirrhotic) Start: ANC > 750×10^6/L (cirrhotic)
Anaemia	Epogen 40 000 units or more weekly as needed Start: haemoglobin < 10 g/dL if asymptomatic Start if decline in haemoglobin is > 3 g/dL ± symptoms Stop/modify dose if haemoglobin > 12.5 g/dL
Thrombocytopenia	No adjunctive therapy available to date Consider low-dose interferon if baseline platelet count < 70×10^9/L at baseline Modify/stop therapy if platelet count < 20×10^9/L; monitor for bleeding

ANC, absolute neutrophil count; NSAIDs, non-steroidal anti-inflammatory drugs.

Fatigue

Fatigue is the most common patient complaint both on and off treatment with interferon monotherapy or interferon/ribavirin combination. The aetiology of treatment-induced fatigue is likely multifactorial given the known neuropsychiatric and endocrine disturbances related to interferon products, and the anaemia related to bone marrow suppression (interferons) and haemolysis (ribavirin). With that said, optimizing fatigue levels on treatment is multifaceted.

Anecdotal evidence suggests that conservative measures such as good sleep hygiene, avoidance of caffeine and nicotine, and increased hydration and exercise, to avoid muscle atrophy, are beneficial. Care must be taken to identify if

fatigue both on and off therapy is related to depression, in which case antidepressant therapy with a selective serotonin reuptake inhibitor (SSRI) or bupropion is favoured. Correction of anaemia, albeit with the use of erythropoietin or dose reductions of ribavirin (less favoured), may help to decrease fatigue levels as well.

Finally, modafinil and methylphenidate have been used for off-label treatment of fatigue in the setting of interferon usage and this has achieved modest improvements [4]. Otherwise, limited data exist to support the use of methylphenidate and modafinil for the treatment of fatigue associated with HCV infection both on and off therapy. Information has been largely borrowed to support their clinical use from response rates in patients suffering from profound fatigue related to multiple sclerosis and primary biliary cirrhosis [5,6]. The physiological effects of modafinil differ from those of methylphenidate in that the former shows greater inhibition of observed and reported sleep, less facilitation of orthostatic tachycardia and less reduction of caloric intake. These findings are consistent with pharmacological data suggesting that modafinil has wake-promoting actions similar to sympathomimetic agents such as amphetamine and methylphenidate, although the pharmacological profile is not identical [7]. Thus modafinil may arguably be a less addictive and more attractive agent for treatment of fatigue in patients with a history of substance abuse, which is commonly encountered in the HCV-infected population or those afflicted with weight loss and anorexia associated with interferon usage. However, modafinil has been associated cutaneous reactions including drug rash with eosinophilia.

Neuropsychiatric symptoms

Neuropsychiatric complaints are associated with chronic HCV infection *per se*. It is estimated that nearly 30% of patients infected with HCV who are new to interferon treatment suffer from neuropsychiatric problems [6]. Moreover, the rate of depressive disorders as defined by the *Diagnostic and Statistical Manual of Mental Disorders* (DSM)-IV ranges from 25 to 70%, in contrast to 6–10% in the general population. *De novo* complaints such as depressed mood, fatigue, sleep changes, anorexia, anhedonia, anxiety, irritability, suicidal/homicidal ideation and in rare cases psychosis are also well described in patients receiving interferon-based therapies [8,9]. Major registration treatment trials investigating peginterferon alfa plus ribavirin in the treatment of chronic HCV infection have reported neuropsychiatric changes in upwards of 35% of patients receiving treatment [10,11].

Identifying and optimizing baseline depression is vital to the control of depressive symptomatology on and off therapy. DSM-IV, along with depression screening tools such as Beck's Depression Inventory and the Hamilton Depression Rating Scale, may be helpful diagnostic tools (particularly in clinical research trials) but often pragmatic and interactive discussions between the treating clinician, the patient and the patient's support systems will suffice. Pharmacological therapy is often tailored to the patient's most dominant neuropsychiatric complaints related to interferon. Despite the numerous antidepressant and anxiolytic agents available on the market, SSRIs are deemed the most appro-

priate choice for interferon-induced depressive symptoms given their ability to modulate the serotonergic system. Citalopram, escitalopram and sertraline all appear to be the most suitable agents given their accepted efficacy, minimal to no hepatic toxicity and limited drug–drug interactions. An improvement in depression scores was noted as early as week 2 on peginterferon therapy in a prospective trial investigating the efficacy of citalopram versus placebo [12]. Pre-emptive treatment of depression with paroxetine has also been examined; however, no significant difference was noted compared with the control group yet the study appeared to be limited by population size and drop-out rates [13]. Finally, mirtazapine and trazodone appear to be accepted for the treatment of interferon-induced depression and have added benefits of sedation for insomnia-related complaints and, in the case of mirtazapine, increased appetite, which may be an added advantage for those patients suffering from anorexia induced by interferon. Psychiatric consultation is recommended if the severity of symptoms is outside the treating clinician's scope of practice and highly recommended at baseline for those patients with a history of bipolar disease, schizophrenia or schizoaffective disorder. Patients who develop *de novo* mania on HCV therapy warrant treatment discontinuation and referral to psychiatry thereafter for close monitoring and/or treatment.

Anaemia

Apart from side effects related to interferon, ribavirin is also a significant contributor to on-treatment symptoms in chronic HCV infection given its ability to induce haemolytic anaemia. Approximately 25% of patients receiving weight-based ribavirin dosing in the registration trial investigating peginterferon alfa-2a in combination with ribavirin 1000–1200 g daily experienced clinically significant anaemia [9]. Clinically, patients will often complain of worsening fatigue levels, exertional dyspnoea and chest tightness. The off-label use of subcutaneous injections of recombinant epoetin alfa 20 000–40 000 units weekly or darbepoetin 200–300 µg every other week is widely accepted by clinicians in the field as improving haematocrit levels, quality of life and symptoms while on HCV therapy. While the use of growth factors for symptom relief is not generally recommended, a reasonable approach would be to treat anaemia when haemoglobin is below 10 g/dL. Also, it is important that the dose and frequency be titrated to improve haemoglobin to around 12 g/dL, as a significant increase above this might potentially increase the risk of thromboembolic phenomena. There are no convincing results to suggest that the use of growth factors increases sustained virological response (SVR) on therapy; however, an impressive amount of data demonstrates improved SVR rates with adherence to ribavirin and increased rates of relapse with dose reductions of ribavirin [14].

Skin manifestations

Dermatopathic findings and associated symptoms of pruritus are also associated with chronic HCV infection. Lichen planus is a violaceous plague-like eruption often found on extensor surfaces, genitalia and occasionally mucous membranes. Although not specific to HCV infection, it is often associated with the disease [15]. Treatment is often supportive with topical corticosteroids and, for severe cases, treatment with calcineurin inhibitors or psoralen with UV-A (PUVA) may be considered. Ribavirin may induce a maculopapular rash with pruritus or sensations of burning. Anecdotally, this rash subsides with the use of topical steroids in combination with oral antihistamines such as Benadryl or hydroxyzine 25 mg four times daily. There is little evidence to support the view that dose reduction improves rash given its often transient nature and lack of dose dependence correlation. Likewise, interferon-induced rash is often appreciated and resembles psoriatic plagues which may be optimized with topicals as well. Further interferon therapy almost invariably worsens pre-existing psoriasis and certainly deserves discussion with the patient prior to initiation of interferon-based therapy.

Other

A broad spectrum of additional physical, psychosomatic and emotional symptoms may be encountered clinically in chronic HCV infection. Symptoms encountered on interferon and ribavirin-based therapy may include gastrointestinal complaints, upper respiratory complaints, migraine headaches, alopecia, visual disturbances and manifestations of thyroid dysfunction. Treatment is often supportive in nature (antiemetics, antidiarrhoeals, analgesics, antitussives) and are anecdotal at best. Correction of underlying thyroid dysregulation at baseline or experienced on chronic HCV therapy are standard of care (i.e. levothyroxine). Upper respiratory complaints should be evaluated thoroughly to rule out concomitant sinus infection or, in rare cases, pulmonary infiltrates/interstitial pneumonitis associated with ribavirin or interferon use, which would prompt therapy discontinuation in the case of the latter.

Summary

A number of physical and psychosomatic side effects can be encountered in the chronically infected patient on or off treatment. A thorough baseline assessment comprising history and physical and laboratory work-up is recommended to identify static versus dynamic patient predictors that will impact treatment success. This, combined with patient counselling about the potential for side effects and identification of a patient support network, is essential. Typically, clinicians will need two or more consultations with the patient to adequately achieve this prior to therapy initiation. Ongoing monthly to bimonthly in-office assessments with frequent laboratory surveillance are needed to effectively impact patient motivation and implement reasonable adjuvant therapy. Finally, and to paraphrase Theophrastus, an ancient Greek philosopher, regardless of the clinician's ability to absolve patients of their HCV symptoms, treatment-induced side effects or achieve SVR with HCV therapy, time spent with the patient and the support network both on and off therapy is invaluable.

References

1. Ware JE Jr, Bayliss MS, Mannocchia M, Davis GL. Health-related quality of life in chronic hepatitis C: impact of disease and treatment response. *Hepatology* 1999;30:550–555. **A compelling publication examining the qualify-of-life scores in patients chronically infected with HCV.** 🔑

2. Dalgard O, Egeland A, Skaug K, Vilimas K, Steen T. Health-related quality of life in active injecting drug users with and without chronic hepatitis C virus infection. *Hepatology* 2004;39:74–80.

3. Spiegel BM, Younossi ZM, Hays RD, Revicki D, Robbins S, Kanwal F. Impact of hepatitis C on health related quality of life: a systematic review and quantitative assessment. *Hepatology* 2005;41:790–800.

4. Martin KA, Krahn LE, Balan V, Rosati MJ. Modafinil's use in combating interferon-induced fatigue. *Digestive Diseases and Sciences* 2007;52:893–896.

5. Jones DE, Newton JL. An open study of modafinil for the treatment of daytime somnolence and fatigue in primary biliary cirrhosis. *Alimentary Pharmacology and Therapeutics* 2007;25:471–476.

6. Rammohan KW, Rosenberg JH, Lynn DJ, Blumenfeld AM, Pollak CP, Nagaraja HN. Efficacy and safety of modafinil

(Provigil) for the treatment of fatigue in multiple sclerosis: a two centre phase 2 study. *Journal of Neurology, Neurosurgery and Psychiatry* 2002;72:179–183.

7. Jasinski DR. An evaluation of the abuse potential of modafinil using methylphenidate as a reference. *Journal of Psychopharmacology* 2000;14:53–60.

8. Fontana R, Hussain K, Schwartz S, Moyer C, Su G, Lok A. Emotional distress in chronic hepatitis C patients not receiving antiviral therapy. *Hepatology* 2002;36:401–407.

9. Dieperink E, Willenbring M, Ho S. Neuropsychiatric symptoms associated with hepatitis C and interferon alpha: a review. *American Journal of Psychiatry* 2000;157:867–876.

10. Manns M, McHutchison J, Gordon S. Peginterferon alfa-2b plus ribavirin compared with interferon alfa-2b plus ribavirin for initial treatment of chronic hepatitis C: a randomised trial. *Lancet* 2001;358:958–965. **Pivotal registration trial data examining effectiveness and potential side effects of peginterferon alfa-2b plus ribavirin.**

11. Fried M, Shiffman M, Reddy R. Peginterferon alfa-2a plus ribavirin for chronic hepatitis C virus. *New England Journal of Medicine* 2002;347:975–982. **Pivotal registration trial data examining effectiveness and potential side effects of peginterferon alfa-2a plus ribavirin.**

12. Kraus MR, Schafer A, Schottker K *et al.* Therapy of interferon-induced depression in chronic hepatitis C with citalopram: a randomised, double-blind, placebo-controlled study. *Gut* 2008;57:531–536. **One of few published papers prospectively examining effects of prophalactic use of SSRI for interferon-induced depression.**

13. Raison CL, Woolwine BJ, Demetrashvili MF *et al.* Paroxetine for prevention of depressive symptoms induced by interferon-alpha and ribavirin for hepatitis C. *Alimentary Pharmacology and Therapeutics* 2007;25:1163–1174.

14. Reddy KR, Shiffman ML, Morgan TR *et al.* Impact of ribavirin dose reductions in hepatitis C virus genotype 1 patients completing peginterferon alfa-2a/ribavirin treatment. *Clinical Gastroenterology and Hepatology* 2007;5:124–129.

15. Chuang TY, Stitle L, Brashear R, Lewis C. Hepatitis C virus and lichen planus: a case-control study of 340 patients. *Journal of the American Academy of Dermatology* 1999;41:787–789.

Complementary therapies in chronic HCV: exploitation or something to offer?

Kelly C. Vranas, K. Rajender Reddy

University of Pennsylvania, Philadelphia, Pennsylvania, USA

LEARNING POINTS

- Many complementary and alternative therapies are currently used worldwide to treat HCV infection with potential but unproven benefits.

- Oral silymarin, glycyrrhizin, HM861, TJ-9 and various other compounds are commonly used for their touted benefit as antioxidants. Intravenous silymarin has been observed in a preliminary study to have antiviral effect.

- There is a specific need to develop methods of standardization in the production of these preparations.

- Once appropriate regulations regarding the production of these preparations have been developed, further randomized clinical trials are necessary in order to better assess their safety and efficacy.

- At this time, complementary and alternative therapies cannot be firmly recommended for the treatment of HCV.

Hepatitis C virus (HCV) is a major cause of mortality and morbidity worldwide. Globally, an estimated 170 million people have HCV infection and the majority of these will go onto develop chronic hepatitis C [1]. Standard treatment of HCV infection includes combination standard interferon or peginterferon plus ribavirin therapy, which are costly, limited in their efficacy and carry the risk of adverse events. Consequently, patients with HCV infection often seek alternative treatments to either complement or replace standard therapy. Some of the more common alternative therapies used in the treatment of HCV include silymarin

Clinical Dilemmas in Viral Liver Disease, 1st edition. Edited by Graham R. Foster and K. Rajender Reddy. © 2010 Blackwell Publishing.

(milk thistle), antioxidants such as N-acetylcysteine (NAC) and vitamin E, glycyrrhizin (liquorice root), Chinese traditional medicine, Japanese Kampo medicine, and thymic extracts. Given the extent of patients' utilization of these complementary treatments, it is important to determine their efficacy, if any, and also understand their mechanisms of action in the treatment of chronic liver disease secondary to HCV via their potential antioxidant, antifibrotic or immunomodulatory activities (Table 23.1).

Silymarin, an extract of *Silybum marianum* (milk thistle), is the most commonly used alternative treatment of HCV infection in the USA. It is found commonly throughout Europe, Asia and North America and has been available in the form of highly purified extracts since the 1960s [2]. Silymarin contains multiple biologically active compounds, including the flavonoid silibinin which accounts for 90% of the herb's components in most preparations [2]. It has been used as therapy for liver disease and jaundice since the sixteenth century and more recently in the treatment of *Amanita phalloides* poisoning [2]. In the laboratory, silymarin has been shown to have antifibrotic effects. Specifically, it interferes with leukotriene formation in Kupffer cell cultures and may thereby inhibit hepatic stellate cell activation, a crucial event in fibrogenesis [3]. Moreover, it has been demonstrated to block the proliferation of hepatic stellate cells and their transformation to myofibroblasts [4].

A 2007 study evaluated the anti-inflammatory and antiviral effects of a highly standardized silymarin extract (MK-001) in human cells. Specifically, human peripheral blood mononuclear cells obtained from two healthy donors were stimulated with plate-bound anti-CD3 in the presence and absence of MK-001. The secretion of tumour necrosis factor (TNF)-α, an inflammatory cytokine, was markedly reduced in the presence of MK-001, while the silymarin extract had no effect when tested in the absence of anti-CD3

TABLE 23.1 Summary of mechanisms of action and side effects of various complementary therapies used in the treatment of hepatitis C.

Alternative therapy	Mechanism of action	Side effects
Antioxidants	Inhibits the production of inflammatory cytokines	Well tolerated
Silymarin (milk thistle)	Antifibrotic effects via inhibition of leukotriene formation in Kupffer cells, hepatic stellate cell activation, and the proliferation of hepatic stellate cells; anti-inflammatory effects via inhibition of both NF-κB-induced transcription in human hepatoma cells and inflammatory cytokine induction; questionable antiviral effects	Well tolerated
Glycyrrhizin (extract of liquorice root)	Antioxidant activity via the induction of glutathione-S-transferase and catalase activity	Mineralocorticoid activity which causes sodium and fluid retention, elevated blood pressure, and hypokalaemia
CH-100 (blend of 19 herbs used in Chinese traditional medicine)	Unknown	Possible hepatotoxic effects of the herbal compound's active constituents
Sho-saiko-to (a form of Japanese Kampo medicine, also known as TJ-9)	Antifibrotic effects via the inhibition of action of hepatic stellate cells	Has been associated with interstitial pneumonitis in case reports
Thymic extracts	Suggested increase in Th1 response and decrease in Th2 response	Well tolerated

stimulation. Moreover, T cells obtained from four HCV-infected subjects also demonstrated pronounced decreases in secretion of TNF-α on treatment with MK-001 (mean fold change 6.5, range 1.7–11.7) [5].

Because TNF-α signals through NF-κB, the effect of MK-001 on TNF-α activation of NF-κB transcription in human hepatoma cells was also evaluated. MK-001 was found to dose-dependently inhibit TNF-α induction of NF-κB transcription [5]. To determine the effect of MK-001 on HCV infection, human hepatoma cells were treated with various doses of MK-001 and then infected with the JFH-1 virus, an infection culture system derived from a genotype 2a genome isolated from a Japanese patient with fulminant hepatitis. Pretreatment of the human hepatoma cells with MK-001 dose-dependently inhibited HCV infection, indicating a prophylactic effect of silymarin against the virus. Finally, human hepatoma cells already infected with the JFH-1 virus were subsequently treated with MK-001 or interferon for 24 hours; MK-001 demonstrated pronounced antiviral effects to an almost similar extent as interferon. When combined with interferon, HCV replication was inhibited to a greater extent than with interferon treatment alone [5]. These data confirmed the anti-inflammatory

actions via the inhibition of both NF-κB-induced transcription in human hepatoma cells and inflammatory cytokine induction in human peripheral blood mononuclear cells. They also revealed both prophylactic and therapeutic effects of silymarin against HCV infection, particularly in combination with interferon treatment [5].

However, the clinical benefits of silymarin are uncertain given inconsistent results of clinical trials, most likely due to the lack of a standardized product [5]. The first long-term, double-blind, randomized controlled trial comparing silymarin with a placebo vitamin in 170 patients with cirrhosis of diverse causes was conducted in 1971. Although this study was designed before the discovery of HCV, it showed a significant difference in survival between patients treated with silymarin and those treated with placebo (77% vs. 67% at 2 years, and 58% vs. 39% at 4 years, respectively) [6]. Subgroup analysis identified patients with Child A cirrhosis and those with alcoholic cirrhosis to particularly benefit, and silymarin did not have any associated side effects. However, the study had several weaknesses: lack of reported histological data, high drop-out rate, uneven randomization showing more severe liver damage in the placebo group, and lack of control for alcohol consumption during the trial [7]. Despite these weaknesses, the results of this trial fuelled the widespread use of silymarin by patients with chronic liver disease in Europe during the last several decades.

In a 2002 meta-analysis of nine trials that studied the use of silymarin in chronic liver disease, the overall odds ratio for mortality in the silymarin group compared with placebo was 0.9 (CI 0–1.5; $P = 0.6$). Overall no differences were observed in transaminases, serum albumin, or prothrombin time, and no improvement in histology was noted among patients assigned to the silymarin group compared with those receiving placebo [8]. More recently, a randomized, double-blind, placebo-controlled cross-over study was conducted in 24 patients with chronic hepatitis C who received 12 weeks of oral milk thistle and placebo separated by a 4-week washout interval. In the 17 patients who completed the trial, mean changes in HCV RNA titres and serum alanine aminotransferase (ALT) levels were not significantly different for those who received silymarin versus placebo [9]. These findings were confirmed in the 2008 Hepatitis C Anti-viral Long-Term Treatment Against Cirrhosis (HALT-C) Trial, in which 1145 patients with biopsy-confirmed fibrosis or cirrhosis secondary to HCV who had previously failed antiviral treatment volunteered to participate in a trial of long-term interferon-based therapy for histologically advanced hepatitis C. As part of the study these patients were questioned regarding their use of herbal supplements in the treatment of their chronic liver disease. Of the 1145 patients interviewed, 195 were actively taking silymarin. Statistical comparisons made between those who used silymarin and those who did not revealed no significant difference in HCV RNA levels; similarly, no significant difference between silymarin users and non-users was noted for mean aspartate aminotransferase (AST) or total serum bilirubin levels [10]. In contrast, the mean ALT level was significantly lower in non-users, whereas the mean serum alkaline phosphatase level was significantly lower in users. Silymarin users were found to have significantly lower levels of fatigue, nausea, pain at the site of the liver, anorexia, headaches, and muscle and joint pains [10].

The majority of published data on silymarin in the treatment of hepatitis C (although limited in their scope and quality) provide little convincing support for its efficacy. Yet a recent study conducted in patients with chronic hepatitis C who were previous non-responders to full-dose interferon/ribavirin therapy revealed that high dose *intravenous* silymarin acted as a potent antiviral agent in this setting and was well tolerated with no serious adverse effects. Intravenous administration of a standardized formulation

of silymarin allowed higher doses to be given with increased bioavailability, in contrast to the oral forms of silymarin used in past studies that varied in their formulations and which had limited bioavailability secondary to their poor water solubility [11]. Several additional randomized controlled trials are currently being conducted with standardized doses, formulations and routes of administration in order to better assess whether silymarin is of benefit in patients with hepatitis C, either by itself or in conjunction with standard antiviral treatment [10,11].

Complex immune mechanisms are involved in the response to HCV infection. Although the mechanisms of liver damage by HCV are not completely understood, it is thought that the immune response to the infection contributes to the inflammatory infiltration seen on liver biopsy, which then leads to fibrosis and chronic liver disease [1,12]. In healthy individuals, the T helper 2 (Th2) component of the immune system is responsible for cell-mediated immunity, while T helper 1 (Th1) cells promote cell-mediated defence. These two systems are mutually inhibitory and act to balance cell-mediated and humoral immunity [1]. However, in the setting of HCV infection, the Th2 system dominates, leading to the overproduction of TNF-α and other proinflammatory cytokines. In this setting, the Th1 system is suppressed, resulting in decreased natural killer cell activity (cells that directly inactivate the virus) [1]. Antioxidants such as NAC and vitamin E inhibit cytokine production and may be useful in preventing or delaying the inflammation that leads to hepatocyte necrosis and subsequent fibrosis observed in HCV infection.

Several randomized clinical trials have assessed the efficacy of antioxidant therapy with NAC and/or vitamin E in combination with interferon alfa in patients with hepatitis C [13]. A systematic review of six such trials, which included a total of 463 patients, revealed no significant differences in virological response between treatment regimens [13]. In a separate randomized double-blind trial studying the effect of 800 IU of vitamin E daily in 23 patients with hepatitis C who had failed interferon therapy, significant reductions in ALT and AST were noted in 48% of subjects, although HCV RNA remained detectable in the serum of all patients at the conclusion of the trial and transaminases returned to near pretreatment values after cessation of vitamin E treatment [14]. Although antioxidants are generally well tolerated, at present there is insufficient evidence to support their use in the treatment of hepatitis C [13].

Glycyrrhizin is an aqueous extract of liquorice root, which has been used for centuries in traditional medicines to treat cough, bronchitis, gastritis and liver inflammation [7]. In Japan it has been developed into a standardized extract called Stronger Neominophagen C (SNMC) which has been used for over 20 years in the treatment of chronic hepatitis. In animal models, glycyrrhizin has been shown to modify arachidonic acid metabolism and inhibit the activity of 11β-hydroxysteroid dehydrogenase and PGE_2 production by macrophages [15]. It also has antioxidant activity via the induction of glutathionine-S-transferase and catalase activity and has been shown to blunt ALT elevations and impede fibrosis in animals [15,16]. In a Japanese study of SNMC in patients with hepatitis C, cirrhosis developed after 15 years in 21% of treated patients compared with 37% of untreated controls; hepatocellular carcinoma arose in 12% of those treated versus 25% of controls [2,17]. However, this trial was neither prospective nor randomized; varying doses of SNMC were used; HCV RNA levels, biochemical tests and liver histology were not reported; and some patients simultaneously received other unknown herbal therapies [2].

To date, four randomized trials of glycyrrhizin (all administered as SNMC) have been identified. In two of these trials, there was no significant difference in the biochemical or virological response of patients who received SNMC in combination with interferon therapy versus those who had received interferon alone [13]. In the third trial, reductions in ALT levels were seen in patients who received SNMC versus placebo, but this was not sustained after the cessation of treatments and there were no significant effects on HCV RNA levels. In the final trial, significant differences existed in transaminase levels between treatment groups, although these were not sustained at follow-up and there were no virological effects observed [13]. Given the mineralocorticoid activity of glycyrrhizin, treatment with it is also not without side effects: patients can experience worsening complications of cirrhosis, including sodium and fluid retention, elevated blood pressure and hypokalaemia [2,13].

Chinese traditional medicine has been practised for roughly two millennia and comprises multiple forms of ritualistic healing practices, including acupuncture, herbal therapy, massage, and exercise therapy [2]. *Plantago asiatica* is one of the more common Chinese herbal remedies used in the treatment of chronic liver disease, although its use has been studied mainly in the context of hepatitis B. A second combination of 10 herbs known as Compound 861 has been shown *in vitro* (using human stellate cells) and *in vivo* (using animal models of fibrosis) to block cyclin/cyclin-dependent kinase activity in the cell cycle, thereby inhibiting stellate cell activation and even reversing early stages of cirrhosis via the reduction of collagen and transforming growth factor (TGF)-β transcripts while increasing that of matrix metalloproteinase I [2,18]. However, neither *Plantago asiatica* or Compound 861 have been evaluated in the treatment of hepatitis C.

CH-100, another form of Chinese traditional medicine, is a combination of 19 herbs that has been used to treat chronic hepatitis C. In a double-blind placebo-controlled trial involving patients with the virus, treatment with CH-100 was associated with a significant reduction in ALT levels, although no person treated cleared the virus [19]. Several other formulations of Chinese traditional medicine also exist that may be useful in the treatment of hepatitis C, either as alternatives or supplements to standard treatments, or to ameliorate side effects of traditional therapy. However, further studies are necessary since pharmacologically active constituents of these herbal compounds are ill-defined, interactions between multiple compounds may occur, and many of these compounds may in themselves be hepatotoxic [7].

Kampo medicine is the Japanese study and adaptation of traditional Chinese medicine. Unlike the USA, herbal medicines in Japan are regulated as pharmaceutical preparations and as such have been integrated into Japan's national medical system [2]. Hundreds of Kampo extracts are currently approved for use. Sho-saiko-to (also known as TJ-9) is one of the most common herbal medicines used in Japan to treat chronic hepatitis. It has been shown *in vitro* and in animal studies to inhibit the action of hepatitic stellate cells, thus slowing the process of fibrosis [20]. However, very few clinical data exist on the safety and efficacy of TJ-9 in the treatment of hepatitis C.

Thymic extracts have also been recognized as a potential complementary treatment of hepatitis C. A 2004 review of complementary and alternative therapies in the treatment of hepatitis C identified five trials in which thymic extracts were used. In three of these trials, synthetic thymosin alpha 1 (Tα1) was given in combination with interferon; the number of patients who experienced a complete virological or biochemical response at the end of treatment was significantly higher in the group receiving both interferon and Tα1 versus those who received either interferon alone or placebo [13]. These differences were sustained at 6 and 12 months after cessation of treatment, and thymic extracts were generally well tolerated. However, no significant difference in biochemical or virological response occurred when patients received thymic extract alone [13]. Current data on the use of thymic extracts in the treatment of hepatitis C are limited, although further randomized trials are warranted to better assess the safety and efficacy of this alternative therapy.

In summary, numerous compounds have been used worldwide in the treatment of hepatitis C. Many of these compounds have been shown to protect against experimental liver disease *in vitro* or in animal models. None, however, have been shown to be consistently effective in ameliorating the course of hepatitis C in properly conducted randomized controlled trials [2]. Moreover, patients must be made aware that the production of herbal products is not regulated in the same manner as pharmaceuticals. Yet, as these products continue to become more mainstream, methods to test their safety and efficacy will need to be established. Only with such a system in place can randomized controlled trials be appropriately designed and conducted in order to better assess the safety and efficacy of these preparations prior to their integration into the common practice of Western medicine for the treatment of hepatitis C [2].

References

1. Patrick, L. Hepatitis C: epidemiology and review of complementary/alternative medicine treatments. *Alternative Medicine Review* 1999;4:220–238.

2. Seeff LB, Lindsay KL, Bacon BR, Kresina TF, Hoofnagle JH. Complementary and alternative medicine in chronic liver disease. *Hepatology* 2001;34:595–603.

3. Dehmlow C, Erhard J, de Groot H. Inhibition of Kupffer cell functions as an explanation for the hepatoprotective properties of silibinin. *Hepatology* 1996;23:749–754.

4. Fuchs EC, Wehenmeyer R, Weiner OH. Effects of silibinin and of a synthetic analogue on isolated rat hepatic stellate cells and myofibroblasts. *Arzneimittelforschung* 1997;12:1383–1387.

5. Polyak SJ, Morishima C, Shuhart MC, Wang CC, Lu Y, Lee DY. Inhibition of T-cell inflammatory cytokines, hepatocyte NF-κB signaling, and HCV infection by standardized silymarin. *Gastroenterology* 2007;132:1925–1936.

6. Ferenci P, Dragosic B, Dittrich H *et al.* Randomized controlled clinical trial of silymarin treatment in patients with cirrhosis of the liver. *Journal of Hepatology* 1989;9:105–113.

7. Stickel F, Schuppan D. Herbal medicine in the treatment of liver diseases. *Digestive and Liver Disease* 2007;39:293–304. **A comprehensive review.** 🔑

8. Jacobs B, Dennehy C, Ramirez G, Sapp J, Lawrence VA. Milk thistle for the treatment of liver diseases: a systematic review and meta-analysis. *American Journal of Medicine* 2002;113:506–515.

9. Gordon A, Hobbs DA, Bowden DS *et al.* Effects of *Silybum marianum* on serum hepatitis C virus RNA, alanine aminotransferase levels, and well-being in patients with chronic hepatitis C. *Journal of Gastroenterology and Hepatology* 2006;21:275–280.

10. Seeff LB, Curto TM, Szabo G *et al.* Herbal product use by persons enrolled in the hepatitis C antiviral long-term treatment against cirrhosis (HALT-C) trial. *Hepatology* 2008;47:605–612. **A post-hoc analysis on the use and impact of herbal products on clinical and biochemical parameters in US patients with advanced fibrosis/cirrhosis due to chronic HCV.** 🔑

11. Ferenci P, Scherzer TM, Kerschner H *et al.* Silibinin is a potent antiviral agent in patients with chronic hepatitis C not responding to pegylated interferon/ribavirin therapy. *Gastroenterology* 2008;135:1561–1567.

12. Gonzales-Peralta RP, Lau JY. Pathogenesis of hepatocellular damage in chronic hepatitis C virus infection. *Seminars in Gastrointestinal Disease* 1995;6:28–34.

13. Coon JT, Ernst E. Complementary and alternative therapies in the treatment of chronic hepatitis C: a systematic review. *Journal of Hepatology* 2004;40:491–500. **A systematic review on complementary and alternative therapies.** 🔑

14. von Herbay A, Stahl W, Niederau C, Sies H. Vitamin E improves the aminotransferase status of patients suffering from viral hepatitis C: a randomized, couble-blind, placebo-controlled study. *Free Radical Research* 1997;27:599–605.

15. Shaikh ZA, Vu TT, Zaman K. Oxidative stress as a mechanism of chronic cadmium-nduced hepatotoxicity and renal toxicity and protection by antioxidants. *Toxicology and Applied Pharmacology* 1999;154:256–263.

16. Wang JY, Guo JS, Li H, Liu SL, Sern MA. Inhibitory effects of glycyrrhizin on NF-kappa B binding activity in CCl_4-plus ethanol-induced liver cirrhosis in rats. *Liver* 1998;18:180–185.

17. Arase Y, Ikeda K, Murashima N. The long term efficacy of glycyrrhizin in chronic hepatitis C patients. *Cancer* 1997;79:1491–1500.

18. Batey RG, Bensousson A, Fan YY, Bollipo S, Hossain M. Preliminary report of a randomized, double-blind placebo-controlled trial of a Chinese herbal medicine preparation CH100 in the treatment of chronic hepatitis C. *Journal of Gastroenterology and Hepatology* 1998;13:244–247.

19. Shimizu I, Ma YR, Mizobuchi Y *et al.* Effects of sho-saiko-to, a Japanese herbal medicine, on hepatic fibrosis in mice. *Hepatology* 1999;29:149–160.

24 HCV in liver transplant recipients: how do you approach them?

Brett E. Fortune, Lisa M. Forman

University of Colorado Denver, Gastroenterology and Hepatology Division, Aurora, Colorado, USA

LEARNING POINTS

- HCV-infected patients have lower survival rates than non-HCV-infected patients after liver transplantation.

- Pre-emptive therapy is not well tolerated in the post-liver transplant population.

- Consider treatment of recurrent HCV in patients with biopsy-proven advanced fibrosis and/or increased hepatic venous pressure gradient.

- Treatment using combination of peginterferon and ribavirin in patients with confirmed HCV recurrence can improve allograft and patient survival.

- Barriers to treatment include patient tolerance due to adverse effects of antiviral therapy, risk of cellular rejection, and risk of alloimmune hepatitis.

Introduction

Hepatitis C virus (HCV) is one of the leading indications for liver transplantation (LT) worldwide. With recurrence of HCV being universal and a significant percentage developing severe histological recurrence, recurrent HCV infection represents one of the most significant issues facing the transplant physician today. Treatment of HCV in the transplant setting is challenging given the limited applicability, reduced tolerability and lower efficacy in comparison with the non-transplant setting.

Natural history of recurrent HCV

Recurrent HCV after LT has been shown to be accelerated and more aggressive when compared with HCV infection in the non-transplant setting. Up to 40% of patients transplanted for HCV develop allograft cirrhosis in 5 years, in contrast to 5–20% at 20 years in the non-transplant setting [1,2]. Once allograft failure occurs, decompensation occurs in up to two-thirds of patients within 3 years. In addition, it has been demonstrated that 5-year survival rates after LT in HCV-positive patients are diminished compared with HCV-negative patients (56.7% vs. 65.6%; $P < 0.05$) (Figure 24.1) [3]. Factors associated with severe HCV recurrence include advanced donor age, female gender, viral load, genotype, cytomegalovirus infection and the treatment of rejection.

Treatment of recurrent HCV

Given the high prevalence of HCV recurrence, one must decide if and when to start antiviral treatment. Considerations include presence of viraemia, degree of allograft damage as well as recipients' psychosocial status. The post-LT treatment

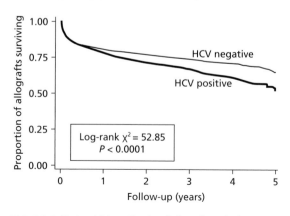

FIG. 24.1 Kaplan–Meier estimates of allograft survival according to HCV status. (From Forman *et al.* [3] with permission from Elsevier.)

Clinical Dilemmas in Viral Liver Disease, 1st edition. Edited by Graham R. Foster and K. Rajender Reddy. © 2010 Blackwell Publishing.

of HCV has improved over the past decade with the best results obtained using the combination of peginterferon and ribavirin [4]. However, sustained virological response (SVR) rates are much lower than those achieved in immuno-competent HCV-infected patients (on average 20–25% less). Positive predictors for SVR include early virological response (> 2 log reduction in HCV RNA at 12 weeks), non-genotype 1 virus, adherence to therapy and lower levels of baseline viraemia.

Pre-emptive antiviral treatment

Pre-emptive treatment refers to early antiviral therapy days to weeks after LT, prior to the development of histological recurrence. Several hypothesized advantages with this approach include low HCV RNA levels and the absence of histologically advanced disease. However, from a clinical standpoint, this timing of treatment is most challenging due to poor performance status, cytopenias from maximal immunosuppression, and higher rates of rejection and infection. Based on limitations due to antiviral toxicity, it has been estimated that only 60% of LT recipients are eligible for pre-emptive therapy and half will require the need for dose reduction [5]. From the only published randomized trial investigating efficacy of pre-emptive HCV therapy (Table 24.1), 41% of patients were eligible and achieved

an SVR of only 9% [6]. Hence, the efficacy of pre-emptive antiviral therapy remains poorly defined. We do not favour this approach due to the lack of proven benefit. However, this approach could be considered in patients undergoing re-transplantation for rapidly progressive recurrent HCV or in patients (e.g. living donor recipients) who were transplanted with lower Model for End-stage Liver Disease (MELD) scores. Regarding the latter, these patients are relatively 'healthier' and therefore may be able to better tolerate treatment [7].

Treatment of established recurrent HCV

Given the lack of efficacy and limitations of pre-emptive therapy, most hepatologists have opted to delay treatment until patients develop significant recurrent disease. This approach selectively targets those likely to achieve most benefit with antiviral therapy and avoids unnecessary toxicity in those without significant disease recurrence.

There have been multiple published studies evaluating the efficacy of recurrent HCV therapy. However, these studies are difficult to compare as a wide variety of study designs and end-points (SVR, histological improvement, allograft and patient survival) have been used (Table 24.1). The majority of these studies have shown that SVR leads to histological improvement or reduction of fibrosis progression and improved allograft and patient survival [4,8–11].

TABLE 24.1 Published controlled trials utilizing antiviral therapy for pre-emptive treatment or for recurrent HCV.

Reference	Type of trial	No. of patients	Antiviral regimen α-2b C/R	SVR
Castells *et al.*, 2005 [10]	NRT Post-LT HCV recurrence	48	Peginterferon α-2b (1.5 μg/kg per week) + ribavirin (600–800 mg/day) for 24 weeks + 24 weeks if RNA negative	33%
			No treatment	0%
Bizollon *et al.*, 2007 [11]	NRT Post-LT HCV recurrence	48	Peginterferon α-2b (1.5 μg/kg per week) + ribavirin (800–1000 mg/day)	30%
			No treatment	0%
Carrion *et al.*, 2007 [9]	RCT Post-LT HCV recurrence	54	Peginterferon α-2b (1.5 μg/kg per week) + ribavirin (800–1200 mg/day)	48%
			No treatment	0%
Shergill *et al.*, 2005 [6]	RCT Pre-emptive	51	Interferon α-2b (3 MU three times per week) or peginterferon α-2b (1.5 μg/kg per week) or peginterferon α-2b (1.5 μg/kg per week) + ribavirin (600–1200 mg/day)	9%
			No treatment	0%

LT, liver transplantation; MU, million units; NRT, non-randomized trial; RCT, randomized controlled trial; SVR, sustained virological response.

Castells *et al.* [10] studied 24 patients receiving peginterferon alfa-2b (1.5 µg/kg per week) and ribavirin (600–800 mg/day) for 48 weeks (if HCV RNA undetectable at 24 weeks) and 24 consecutive untreated controls. Overall SVR was 33% in the treatment group and 0% in controls. On univariate analysis, SVR was associated with absence of corticosteroid administration to treat rejection ($P = 0.01$), presence of early virological response ($P = 0.002$) and absence of cytomegalovirus infection ($P = 0.001$).

Bizollon *et al.* [11] studied 27 patients with established recurrent HCV (median 10 months after LT) receiving peginterferon alfa-2b (1.5 µg/kg per week) and ribavirin (800–1000 mg/day) for 48 weeks and compared them to 21 consecutive untreated controls. SVR was 30% in the treatment group and 0% in controls. All eight patients achieving SVR had improvement in histology. Based on univariate analysis, the use of cyclosporine ($P = 0.03$) and early virological response ($P = 0.02$) were associated with SVR.

Carrion *et al.* [9] have published the only randomized study to date. In this study, 54 patients with mild HCV recurrence at least 6 months after LT were randomized to either peginterferon alfa-2b (1.5 µg/kg per week) and ribavirin (800–1200 mg/day) for 48 weeks or no treatment. Overall SVR in the treatment group was 48%. Histological response was seen in 74% of the treated compared with 30% of controls, with all patients achieving SVR having a histological response.

Given the supportive data for treatment in patients with biopsy-proven HCV recurrence, there remains the question of how to approach the timing of therapy. One approach initiates antiviral treatment at the time of initial diagnosis of acute recurrent hepatitis, utilizing liver biopsy to exclude other causes for elevated liver enzymes such as acute cellular rejection. The second approach is to initiate antiviral therapy when clinically significant fibrosis exists based on predetermined protocol liver biopsies.

The 12-month post-LT liver biopsy has the capability to stratify fibrosis progression among patients transplanted for HCV and to help determine whether to initiate antiviral therapy. Patients whose biopsies show severe disease recurrence within the first year after transplant are at a higher chance of progressing to allograft failure and should be considered for antiviral therapy [12]. Another option for monitoring post-LT patients with HCV is measurement of the hepatic venous pressure gradient (HVPG). This appears to have some benefit in the assessment of progressive fibrosis from recurrent HCV [13]. Elevated HVPG at 1 year after

LT has been shown to be superior to liver biopsy in accurately predicting clinical decompensation. Similar studies have also shown strong correlation between HVPG measurements and histological response after treatment with antivirals [10].

We recommend that patients with recurrent HCV-related fibrosis (Metavir stage ≥ 2), severe inflammation (Metavir grade ≥ 3), evidence of significant hepatic dysfunction (elevated bilirubin, prolonged prothrombin time), or elevated HVPG gradients should be evaluated for antiviral therapy [7]. Overall, treatment of appropriately selected patients with HCV recurrence and confirmed progressive histological disease has been shown to reduce or possibly reverse progression of fibrosis, decrease the risk of allograft failure, and improve patient survival.

Barriers and limitations to antiviral treatment

There are several limitations or barriers to antiviral therapy in patients with recurrent HCV. SVR rates in these patients are significantly less than in non-transplant patients due to a higher percentage of genotype 1 patients, poor patient tolerability, and lower drug dosing secondary to drug toxicity and the possibility of interferon-induced acute cellular rejection.

Patient tolerance of antiviral medications is a major limitation for treatment success. Patients may not be able to tolerate the major adverse effects of peginterferon or ribavirin at therapeutic doses, especially cytopenias. During the post-LT period, immunosuppression can lead to severe reduction in bone marrow production of white blood cells as well as production of red blood cells. Antiviral therapy may further reduce these cell lines, leading to serious complications such as infection or sepsis. However, with the addition of medications that stimulate red cell and white cell production, more patients may be able to tolerate antivirals at higher doses and for longer periods of time. Another option is to use a low-accelerating dose regimen (LADR) to help increase patient tolerance and assist with improved survival after transplantation. Using LADR, Everson *et al.* [14] achieved an overall SVR rate of 24%; tolerance was much improved and patients required less dose reduction and/or discontinuation.

A potentially serious and controversial complication of antiviral therapy unique to the post-transplant population is interferon-induced rejection. Studies using peginterferon and ribavirin have yielded conflicting results [9], but the trend for acute rejection has been observed and cannot be dismissed. Another concern is the development of chronic cellular rejection due to the patient having repeated episodes of acute cellular rejection. In addition, calcineurin inhibitor levels must be monitored during antiviral therapy; a greater proportion of antiviral responders experienced a greater reduction in immunosuppression levels than non-responders. This is presumably due to improved hepatic function leading to enhanced biotransformation and lower immunosuppression levels and may play a key role in predisposing these patients to rejection.

Another potential complication from antiviral therapy is alloimmune hepatitis, a condition characterized by biopsy findings of severe interface hepatitis with plasmacellular infiltration and rosettes [15]. A positive predictor for the occurrence of alloimmune hepatitis includes the use of anti-lymphocyte antibodies for immunosuppression induction. A protective variable is the use of granulocyte colony-stimulating factor. Unfortunately, due to a small sample size, it is difficult to determine the clinical significance of these findings, but alloimmune hepatitis as a potential complication of peginterferon-based therapy cannot be dismissed. There should be a high suspicion for either alloimmune hepatitis or acute cellular rejection in patients on antiviral therapy who have worsening liver enzymes in the setting of undetectable HCV RNA.

Liver biopsy is important for differentiating rejection, HCV recurrence or alloimmune hepatitis. This is extremely important since the treatment of rejection/alloimmune hepatitis with OKT3 and steroids can lead to rapid progression of HCV-induced allograft injury. Of course, a greater challenge for the clinician is how to treat the patient with simultaneous acute rejection and HCV recurrence. This remains a much-debated topic and thus far no conclusions can be made.

Summary

HCV recurrence is frequent and leads to a significant reduction in patient and allograft survival as well as fibrosis progression after transplantation. SVR is achievable, but challenging, with the use of combined peginterferon and ribavirin. Several obstacles remain for the transplant physician and include patient tolerance, risk of rejection and the development of alloimmune hepatitis. Moreover, during this time after transplantation, social and psychiatric factors may also add into the equation of selecting which patients would be capable of tolerating these medications.

Based on our experience, we do not endorse pre-emptive treatment due to the lack of proven efficacy. However, this approach could be used in the future for living-donor LT and other patients with 'lower' MELD scores, depending on the presence of future supportive data. We do advocate using protocol liver biopsies or biopsy when liver tests are abnormal. If these biopsies show any advanced histological changes due to HCV recurrence, we would consider using the LADR approach consisting of peginterferon and ribavirin. We would also use the trend of HCV RNA levels and liver tests to assist with efficacy of treatment as well as titration of antiviral dosing. There may be a need to re-biopsy if liver tests continue to remain elevated during treatment in order to evaluate for superimposed acute cellular rejection and/or alloimmune hepatitis. If alloimmune hepatitis or rejection develops, HCV therapy may need to be held or possible additional immunosuppression added to antiviral treatment. Treatment of recurrent HCV is challenging and remains a major clinical dilemma in LT. Future trials and protocols will need to be developed in order to improve our management of these patients.

References

1. Gane EJ, Portmann BC, Naoumov NV *et al*. Long-term outcome of hepatitis C infection after liver transplantation. *New England Journal of Medicine* 1996;334:815–820.

2. Berenguer M, Prieto M, Rayon JM *et al*. Natural history of clinically compensated HCV-related graft cirrhosis following liver transplantation. *Hepatology* 2000;32:852–858.

3. Forman LM, Lewis JD, Berlin JA *et al*. The association between hepatitis C infection and survival after orthotopic liver transplantation. *Gastroenterology* 2002;122:889–896. **Pivotal study demonstrating the diminished survival of HCV patients after LT.** 🔑

4. Xirouchakis E, Triantos C, Manousou P *et al*. Pegylated-interferon and ribavirin in liver transplant candidates and recipients with HCV cirrhosis: systematic review and meta-analysis of prospective controlled studies. *Journal of Viral Hepatitis* 2008;15:699–709. **Meta-analysis providing a review of the major trials involving pre-emptive and recurrent HCV therapy to date.** 🔑

5. Terrault NA. Prophylactic and preemptive therapies for hepatitis C virus-infected patients undergoing liver transplantation. *Liver Transplantation* 2003;9:S95–S100.

6. Shergill AK, Khalili M, Straley S *et al*. Applicability, tolerability, and efficacy of preemptive antiviral therapy in

hepatitis C-infected patients undergoing liver transplantation. *American Journal of Transplantation* 2005;5: 118–124.

7. Wiesner RH, Sorrell M, Villamil F, International Liver Transplant Society Expert Panel. Report of the first International Liver Transplant Society expert panel consensus conference on liver transplantation and hepatic C. *Liver Transplantation* 2003;9:S1–S9.

8. Triantos C, Samonakis D, Stigliano R *et al.* Liver transplantation and hepatitis C virus: systematic review of antiviral therapy. *Transplantation* 2005;79:261–268.

9. Carrion JA, Navasa M, Garcia-Retortillo M *et al.* Efficacy of antiviral therapy on hepatitis C recurrence after liver transplantation: a randomized controlled study. *Gastroenterology* 2007;132:1746–1756.

10. Castells L, Vargas V, Allende H *et al.* Combined treatment with pegylated interferon (alpha-2b) and ribavirin in the acute phase of hepatitis C virus recurrence after liver transplantation. *Journal of Hepatology* 2005;43:53–59.

11. Bizollon T, Pradat P, Mabrut JY *et al.* Histological benefit of retreatment by pegylated interferon alpha-2b and ribavirin in patients with recurrent hepatitis C virus infection post-transplantation. *American Journal of Transplantation* 2007;7:448–453.

12. Firpi RJ, Abdelmalek MF, Soldevila-Pico C *et al.* One-year protocol liver biopsy can stratify fibrosis progression in liver transplant recipients with recurrent hepatitis C infection. *Liver Transplantation* 2004;10:1240–1247.

13. Samonakis D, Cholongitas E, Thalheimer U *et al.* Hepatic venous pressure gradient to assess fibrosis and its progression after liver transplantation for HCV cirrhosis. *Liver Transplantation* 2007;13:1305–1311.

14. Everson GT, Trotter J, Forman L *et al.* Treatment of advanced hepatitis C with a low accelerating dosage regimen of antiviral therapy. *Hepatology* 2005;42:255–262.

15. Berardi S, Lodato F, Gramenzi A *et al.* High incidence of allograft dysfunction in liver transplanted patients treated with pegylated-interferon alpha-2b and ribavirin for hepatitis C recurrence: possible de novo autoimmune hepatitis? *Gut* 2007;56:237–242.

25 HCV in patients with advanced disease: do you treat them and do you have any caveats?

Gregory T. Everson

University of Colorado School of Medicine, University of Colorado Health Sciences Center, Transplant Center and Hepatology, Aurora, Colorado, USA

LEARNING POINTS

- An increasing number of patients with advanced hepatitis C are presenting to clinics for treatment of chronic hepatitis C.

- The clinician must characterize the severity of the underlying liver disease before recommending or embarking on a course of antiviral therapy. In general, the Child–Turcotte–Pugh classification is useful for defining compensated (class A) and decompensated (class B or C) cirrhosis.

- Compensated patients have reasonably good chances for SVR and are less prone to severe adverse events or complications.

- Decompensated patients are difficult to treat and difficult to cure and should be managed primarily by physicians or care providers experienced in the treatment of HCV and management of cirrhosis.

- Rendering blood free of HCV RNA prior to liver transplantation reduces the rate of post-transplant recurrence of hepatitis C.

- These patients are prone to cytopenias, which worsen with treatment: growth factors such as G-CSF and erythropoietin analogue are often required.

- The clinician is required to monitor these patients carefully to detect and manage treatment-emergent adverse events or complications.

Clinical Dilemmas in Viral Liver Disease, 1st edition. Edited by Graham R. Foster and K. Rajender Reddy. © 2010 Blackwell Publishing.

Natural history after development of cirrhosis

Clinically, cirrhosis due to hepatitis C virus (HCV) progresses from compensation to decompensation. The term 'compensation' defines patients with Child–Turcotte–Pugh (CTP) class A or score 6 or less, low MELD (Model for End-stage Liver Disease) score, and no history of clinical complications. Despite relative clinical stability at time of presentation, patients with compensated cirrhosis are at risk for progression of disease and clinical deterioration. Estimated rates for development of clinical deterioration (decompensation), hepatoma and death from liver disease in patients with compensated cirrhosis are 3.6–6.0% per year, 1.4–3.3% per year, and 2.6–4.0% per year, respectively [1–7]. Patients with hepatitis C and cirrhosis who experience decompensation have a 5-year survival of only 50% [3].

Goals of antiviral therapy

Disease progression is driven by ongoing active viral replication. Sustained virological response (SVR) to antiviral therapy reduces the risk of progression of fibrosis to cirrhosis [8] and, in patients with compensated cirrhosis, reduces the risk of decompensation, liver-related death and hepatoma [9,10]. SVR may even improve outcomes in patients with decompensated cirrhosis [11]. Thus, the main goal of treatment of cirrhosis, compensated or decompensated, is SVR. In patients on transplant waiting lists, another goal is rendering the patient's blood negative for HCV RNA prior to transplantation to prevent post-transplant HCV recurrence and allograft hepatitis [12–14].

Antiviral therapy in naive compensated patients

The large randomized controlled trials of interferon-based therapy included a small percentage of patients with either advanced bridging fibrosis or compensated cirrhosis [15–22]. All patients with cirrhosis who enrolled into these trials had well-compensated disease, i.e. normal or nearly normal laboratory tests and absence of history of clinical decompensation. Although entry criteria allowed platelet counts as low as $90–100 \times 10^9$/L, average platelet counts were within the normal range. In all these trials SVR was 5–10% lower in patients with advanced fibrosis or cirrhosis compared to patients with lesser degrees of fibrosis. SVRs were 5–15% for interferon monotherapy, 20–30% for peginterferon monotherapy, 30–40% for interferon plus ribavirin, and 40–50% for peginterferon plus ribavirin. Response was lowest in patients with genotype 1 infection, particularly those with high viral load. In the study by Hadziyannis et al. [22], SVR was 41% in genotype 1 infection and 73% in genotype 2 and 3 infection with bridging fibrosis or cirrhosis. Helbling et al. [23] randomized 124 patients with advanced fibrosis or compensated cirrhosis to peginterferon with either standard or low-dose ribavirin. Overall SVR was 58% for patients infected with HCV genotypes 2 or 3, and 32% for patients infected with HCV genotype 1.

Antiviral therapy in treatment-experienced compensated patients

In the lead-in phase of the Hepatitis C Antiviral Long-Term Treatment against Cirrhosis (HALT-C) trial, 1145 prior non-responders to interferon or interferon/ribavirin with advanced fibrosis or cirrhosis were retreated with peginterferon/ribavirin [24,25]. The overall rate of SVR was 18% and was related to type of prior therapy: SVR was 27% when prior therapy was interferon monotherapy, 34% when peginterferon monotherapy, 13% when interferon/ribavirin, and 11% when peginterferon/ribavirin. SVR correlated with HCV genotypes 2 or 3, higher platelet count and lower fibrosis score and was compromised by dose reduction.

SVR declined from 23% in least severe disease to 9% in most severe disease independently of dose reductions [25]. Patients with least severe disease were defined by fibrosis and platelet count in excess of 125×10^9/L and patients with most severe disease as those with cirrhosis and platelet count of 125×10^9/L or less. Reduction in SVR, independent of dose reductions and other factors predicting response, indicates that patients with cirrhosis are not only difficult to treat but also relatively resistant to peginterferon/ribavirin and therefore difficult to cure.

Patients with cirrhosis infected with HCV genotypes 2 or 3 are much more likely to experience SVR than patients infected with HCV genotype 1 when retreated with peginterferon/ribavirin. In the EPIC trial [26], 2333 prior non-responders or relapsers to either interferon/ribavirin or peginterferon/ribavirin were retreated with peginterferon/ribavirin. Rates of SVR in the patients with compensated cirrhosis retreated with peginterferon/ribavirin are shown in Table 25.1. Rates of SVR were higher in relapsers compared with non-responders across all genotypes.

Outcome after SVR in compensated patients

Hepatic fibrosis reverses and clinical outcome improves after SVR. Camma et al. [27] performed a meta-analysis of 1013 patients enrolled in three randomized trials of interferon or peginterferon spanning the spectrum from mild fibrosis to cirrhosis who had liver biopsies at baseline and after 6 months of treatment. SVR was associated with a −0.59 reduction in fibrosis score (4-point scale). In another study, SVR was associated with a −1.0 reduction in fibrosis score and a −0.65 reduction in inflammation score [28]. In multivariate analysis, the only factors associated with histological improvement in the cohort was SVR and lower body weight.

TABLE 25.1 Rates of SVR (%) in patients with compensated cirrhosis retreated with peginterferon/ribavirin.

	Previous therapy	
	Interferon/ribavirin	Peginterferon/ribavirin
HCV genotype 1	11	9
HCV genotype 2 or 3	50	45

Veldt *et al.* [9] studied 479 patients with a median follow-up of 2.1 years (range 0.8–4.9 years); 142 patients experienced SVR and outcome was compared to the 337 without SVR. SVR was associated with reduction in a composite end-point of clinical decompensation, liver transplantation and mortality: the improvement in outcome was mainly related to decrease in risk of liver-related death. Bruno *et al.* [10] studied 883 patients with biopsy-proven cirrhosis with a mean follow-up of 96.1 months (range 6–167 months). There were no liver-related complications, and rates of hepatocellular carcinoma (HCC) and liver-related death were significantly lower in the 124 patients who experienced SVR. Thus, SVR halts or reverses fibrosis, preventing disease progression, and reduces rates of clinical outcomes in patients with advanced fibrosis or cirrhosis.

Although the patient with compensated cirrhosis may be difficult to treat and difficult to cure, achievement of SVR yields significant long-term clinical benefits that clearly warrant an attempt at antiviral therapy.

The decompensated patient: selection criteria

Treatment of patients with clinical decompensation using peginterferon/ribavirin is problematic: virological response is lower and severe complications, some life-threatening, may occur. In addition, several characteristics of these patients impair virological response (Table 25.2). Careful selection of candidates may yield greatest chance for SVR and limit risk.

TABLE 25.2 Factors impairing virological response to peginterferon/ribavirin in patients with advanced fibrosis or compensated cirrhosis.

Genotype 1 HCV (especially high viral load)

Increasing disease severity defined by increasing fibrosis (Ishak 5 or 6) and decreasing platelet count (cut-off 125×10^9/L)

Reduction in doses of peginterferon or ribavirin

Discontinuation of peginterferon/ribavirin

Severe hepatic impairment

Prior non-response or relapse with interferon or peginterferon plus ribavirin

Intolerant of side effects

Cytopenia

Patients experiencing decompensation are typically evaluated for liver transplantation and, if candidacy is confirmed, they may be listed. Approximately 40% of the patients listed for liver transplantation in the USA have either a primary or secondary diagnosis of hepatitis C (Organ Procurement and Transplantation Network data, http://www.OPTN.org/LatestData/rptData.asp). Because these patients may decompensate further during treatment, many centres restrict treatment of decompensated patients to those who are candidates or listed for liver transplantation [29].

The Consensus Development Conference on Liver Transplantation and Hepatitis C suggested that patients on the waiting list with MELD scores 18 or less could be considered for treatment [30]. In addition, the American Association for the Study of Liver Diseases (AASLD) practice guidelines state that patients referred for liver transplantation with a mild degree of hepatic compromise could be considered for antiviral therapy, initiated at low dose, 'as long as treatment is administered by experienced clinicians, with vigilant monitoring for adverse events' [31].

Given these guidelines, the characteristics of patients who may be potential candidates for antiviral therapy include:

- MELD score 18 or less;
- living donor recipients;
- MELD upgrade for HCC.

In the USA, the average MELD score at time of transplantation is typically greater than 25. These patients may be too sick to treat. Patients who undergo living donor liver transplantation typically have less severe disease and lower MELD score at time of transplantation, compared with patients who wait for a liver graft from a deceased donor. Also, patients who receive MELD upgrade points for early HCC can have relatively mild liver disease. MELD scores based on severity of liver disease prior to MELD upgrade for underlying HCC are typically less than 18.

Results of antiviral therapy

There are two goals in treating patients with decompensated cirrhosis. The first is to achieve SVR with the potential that SVR could stabilize or reverse disease progression and eliminate the need for transplantation. The second goal, in patients listed for transplantation, is to render the recipient's blood negative for HCV RNA prior to transplantation to prevent post-transplant recurrence of HCV infection.

TABLE 25.3 SVR in decompensated cirrhosis.

Reference	No. of patients	Treatment	RNA negative at end of treatment (%)	SVR (%)
Iacobellis et al. [11]	66	PEG/RBV	49	20
Forns [43]	51	PEG/RBV	29	20
Tekin et al. [39]	20	PEG/RBV	45	30
Annicchiarico et al. [38]	15	PEG/RBV	47	20
Lim/Imperiale [unpublished]	32	IFN, PEG/RBV	–	31
Everson et al. [32]	124	IFN/RBV	46	24
Forns et al. [33]	30	IFN/RBV	30	20
Thomas et al. [34]	20	IFN	60	20
Amarapurkar et al. [37]	18	IFN ± RBV	61	38
Crippin et al. [35]	15	IFN ± RBV	33	0
Total	391		44	23

SVR, sustained virological response (defined as HCV RNA negative 6 months or more after discontinuation of treatment); PEG, peginterferon; RBV, ribavirin; IFN, non-pegylated interferon.

Halting disease progression

The published experience with antiviral therapy of decompensated cirrhosis is given in Table 25.3. Except for the study by Iacobellis et al. [11], most series represented single-centre experiences, were non-randomized uncontrolled trials, and patients selected for treatment were candidates or listed for transplantation [32–39].

Iacobellis et al. [11] randomized 129 patients with decompensated cirrhosis due to HCV who were not candidates for liver transplantation to either peginterferon/ribavirin ($N = 66$) or no treatment ($N = 63$). The patients selected for this trial had had hospital admissions for ascites, variceal bleeding or encephalopathy, were naive to interferon/ribavirin or peginterferon/ribavirin, and lacked overt liver failure. Approximately 75% were classified as Child–Pugh class A or B and average MELD score was 14. Two-thirds were infected with HCV genotype 1 and average platelet count was 86×10^9/L. Rates of SVR were 43.5% and 7.0% for patients infected with HCV genotypes 2 or 3 and HCV genotype 1, respectively. The outcome of patients achieving SVR was favourable and included marked reduction in risk for decompensation, complications, and death related to liver disease. The results suggested that clearance of HCV with antiviral therapy may reduce disease progression and potentially be life-saving in patients with decompensated cirrhosis. However, the low response in HCV genotype 1 infection coupled with adverse and serious adverse events indicates limited application of this strategy.

Patients with cirrhosis need ongoing monitoring, even after SVR. We have examined the long-term outcome of 18 patients who experienced SVR but who did not undergo transplantation (unpublished data). These patients have experienced reduction in risk of liver-related complications and mortality, but four have expired from HCC. Despite SVR and stabilization of hepatic disease, patients with cirrhosis should continue to undergo frequent monitoring for development of HCC.

We reported our experience treating 124 patients with advanced hepatitis C with a low accelerating dose regimen (LADR) of interferon (or peginterferon) plus ribavirin [32]; 80% were classified as Child–Pugh class A or B, average CTP score was 7.4 ± 2.3 and average MELD score was 11.0 ± 3.7. SVR was 13% and relapse 65% in patients with genotype 1 HCV and 50% and 42% in patients with genotype 2 or 3 HCV. There have now been additional reports [32–39] in the literature encompassing a total of 391 patients, yielding a pooled SVR of 23% (Table 25.3).

In our experience, side effects and adverse events were common. During treatment, 56% developed anaemia (haemoglobin < 12 g/dL), 49% leucopenia (absolute neutrophil

TABLE 25.4 Prevention of post-transplant recurrence.

Reference	No. of patients	RNA negative on day of transplant (%)	Post-transplant virological response (%)*
Forns [43]	51	29	20
Everson [32]	47	32	26
Forns [33]	30	30	20
Thomas [34]	20	60	20
Crippin [35]	2	0	0
Everson (LADR-A2ALL)† [unpublished]	79	46 to 69	G1 18 G2/3 39
Total	150	34	21

* Defined as HCV RNA negative for 6 months or more after transplantation.
† Randomized controlled trial submitted to AASLD 2009. LADR-A2ALL, low accelerated dose regimen of peginterferon/ribavirin conducted as a substudy of the NIH-sponsored Adult-to-Adult Living Donor Liver Transplantation (A2ALL) study. Patients infected with genotypes 1, 4, 5 and 6 were randomized 2 : 1 treatment to control, and patients infected with genotypes 2 or 3 were treated.

count $< 1000 \times 10^6/L$) and 33% significant thrombocytopenia ($< 50 \times 10^9/L$). Of 22 serious complications, 21 occurred in 14 patients with CTP class B or C cirrhosis; complications included encephalopathy, ascites, infection, gastrointestinal bleeding, diabetes mellitus and venous thrombosis. Overall there were seven deaths, two during antiviral therapy.

Preventing post-transplant recurrence of HCV

As stated above, one of the goals of treating decompensated patients who are on the waiting list is to render their blood free of HCV RNA in order to prevent reinfection of the liver graft with HCV (Table 25.4). In our published experience, we have transplanted 47 patients, 32 of whom were HCV RNA positive and 15 who were HCV RNA negative at the time of transplantation [32]. All of the 32 who were HCV RNA positive before transplantation had recurrence of HCV after transplantation. In contrast, 12 of the 15 who were HCV RNA negative at the time of transplantation remained free of HCV after transplantatin. These results prove the concept that effective suppression of HCV RNA prior to liver transplantation can potentially eliminate post-transplant recurrence. Similar results were reported by Forns et al. [33], who treated 30 patients with hepatitis C and cirrhosis awaiting liver transplantation with an estimated time to transplantation of 5 months or less. Nine patients (30%) achieved on-treatment clearance of HCV RNA from blood and six (20%) remained free of HCV after transplantation. Very early virological response ($\geq 2 \log_{10}$ at week 4) was the strongest predictor of SVR. Overall, the published experience suggests that post-transplant recurrence may be prevented in 21% of patients selected for this treatment (Table 25.4).

The most recent experience from Barcelona highlights the advantages and disadvantages of pretransplant antiviral therapy [36]. On the plus side, treatment was associated with SVR of 20%, early virological response and non-genotype 1 HCV being predictive of SVR. In contrast, negative aspects of treatment included higher rates of side effects and incidence of bacterial infections compared with case-controls (17 vs. 3 episodes; $P = 0.0016$). As a result of this experience, the authors recommended antibiotic prophylaxis during antiviral therapy for this patient population.

It is currently recommended that patients with decompensated cirrhosis should only be treated with antiviral therapy by experienced clinicians or in the setting of a clinical trial [40].

Growth factors

Many patients with cirrhosis may have neutropenia, thrombocytopenia and anaemia prior to institution of treatment. Use of interferon and ribavirin in this population will tend to worsen or precipitate cytopenias. Treatment-related neutropenia and thrombocytopenia are more common and severe with peginterferon compared with non-pegylated interferon. The benefit of higher virological response rates with peginterferon may be counterbalanced by complications related to cytopenias.

Two strategies are used to control these side effects: dose reduction or use of growth factors such as granulocyte colony-stimulating factor (G-CSF) and erythropoietin analogues. The value of either G-CSF or erythropoietin in preventing complications or enhancing virological response is unknown. However, the alternative strategy, dose reduction, may compromise the primary objective of achieving the highest rate of virological response. Dietrich *et al.* [41] have demonstrated that use of erythropoietin during treatment of chronic hepatitis C with interferon plus ribavirin can increase haemoglobin concentrations and maintain higher doses of ribavirin. For these reasons, use of growth factors is favoured over dose reduction in the management of cytopenias.

Management of the patient who fails to respond

The primary goal of antiviral therapy, sustained viral clearance, can be achieved in only a minority of patients with cirrhosis, especially those with more severe disease or decompensation. In the absence of SVR, suppression of disease activity and monitoring patients for disease progression and development of HCC are secondary goals.

Maintenance therapy with low-dose peginterferon was suggested as one means of controlling disease progression. However, the recently published results of 1050 patients (622 with advanced fibrosis and 428 with cirrhosis) from the HALT-C trial indicate that this type of maintenance therapy is ineffective [42]. In HALT-C, 517 patients received low-dose peginterferon monotherapy for 3.5 years and 533 were not treated but served as controls. Although alanine aminotransferase (ALT), HCV RNA level and hepatic inflammation were significantly lower in patients receiving peginterferon, there was no difference in the rate of any clinical outcome (34.1% in the treatment group and 33.8% in the control group). Clinical outcomes included death, HCC, hepatic decompensation, or progression of fibrosis to cirrhosis. There was a trend towards higher rates of serious adverse events in the treated group ($P = 0.07$). Unpublished results from COPILOT and EPIC, other trials of maintenance low-dose peginterferon, also failed to demonstrate improvement in clinical outcome, although events related to portal hypertension, such as variceal haemorrhage, were lower in patients treated with peginterferon. The conclusion from these trials is that maintenance therapy is not likely of benefit in reducing rates of clinical outcomes.

Given the absence of effective therapy to suppress disease progression, patients with cirrhosis must be monitored for complications of liver disease and development of HCC. Screening protocols to detect and manage oesophageal varices and HCC are warranted. Although screening is particularly relevant for the patient who has failed antiviral therapy and who remains positive for HCV, patients with cirrhosis who have achieved SVR can still develop HCC and should be monitored.

Summary

Antiviral therapy for patients with chronic hepatitis C and compensated cirrhosis, decompensated cirrhosis or patients on the waiting list for liver transplantation is evolving. Current data from existing clinical trials suggest that about one-third of naive patients with genotype 1 HCV and two-thirds of naive patients with genotype 2 and 3 HCV with advanced fibrosis or early compensated cirrhosis can achieve SVR. These results have prompted many to advocate aggressive therapy in well-compensated cirrhotics (CTP Class A) who lack evidence of clinical decompensation. However, the response of cirrhotics to antiviral therapy declines with severity of liver disease and non-response to prior interferon-based treatments. The pooled experience from the published literature indicates that only 23% of patients with decompensated cirrhosis can achieve SVR with current therapies. SVR in patients with HCV genotype 1 infection range from 5 to 20%. In contrast, SVR in genotypes 2 and 3 are approximately 50%. The low rate of SVR in decompensated patients is related to high prevalence of genotype 1 HCV, inability to achieve full doses of interferon and ribavirin due to side effects and dose-limiting cytopenias, and risk of complications related to deteriorating liver function. Despite the low rates of SVR, on-treatment clearance of HCV from blood occurs in approximately 30% of genotype 1 patients and 80% of genotype 2 and 3 patients; these patients have retained some level of response to interferon/ribavirin. In addition, pretransplant clearance of HCV RNA from blood may reduce the risk of post-transplant recurrence of hepatitis C. Addition of highly active anti-HCV therapies either alone or in combination with peginterferon/ribavirin may significantly improve outcomes in cirrhosis and reduce rates of HCV recurrence after transplantation. Carefully controlled trials of current and emerging antiviral therapies are critically in need for these difficult-to-treat and difficult-to-cure patients.

References

1. Tong MJ, el-Farra NS, Reikes AR, Co RL. Clinical outcomes after transfusion-associated hepatitis C. *New England Journal of Medicine* 1995;332:1463–1466.

2. Kiyosawa K, Umemura T, Ichijo T *et al.* Hepatocellular carcinoma: recent trends in Japan. *Gastroenterology* 2004;127(5 Suppl 1):S17–S26.

3. Fattovich G, Giustina G, Degos F *et al.* Morbidity and mortality in compensated cirrhosis type C: a retrospective follow-up study of 384 patients. *Gastroenterology* 1997;112:463–472.

4. Serfaty L, Aumaitre H, Chazouilleres O *et al.* Determinants of outcome of compensated hepatitis C virus-related cirrhosis. *Hepatology* 1998;27:1435–1440.

5. Hu KQ, Tong MJ. The long-term outcomes of patients with compensated hepatitis C virus-related cirrhosis and history of parenteral exposure in the United States. *Hepatology* 1999;29:1311–1316.

6. Khan MH, Farrell GC, Byth K *et al.* Which patients with hepatitis C develop liver complications? *Hepatology* 2000;31:513–520.

7. Lok AS, Seeff LB, Morgan TR *et al.* Incidence of hepatocellular carcinoma and associated risk factors in hepatitis C-related advanced liver disease. *Gastroenterology* 2009;136:138–148.

8. Huang JF, Yu ML, Lee CM *et al.* Sustained virological response to interferon reduces cirrhosis in chronic hepatitis C: a 1386-patient study from Taiwan. *Alimentary Pharmacology and Therapeutics* 2007;25:1029–1037.

9. Veldt BJ, Heathcote EJ, Wedemeyer H *et al.* Sustained virologic response and clinical outcomes in patients with chronic hepatitis C and advanced fibrosis. *Annals of Internal Medicine* 2007;147:677–684. **Sustained virological response in patients with advanced hepatitis C was associated with reduced risk for clinical decompensation or liver-related death.** ⊙━

10. Bruno S, Stroffolini T, Colombo M *et al.* Sustained virologic response to interferon-α is associated with improved outcome in HCV-related cirrhosis: a retrospective study. *Hepatology* 2007;45:579–587. **Sustained virology response in patients with cirrhosis was associated with reduced risk for clinical decompensation or liver-related death.** ⊙━

11. Iacobellis A, Siciliano M, Perri F *et al.* Peginterferon alfa-2b and ribavirin in patients with hepatitis C virus and decompensated cirrhosis: a controlled study. *Journal of Hepatology* 2007;46:206–212.

12. Everson GT. Management of cirrhosis due to chronic hepatitis C. *Journal of Hepatology* 2005;42:S65–S74.

13. Everson GT. Should we treat patients with chronic hepatitis C on the waiting list? *Journal of Hepatology* 2005;42:456–462.

14. Everson GT, Kulig CC. Antiviral therapy for hepatitis C in the setting of liver transplantation. *Current Treatment Options in Gastroenterology* 2006;9:520–529.

15. Davis GL, Balart LA, Schiff ER *et al.* Treatment of chronic hepatitis C with recombinant interferon alfa. A multicenter randomized, controlled trial. *New England Journal of Medicine* 1989;321:1501–1506.

16. Di Bisceglie AM, Martin P, Kassianides C *et al.* Recombinant interferon alfa therapy for chronic hepatitis C. A randomized, double-blind, placebo-controlled trial. *New England Journal of Medicine* 1989;321:1506–1510.

17. Hoofnagle JH, Di Bisceglie AM. The treatment of chronic viral hepatitis. *New England Journal of Medicine* 1997;336:347–356.

18. McHutchison JG, Gordon SC, Schiff ER *et al.* Interferon alfa-2b alone or in combination with ribavirin as initial treatment for chronic hepatitis C. *New England Journal of Medicine* 1998;339:1485–1492.

19. Davis GL, Esteban-Mur R, Rustgi V *et al.* Interferon alfa-2b alone or in combination with ribavirin for the treatment of relapse of chronic hepatitis C. *New England Journal of Medicine* 1998;339:1493–1499.

20. Fried MW, Shiffman ML, Reddy KR *et al.* Peginterferon alfa-2a plus ribavirin for chronic hepatitis C infection. *New England Journal of Medicine* 2002;347:975–982.

21. Manns MP, McHutchison JG, Gordon SC *et al.* Peginterferon alfa-2b plus ribavirin compared to interferon alfa-2b plus ribavirin for initial treatment of chronic hepatitis C: a randomized trial. *Lancet* 2001;358:958–965.

22. Hadziyannis SJ, Sette H, Morgan TR *et al.* Peginterferon alfa-2a and ribavirin combination therapy in chronic hepatitis C: a randomized study of treatment duration and ribavirin dose. *Annals of Internal Medicine* 2004;140:346–355.

23. Helbling B, Jochum W, Stamenic I *et al.* HCV-related advanced fibrosis/cirrhosis: randomized controlled trial of pegylated interferon α-2a and ribavirin. *Journal of Viral Hepatitis* 2006;13:762–769.

24. Shiffman ML, Di Bisceglie AM, Lindsay KL *et al.* Peginterferon alfa-2a and ribavirin in patients with chronic hepatitis C who have failed prior treatment. *Gastroenterology* 2004;126:1015–1023.

25. Everson GT, Hoefs JC, Seeff LB *et al.* Impact of disease severity on outcome of antiviral therapy for chronic hepatitis C: lessons from the HALT-C Trial. *Hepatology* 2006;44:1675–1684.

26. Poynard T, Colombo M, Bruix J *et al.* Peginterferon alfa-2b and ribavirin: effective in patients with hepatitis C who failed interferon alfa/ribavirin therapy. *Gastroenterology* 2009;136:1618–1628.

27. Camma C, Di Bona D, Schepis F *et al.* Effect of peginterferon alfa-2a on liver histology in chronic hepatitis C: a meta-analysis of individual patient data. *Hepatology* 2004;39:333–342.

28. Everson GT, Balart L, Lee SS *et al.* Histologic benefits of virologic response to peginterferon alfa-2a monotherapy

in patients with hepatitis C and advanced fibrosis or compensated cirrhosis. *Alimentary Pharmacology and Therapeutics* 2008;27:542–551.

29. Everson GT. Treatment of hepatitis C in the patient with decompensated cirrhosis. *Clinical Gastroenterology and Hepatology* 2005;3:S106–S112.

30. Wiesner RH, Sorrell M, Villamil F. Report of the First International Liver Transplantation Society Expert Panel Consensus Conference on Liver Transplantation and Hepatitis C. *Liver Transplantation* 2003;9(Suppl 3):S1–S9.

31. Strader DB, Wright T, Thomas DL, Seeff LB. AASLD Practice Guideline: diagnosis, management, and treatment of hepatitis C. *Hepatology* 2004;39:1147–1171.

32. Everson GT, Trotter J, Forman L *et al.* Treatment of advanced hepatitis C with a low accelerating dosage regimen of antiviral therapy. *Hepatology* 2005;42:255–262. **This paper describes the results of interferon/ribavirin treatment of 124 patients with advanced hepatitis C. Factors associated with SVR were non-genotype 1 HCV, well-compensated disease (CTP class A), and ability to tolerate full doses and duration of treatment. Recurrence of hepatitis C after liver transplantation was prevented in some patients by rendering the patient negative for HCV RNA prior to transplantation.** ⚷

33. Forns X, García-Retortillo M, Serrano T *et al.* Antiviral therapy of patients with decompensated cirrhosis to prevent recurrence of hepatitis C after liver transplantation. *Journal of Hepatology* 2003;39:389–396. **First report to demonstrate potential benefit of pretransplant antiviral therapy in preventing post-transplant recurrence of hepatitis C.** ⚷

34. Thomas RM, Brems JJ, Guzman-Hartman G, Yong S, Cavaliere P, Van Thiel DH. Infection with chronic hepatitis C virus and liver transplantation: a role for interferon therapy before transplantation. *Liver Transplantation* 2003;9:905–915.

35. Crippin JS, McCashland T, Terrault N, Sheiner P, Charlton MR. A pilot study of the tolerability and efficacy of antiviral therapy in hepatitis C virus-infected patients awaiting liver transplantation. *Liver Transplantation* 2002;8: 350–355.

36. Carrion JA, Martinez-Bauer E, Crespo G *et al.* Antiviral therapy increases the risk of bacterial infections in HCV-infected cirrhotic patients awaiting liver transplantation: a retroprospective study. *Journal of Hepatology* 2009;50:719–728.

37. Amarapurkar DN, Patel ND, Kamani P. Antiviral therapy of decompensated cirrhosis due to hepatitis C viral infection. *Tropical Gastroenterology* 2005;26:119–122.

38. Annicchiarico BE, Siciliano M, Avolio AW *et al.* Treatment of chronic hepatitis C virus infection with pegylated interferon and ribavirin in cirrhotic patients awaiting liver transplantation. *Transplantation Proceedings* 2008;40:1918–1920.

39. Tekin F, Gunsar F, Karasu Z, Akarca U, Ersoz G. Safety, tolerability, and efficacy of pegylated-interferon alfa-2a plus ribavirin in HCV-related decompensated cirrhotics. *Alimentary Pharmacology and Therapeutics* 2008;27:1081–1085.

40. Fontana RJ, Everson GT, Tuteja S, Vargas HE, Shiffman ML. Controversies in the management of hepatitis C patients with advanced fibrosis and cirrhosis. *Clinical Gastroenterology and Hepatology* 2004;2:183–197.

41. Dietrich DT, Wasserman R, Brau N *et al.* Once-weekly epoetin alfa improves anemia and facilitates maintenance of ribavirin dosing in hepatitis C virus-infected patients receiving ribavirin plus interferon alfa. *American Journal of Gastroenterology* 2003;98:2491–2499.

42. DiBisceglie AM, Shiffman ML, Everson GT *et al.* Prolonged therapy of advanced chronic hepatitis C with low-dose peg-interferon. *New England Journal of Medicine* 2008;359:429–441.

43. Carrion JA, Martinez-Bauer E, Crespo G *et al.* Antiviral therapy increases the risk of bacterial infection in HCV-infected patients awaiting liver transplantation: A retrospective study. *J Hepatol* 2009;50:719–728.

Section 2: HBV

26 Management of acute HBV

Dennis A. Freshwater, David J. Mutimer

Liver and Hepatobiliary Unit, Queen Elizabeth Hospital, Birmingham, UK

LEARNING POINTS

- The management of acute HBV infection is controversial.

- There are some data suggesting that nucleoside analogues may be beneficial and may help to prevent progression to liver failure and evolution to chronic hepatitis B. However, the evidence is fragmentary at present.

- The value of therapy with direct-acting antiviral agents in fulminant hepatitis B in order to resolve liver failure and/or in anticipation of liver transplantation is controversial.

Introduction

Most cases of acute hepatitis B virus (HBV) infection in the developed world and other non-endemic countries develop in patients from high-risk groups, such as those who use intravenous drugs or who are sexually promiscuous, as well as in those who are not vaccinated and who live in communities with a large proportion of immigrants from regions where HBV is endemic such as the Indian subcontinent or the Far East. The majority of children with newly diagnosed HBV are immigrants, have immigrant parents, or become exposed through other household contacts [1]. Vaccination programmes have the potential to substantially reduce the frequency of acute and fulminant hepatitis B, and the consequent progression to chronic disease [2]. However, despite vaccination programmes, patients with acute HBV infection continue to present and their management remains challenging.

Clinical Dilemmas in Viral Liver Disease, 1st edition. Edited by Graham R. Foster and K. Rajender Reddy. © 2010 Blackwell Publishing.

Clinical manifestations and natural history

Acute HBV infection has a variable course, ranging from asymptomatic infection to fulminant hepatitis. Fulminant hepatitis is defined as encephalopathy developing within 8 weeks of the onset of jaundice [3]. Approximately 70% of patients with acute hepatitis B have subclinical or anicteric hepatitis, while 30% develop jaundice. Fulminant hepatitis develops in only 0.1–0.5% of patients and is believed to be due to massive immune-mediated lysis of infected hepatocytes. This explains why some patients with fulminant hepatitis B were thought to have no evidence of HBV replication at presentation [4]. Survival without liver transplantation in fulminant hepatitis B has been found to be 17–47% [5–7]. Survival rates following liver transplantation have not been studied in patients with fulminant HBV infection alone, but appear to be much in keeping with those transplanted for other conditions, with 5-year survival being approximately 75% [8]. The rate of progression from acute to chronic hepatitis B is primarily determined by the age at infection, being approximately 90% for perinatally acquired infection, 20–50% for infections acquired between the ages of 1 and 5 years, and less than 5% for adult-acquired infection. Treatment of the acute infection has traditionally been supportive and symptomatic.

Rationale for use of antivirals

The rationale for treatment of fulminant hepatitis B with antiviral therapy is to improve liver function and to prevent death or the need for liver transplantation. In acute hepatitis B, the rationale is to prevent progression to acute liver failure or transition to chronic infection and disease. Early studies of HBV replication in fulminant liver disease suggested that replication stopped after the development of encephalopathy in the majority of cases [9–11], but these studies used HBeAg and insensitive HBV DNA assays. Later studies have used sequential measurements of HBV DNA and more sensitive assays and have showed that progression to chronic HBV infection is characterized by high levels of viral replication appearing early during the acute phase of infection [12] and that faster HBV DNA doubling time during the early infection predicts more severe disease [13].

Fulminant hepatitis B

Early reports of the use of lamivudine to treat acute severe hepatitis B took the form of case reports and small series. The case reports suggested that lamivudine reduced viral load in acute HBV [14,15] and small series of lamivudine therapy in acute severe hepatitis B were similarly hopeful. Schmilovitz-Weiss *et al.* [16] found that encephalopathy disappeared within 3 days of treatment and coagulopathy improved within 1 week. Serum HBV DNA was undetectable within 4 weeks, and serum liver enzyme levels normalized within 8 weeks. HBsAg became undetectable in all tested patients and the authors concluded that lamivudine may prevent the progression of severe acute disease to fulminant or chronic hepatitis and should be considered in selected patients. Tillmann *et al.* [17] reported that use of lamivudine resulted in greater survival without liver transplantation compared with historical controls (82.4 vs. 20%; $P < 0.001$).

More recently, Miyake *et al.* [18] published a retrospective cohort study of 33 patients with fulminant hepatitis B; 10 patients received lamivudine, 23 did not. Baseline characteristics were similar in the two groups. Using a multivariate Cox proportional hazard model the following factors were associated with a fatal outcome: age over 45 years ($P = 0.009$), systemic inflammatory response syndrome ($P = 0.025$) and non-administration of lamivudine ($P = 0.036$). Patients receiving lamivudine had an overall survival of 70% compared with 26% in those who did not receive it [18].

To date there has been only one randomized controlled trial of lamivudine to treat acute hepatitis B, performed by Kumar *et al.* [19]. The group studied 31 patients randomized to receive lamivudine 100 mg daily for 3 months compared with 40 randomized to receive placebo. Baseline characteristics including HBV viral load were similar in both groups, and similar numbers were classified as having 'severe' hepatitis, although the definition of severe was not given. At week 4, HBV DNA levels were significantly lower in the lamivudine group ($P = 0.037$), but thereafter there was no difference between the two groups. There was also no difference in loss of HBsAg at 1 year. There was a slightly lower rate of development of protective anti-HBs in the lamivudine group (67.7%) compared with the placebo group (85%) but this was not significant ($P = 0.096$). No mortality was observed in either group, and there was no significant difference in the clinical outcome between the groups.

Poor prognostic criteria for severe acute hepatitis B have been identified by O'Grady *et al.* [20] and Bernuau *et al.* [5] and these allow stratification of patients into high- and low-risk groups.

- O'Grady: age > 40 years, jaundice to encephalopathy time > 7 days, bilirubin > 17.65 mg/dL (300 μmol/L), prothrombin time > 50 s.
- Bernuau: age > 40 years, cerebral oedema, bilirubin > 15 mg/dL (255 μmol/L), prothrombin time > 25 s more than control.

We cannot directly compare the patients in Kumar's study against these criteria as the details are not published for each individual patient in the trial. However, the summary data for the trial patients are reproduced in Table 26.1 and it can be seen that the median and mean data for these

TABLE 26.1 Baseline characteristics of patients in randomized trial of lamivudine.

Group	Mean age (years)	Median age (years)	Mean INR	Mean bilirubin (mg/dL)	Median bilirubin (mg/dL)
Lamivudine (*N* = 31)	37.2	35	2.0	10.9	1.68
Placebo (*N* = 40)	36.4	36	1.89	12.3	1.74

Source: based on data from Kumar *et al.* [19].

patients do not reach the poor prognostic criteria defined by O'Grady and Bernuau. Thus, the majority of patients reported by Kumar suffered disease with a good prognosis. Under these circumstance, the survival rate in the non-treated group was predictably excellent, and treatment with lamivudine could not be expected to enhance survival in such a cohort. Larger studies that include patients with more severe acute liver disease would be required to examine the putative survival benefit of antiviral therapy in this setting.

Miyake *et al.* [18] argue that the better results seen in their cohort study may be related to the early reduction of viral load in the lamivudine group, preventing the development of systemic inflammatory response syndrome, and it has been shown that systemic inflammatory response syndrome is a poor prognostic marker in fulminant hepatitis B [7]. There is thus evidence that lamivudine in fulminant hepatitis B may improve outcomes, but its use in all cases of acute hepatitis B cannot be recommended.

Prevention of chronic infection

In renal dialysis patients recently infected with HBV, there is a much higher rate of progression to chronic hepatitis, approximately 30–60% [21,22]. Progression to chronic HBV infection is predicted by high peak levels of viral replication and higher peak HBeAg levels [12] and persistence of HBeAg during the acute phase [23]; thus it is tempting to use lamivudine (or other antiviral agent) to try to reduce the viral load and thereby risk of progression to chronic disease in these patients. At present, although there have been some case reports [15], there are no rigorous trials of lamivudine in HBV-exposed dialysis patients and routine use therefore cannot be recommended.

Another group with higher progression to chronic carriage of hepatitis B following acute exposure are immunosuppressed individuals, such as transplant recipients. Data on the use of lamivudine in these groups are similarly very scarce. In a study of 12 patients with *de novo* HBV infection after liver transplantation given lamivudine, 43% became HBsAg negative and negative for HBV DNA by PCR, although viral resistance occurred in 27% [24]. There are, unsurprisingly, no randomized controlled trials in this area. As patients would require lifelong prophylaxis to prevent possible reactivation of HBV in any case, use of nucleoside or nucleotide analogues in acute infection would seem sensible.

Summary

There are data to encourage the use of lamivudine in fulminant HBV and in acute HBV infection of immunosuppressed patients such as transplant recipients, although the data remain patchy. There is no evidence to show that lamivudine is harmful in these settings, so clinicians may choose to use lamivudine for patients with severe acute hepatitis and in the immunosuppressed. Larger studies would be useful, but studies may be difficult to design and conduct. The value of agents other than lamivudine in these settings remains untested and whether the third-generation antivirals with enhanced efficacy and lower resistance profiles will prove to be more effective remains to be determined.

References

1. Ordog K, Szendroi A, Szarka K *et al.* Perinatal and intrafamily transmission of hepatitis B virus in three generations of a low-prevalence population. *Journal of Medical Virology* 2003;70:194–204.

2. Kao JH, Hsu HM, Shau WY, Chang MH, Chen DS. Universal hepatitis B vaccination and the decreased mortality from fulminant hepatitis in infants in Taiwan. *Journal of Pediatrics* 2001;139:349–352.

3. Lee W, Schiodt F. Fulminant hepatic failure. In: Schiff E, Sorrell MF, Maddrey W, eds. *Schiff's Diseases of the Liver.* Philadelphia: JB Lippincott, 1999:879–895.

4. Wright TL, Mamish D, Combs C *et al.* Hepatitis B virus and apparent fulminant non-A, non-B hepatitis. *Lancet* 1992;339:952–955.

5. Bernuau J, Goudeau A, Poynard T *et al.* Multivariate analysis of prognostic factors in fulminant hepatitis B. *Hepatology* 1986;6:648–651.

6. Acharya SK, Dasarathy S, Kumer TL *et al.* Fulminant hepatitis in a tropical population: clinical course, cause, and early predictors of outcome. *Hepatology* 1996;23:1448–1455.

7. Miyake Y, Iwasaki Y, Terada R, Takaguchi K, Sakaguchi K, Shiratori Y. Systemic inflammatory response syndrome strongly affects the prognosis of patients with fulminant hepatitis B. *Journal of Gastroenterology* 2007;42:485–492.

8. Benner A, Lyden E, Rogge J, Weaver L, Mukherjee S. Outcomes of liver transplantation for hepatitis B: a single-center study of 35 patients. *Transplantation Proceedings* 2004;36:2741–2743.

9. Brechot C, Bernuau J, Thiers V *et al.* Multiplication of hepatitis B virus in fulminant hepatitis B. *British Medical Journal* 1984;288:270–271.

10. Fong TL, Akriviadis EA, Govindarajan S, Valinluck B, Redeker AG. Serum hepatitis B viral DNA in acute viral hepatitis B. *Annals of Internal Medicine* 1989;110:936–937.

11. Gimson AE, Tedder RS, White YS, Eddleston AL, Williams R. Serological markers in fulminant hepatitis B. *Gut* 1983;24:615–617.

12. Fong TL, Di Bisceglie AM, Biswas R *et al.* High levels of viral replication during acute hepatitis B infection predict progression to chronicity. *Journal of Medical Virology* 1994;43:155–158.

13. Whalley SA, Murray JM, Brown D *et al.* Kinetics of acute hepatitis B virus infection in humans. *Journal of Experimental Medicine* 2001;193:847–854.

14. Reshef R, Sbeit W, Tur-Kaspa R. Lamivudine in the treatment of acute hepatitis B. *New England Journal of Medicine* 2000;343:1123–1124.

15. Kondili LA, Osman H, Mutimer D. The use of lamivudine for patients with acute hepatitis B (a series of cases). *Journal of Viral Hepatitis* 2004;11:427–431.

16. Schmilovitz-Weiss H, Ben-Ari Z, Sikuler E *et al.* Lamivudine treatment for acute severe hepatitis B: a pilot study. *Liver International* 2004;24:547–551.

17. Tillmann HL, Hadem J, Leifeld L *et al.* Safety and efficacy of lamivudine in patients with severe acute or fulminant hepatitis B: a multicenter experience. *Journal of Viral Hepatitis* 2006;13:256–263. **An important clinical study of therapy in patients with severe acute hepatitis B.** 🔑

18. Miyake Y, Iwasaki Y, Takaki A *et al.* Lamivudine treatment improves the prognosis of fulminant hepatitis B. *Internal Medicine* 2008;47:1293–1299. **An important clinical study of therapy in patients with severe acute hepatitis B.** 🔑

19. Kumar M, Satapathy S, Monga R *et al.* A randomized controlled trial of lamivudine to treat acute hepatitis B. *Hepatology* 2007;45:97–101.

20. O'Grady JG, Alexander GJ, Hayllar KM, Williams R. Early indicators of prognosis in fulminant hepatic failure. *Gastroenterology* 1989;97:439–445.

21. Mazzoni A, Innocenti M, Consaga M. Retrospective study on the prevalence of B and non-A, non-B hepatitis in a dialysis unit: 17-year follow-up. *Nephron* 1992;61:316–317.

22. Saha D, Agarwal SK. Hepatitis and HIV infection during haemodialysis. *Journal of the Indian Medical Association* 2001;99:194–199, 203, 213.

23. Babes VT, Cepanaru S, Cepanaru R, Tanase M. Investigations on HBe antigen. Note II. Dynamics of HBsAg in acute viral hepatitis, according to HBeAg persistence or seroconversion. *Virologie* 1981;32:187–191.

24. Andreone P, Caraceni P, Grazi GL *et al.* Lamivudine treatment for acute hepatitis B after liver transplantation. *Journal of Hepatology* 1998;29:985–989.

27 Rethinking the inactive carrier state: management of patients with low-replicative HBeAg-negative chronic hepatitis B and normal liver enzymes

Ilan S. Weisberg, Ira M. Jacobson

New York Presbyterian Hospital–Weill Cornell Medical Center, Division of Gastroenterology and Hepatology, New York, New York, USA

LEARNING POINTS

- The inactive carrier state is characterized by persistence of HBsAg, absence of HBeAg, low level or absence of HBV DNA, and normal liver function tests.

- ALT can fluctuate widely during the course of chronic HBV infection and therefore serial ALT assessments are required for the correct diagnosis of the inactive carrier state.

- There is a small yet significant increased risk of progressive liver disease, cirrhosis or hepatocellular carcinoma with even the lowest levels of HBV viraemia.

- Individuals with low-level replication (< 2000 IU/mL) should be classified as having low-replicative HBeAg-negative chronic hepatitis B.

Introduction

With nearly 400 million people infected, hepatitis B virus (HBV) is the leading cause of chronic liver disease worldwide. The clinical spectrum of chronic hepatitis B (CHB) ranges widely from subclinical disease to active hepatitis, hepatocellular carcinoma (HCC) and decompensated cirrhosis [1]. Many infected individuals are said to exist in the *inactive carrier state*, characterized by persistence of the hepatitis B surface antigen (HBsAg), low-level or undetectable HBV DNA, normal serum alanine aminotransferase (ALT) and minimal histological disease activity [2].

Clinical Dilemmas in Viral Liver Disease, 1st edition. Edited by Graham R. Foster and K. Rajender Reddy. © 2010 Blackwell Publishing.

Historically, these individuals were referred to as 'healthy' or 'asymptomatic' carriers, which erroneously implied a durable absence of HBV replication or the potential for clinically significant liver disease. Consequently, clinical attention and research on this large CHB population was limited. With improved molecular diagnostic testing, it is clear that the inactive carrier state encompasses a heterogeneous population of patients, including those who are truly inactive and those with low-level viral replication. Moreover, the term 'inactive carrier state' belies the fact that longitudinal natural history studies demonstrate a small but significant risk of progressive liver disease in patients with low-level viraemia, suggesting that these individuals are better classified as having low-replicative HBeAg-negative CHB. In this chapter, we review the natural course of the inactive carrier state and use it as a framework to appraise current management guidelines.

Natural history of chronic HBV infection

From natural history studies, four distinct phases of HBV infection have been defined [3]. During the *immune-tolerant phase*, individuals are asymptomatic, HBeAg is detectable, HBV viral titres are markedly elevated, serum ALT levels are normal or marginally elevated, and histological activity is minimal. Transition to the *immune clearance phase*, or perhaps more descriptively the *immune clearance phase* (HBeAg-positive CHB), is characterized by fluctuations in the ALT and HBV DNA titre with necroinflammatory injury observed on liver biopsy. This phase is highly variable in duration, with persistent injury resulting in progressive necroinflammation and fibrosis.

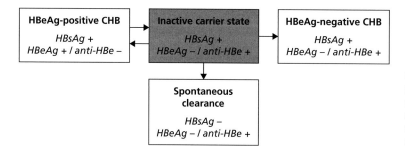

FIG. 27.1 Dynamic nature of the inactive carrier state with potential for reversion to HBeAg-positive hepatitis, spontaneous loss of HbsAg or, more frequently, reactivation to HBeAg-negative chronic hepatitis.

The end of this phase is characterized by HBeAg seroconversion (loss of HBeAg and formation of anti-HBe) and passage into the *inactive carrier state*, a low-replicative phase of chronic HBV infection characterized by the presence of HBsAg and anti-HBe in serum, absence of HBeAg, persistently normal ALT, and markedly reduced (< 2000 IU/mL) or undetectable HBV viral DNA. The inactive carrier state is a potentially dynamic phase in the natural history of chronic HBV infection (Figure 27.1) with the capacity for reversion to HBeAg-positive hepatitis, spontaneous loss of HBsAg or reactivation to *HBeAg-negative chronic hepatitis*, featuring populations with a preponderance of precore and/or core promoter mutations.

Serological and biochemical testing

Serologically, the inactive carrier state is indistinguishable from HBeAg-negative chronic HBV infection; both conditions are characterized by the presence of HBsAg in the serum for at least 6 months, HBeAg negativity and detectable anti-HBe antibodies. These two phases of HBV infection are distinguished by the level of viral replication and the degree of biochemical activity. Recently, the American Association for the Study of Liver Diseases (AASLD) guidelines and a US expert panel algorithm for the treatment of CHB have published updated criteria to better define the inactive carrier state (Table 27.1) [3,4]. Both groups require a single baseline HBV DNA of less than 2000 IU/mL, accompanied by a persistently normal ALT using the recently adopted values for healthy men (< 30 IU/mL) and women (< 19 IU/mL) [5]. Since ALT can fluctuate widely during the course of HBeAg-negative CHB, with long periods of biochemical inactivity [1,2,6], it follows that ALT should be serially assessed every 3 months for the first year to ensure correct identification of inactive disease and every 6 months thereafter to identify reactivation.

TABLE 27.1 Diagnostic criteria for the inactive carrier state of chronic HBV infection.

HBsAg: seropositive for at least 6 months

HBeAg: seronegative

Anti-HBe antibody positive

Persistently normal ALT (≤ 30 IU/mL for men, ≥ 19 IU/mL for women)

Undetectable or low-level HBV DNA (< 2000 IU/mL)

Liver biopsy* findings with minimal activity (necroinflammatory score < 4) and scant fibrosis

* Liver biopsy optional; may be beneficial in indeterminate cases or individuals at risk for progressive liver disease.
Source: adapted from Lok *et al.* [4] and Keeffe *et al.* [3].

Viral load testing

Multiple studies from Asia [7,8] and Europe [5,9–11] have unsuccessfully attempted to identify a baseline viral DNA that reliably distinguishes the inactive carrier state from HBeAg-negative CHB. In 2001, a serum HBV DNA level less than 10^5 copies/mL (20 000 IU/mL) was proposed at the National Institutes of Health workshop to differentiate these two phases of chronic HBV infection [2]. This value reflected the lower detection limit of early non-PCR-based assays rather than patient epidemiological data and has now been replaced by a more stringent value (< 2000 IU/mL) in the newest AASLD and US expert panel treatment guidelines [3,4]. Serial HBV DNA testing has been shown to improve the classification of inactive disease [7,8,11] and accordingly some guidelines advocate serial HBV DNA testing to ensure that the inactive state is maintained [3,12] and when ALT elevations are noted or clinical suspicion of reactivation is raised.

Prognosis

Longitudinal studies of the inactive carrier state are plagued by heterogeneity, both in the diagnostic criteria used to define the state and in the demographic features of the study population. Accordingly, the reported rates of progression to HBeAg-negative CHB or decompensated liver disease vary widely. Although the literature demonstrates that most individuals will have an excellent long-term prognosis, nearly one-third of individuals will progress to active chronic infection. Moreover, most studies demonstrate a small but significant risk of developing cirrhosis or HCC, validating the need for regular follow-up and monitoring.

The long-term outcome of a cohort of 283 Taiwanese patients with well-documented spontaneous HBeAg seroconversion has been described [13]. After a median follow-up of 8.6 years (range 1–18.4), 189 (67%) maintained a sustained remission of the inactive carrier state; 94 (33.2%) relapsed to active hepatitis: 12 (4.2%) reverted to HBeAg-positive CHB, 68 (24%) to HBeAg-negative CHB and 14 (5%) were indeterminate. Patients with pre-existing cirrhosis (4.9% of the total cohort) at time of seroconversion had a 10-fold increased risk of developing HBeAg-negative CHB and a 12-fold risk of reverting to HBeAg-positive CHB compared with patients without significant fibrosis on liver biopsy. Of the 269 patients without pre-existing cirrhosis, 21 (7.8%) developed cirrhosis after seroconversion: 5 of 9 (55%) with reversion to HBeAg-positive CHB, 14 of 62 (23%) with HBeAg-negative CHB, 1 of 14 (7%) with active hepatitis of indeterminate cause, and 1 of 184 (0.5%) with sustained maintenance of the inactive state. Six patients developed HCC 5.3–14.3 years after seroconversion, with an annual incidence of 0.2%: three cases (1.6%) were in long-term inactive carriers and three (4.4%) in patients who reverted to HBeAg-negative CHB.

The same group recently described the risk of relapse to active hepatitis and development of cirrhosis or HCC in a large study of 1965 'asymptomatic' HBsAg-positive blood donors in Taiwan [14]. Relapse to HBeAg-negative CHB occurred in 314 patients. The cumulative rate of relapse was approximately 22% after 25 years of follow-up, with more than 85% of relapse occurring in the first 10 years after enrolment and an annual relapse rate of 1.55%. Men were 2.5 times as likely to relapse as women ($P < 0.0001$). A total of 57 patients developed sonographic or clinical evidence of cirrhosis: 10 of 1651 inactive carriers (0.6%) and 47 of 314 relapsers (15.97%). The risk of developing cirrhosis

was increased in those with advanced age at study entry, male gender, and reactivation to HBeAg-negative chronic hepatitis.

Recently, a cohort of 61 treatment-naive HBeAg-positive Italian patients followed prospectively for more than 20 years after seroconversion to HBeAg-negative CHB has been described [15]. The majority of individuals ($N = 40$, 66%) transitioned to the inactive carrier state with sustained normalization of ALT and undetectable HBV DNA by non-PCR-based detection methods; 21 individuals (34%) progressed to HBeAg-negative active hepatitis. Eleven patients in the cohort had pre-existing cirrhosis at the time of seroconversion. Among the cirrhotics, there was a higher prevalence of progression to HBeAg-negative CHB than transition to the inactive carrier state (50% vs. 17.5%; $P = 0.04$). After a median of 13.8 years (range 1.1–26.9), 18 (45%) of the inactive carriers lost their HBsAg, yielding an HBsAg loss rate of 2.1 per 100 person-years. The cumulative probability of survival at 25 years was significantly lower in the patients who progressed to chronic hepatitis (50%) compared with those who remained in the inactive carrier state (95%) ($P < 0.0001$), and the risk of orthotopic liver transplantation or liver-related mortality was 38-fold higher in those with reversion to CHB compared with those in sustained remission. Despite this excellent prognosis, two individuals (both with pre-existing cirrhosis) in the inactive carrier state developed HCC 7.7 and 9.4 years after seroconversion. Conversely, there were no cases of HCC or liver-related death in the 33 non-cirrhotic inactive patients. As seen in the Asian studies, male gender, older age, presence of cirrhosis and absence of sustained remission were all predictors of increased liver-related mortality.

Liver biopsy

The HBeAg-negative inactive carrier state is defined by ALT and viral load. Under current treatment guidelines (Table 27.1), liver biopsy is an optional assessment reserved for individuals at risk for progressive liver disease or in cases of indeterminate disease activity. However, it is well established that ALT and HBV DNA are imperfect surrogates for determining liver activity and fibrosis. Histological evaluation may therefore be a useful adjunct in selected individuals.

Nguyen et al. [16] demonstrated that up to one-third of patients with persistently normal ALT, particularly those over age 35, have significant liver activity on biopsy. Kumar et al. [17] evaluated 116 HBeAg-negative patients with persistently normal ALT. Of the 58 patients who underwent liver biopsy, the median histological activity index (HAI) and fibrosis scores were 3.0 (1.0–10.0) and 1.0 (1.0–3.0), respectively. Overall, 13.8% had histological evidence of significant fibrosis (stage ≥ 2). Of the patients with a viral load less than 10^5 copies/mL (≤ 20 000 IU/mL), 21% had histologically active liver disease with HAI 3 or more and/or stage 2 or greater fibrosis. Only a small subset of patients with persistently normal ALT and low viral load (< 2000 IU/mL) underwent liver biopsy (9 of 52, 17.3%). However, two of these 'inactive' patients (22.2%) were subsequently found to have active liver disease on biopsy (HAI ≥ 3 and/or ≥ stage 2 fibrosis). Even when the data were reanalysed using the updated norms for ALT (30 IU/mL for men, 19 IU/mL for women), ALT and HBV DNA were inaccurate in distinguishing histologically active and inactive disease. Despite this cautionary report, there is insufficient evidence at this time to recommend routine liver biopsy for low-replicative chronic HBV infection, although it might be considered on an individual basis (e.g. based on ALT or other laboratory parameters or imaging suggesting progressive disease, closeness of HBV DNA to the cut-off of 2000 IU/mL, age). Further histological studies are needed to better define the risk of active disease in low-replicative HBV infection.

Hepatocellular carcinoma screening

The risk of HCC in patients in the inactive carrier state is small. Most, but not all, cases of HCC arise in patients with pre-existing cirrhosis at the time of diagnosing inactive disease [13,15,18,19]. Most published guidelines [3,4,12] do not directly address the issue of HCC screening in the inactive carrier state. In our practice, screening of all adult carriers with periodic abdominal imaging and alpha-fetoprotein is performed despite the absence of proven cost-effectiveness in those with the inactive carrier state. This approach would seem to be supported by the recent report from the REVEAL study in which HBsAg-positive individuals with undetectable (< 300 copies/mL) or low-level viraemia (300–9999 copies/mL) had hazard ratios of 3.0 (1.4–6.3) and 3.3 (1.7–6.6), respectively, for developing HCC compared with HBsAg-negative controls [20,21].

Treatment and surveillance

Currently, patients who meet criteria for the inactive carrier state are not considered candidates for antiviral therapy

[3,4]. However, they should be monitored throughout their lives for progression to HBeAg-negative CHB and for development of progressive liver disease.

Determination of HBV genotype and assessment for the presence of precore or basal core promoter mutations may prove useful for long-term surveillance. It has been shown that genotype C is associated with increased risk of reactivation to HBeAg-negative CHB and progression to cirrhosis [22,23]. Similarly, it has recently been suggested that the addition of the precore (A1896) and basal core promoter (T1762/A1764) mutations into treatment algorithms might assist in the identification of patients at risk for developing HCC [24]. Studies demonstrate that the precore mutation can be detected in 38–99% of patients in the 'inactive state' with detectable virus [17,22,25] and further research is needed to determine if this imparts increased risk of HCC in this population.

Patients should be counselled on lifestyle modifications, including abstinence from alcohol, weight loss and glycaemic control where relevant. Seronegative individuals should be offered vaccination against hepatitis A virus. The risk of transmission should be routinely discussed, and family members and household contacts should be vaccinated against HBV, if not already immune, even if the index patient is HBV negative. Patients in the inactive carrier state should be counselled on the risk of reactivation in the face of immunosuppression (chemotherapy, systemic steroids, anti-TNF-α treatments) and appropriate prophylactic antiviral therapy should be administered.

Summary

- Diagnosis of the inactive carrier state requires repeated assessments of ALT and HBV DNA over at least a 1-year period using the most stringent ALT cut-offs (30 IU/mL in men, 19 IU/mL in women) to truly differentiate from HBeAg-negative CHB.
- ALT and HBV DNA are imperfect surrogates for assessing liver disease; however, liver biopsy is not part of the routine assessment of the inactive carrier state. Histological evaluation may be considered for selected individuals with risk factors for progression, such as male gender, Asian ethnicity, age over 35, genotype C and possibly the presence of precore or basal core promoter mutations.
- Lifelong serial monitoring for prompt diagnosis of viral relapse and initiation of antiviral therapy for individuals

with progression to HBeAg-negative CHB (HBV DNA > 2000 IU/mL, elevation in ALT and/or active necroinflammatory histology on liver biopsy).

- Given the small but significant risk of progressive liver disease, cirrhosis and HCC, the term 'inactive carrier state' should be reconsidered and replaced with 'low-replicative HBeAg-negative CHB' for patients with low-level rather than undetectable HBV DNA.

References

1. McMahon BJ. Epidemiology and natural history of hepatitis B. *Seminars in Liver Disease* 2005;25(Suppl 1):3–8.

2. Lok AS, Heathcote EJ, Hoofnagle JH. Management of hepatitis B: 2000 summary of a workshop. *Gastroenterology* 2001;120:1828–1853.

3. Keeffe EB, Dietrich DT, Han SH *et al*. A treatment algorithm for the management of chronic hepatitis B infection in the United States: 2008 update. *Clinical Gastroenterology and Hepatology* 2008;6:1315–1341. **An update of the US expert panel treatment algorithm for the management of chronic hepatitis B infection.** 🔑

4. Lok AS, McMahon BJ. Chronic hepatitis B. *Hepatology* 2007;45:507–539. **An update of the treatment guidelines from the American Association for the Study of Liver Disease (AASLD).** 🔑

5. Prati D, Taioli E, Zanella A *et al*. Updated definitions of healthy ranges for serum alanine aminotransferase levels. *Annals of Internal Medicine* 2002;137:1–10.

6. Papatheodoridis GV, Manesis EK, Manolakopoulos S *et al*. Is there a meaningful serum hepatitis B virus DNA cutoff level for therapeutic decisions in hepatitis B e antigen-negative chronic hepatitis B infection? *Hepatology* 2008;48:1451–1459.

7. Chu CJ, Hussain M, Lok AS. Quantitative serum HBV DNA levels during different stages of chronic hepatitis B infection. *Hepatology* 2002;36:1408–1415.

8. Seo Y, Yoon S, Truong BX *et al*. Serum hepatitis B virus DNA levels differentiating inactive carriers from patients with chronic hepatitis B. *European Journal of Gastroenterology and Hepatology* 2005;17:753–757.

9. Martinot-Peignoux M, Boyer N, Colombat M *et al*. Serum hepatitis B virus DNA levels and liver histology in inactive HBsAg carriers. *Journal of Hepatology* 2002;36:543–546.

10. Manesis EK, Papatheodoridis GV, Hadziyannis SJ. Serum HBV-DNA levels in inactive hepatitis B carriers. *Gastroenterology* 2002;122:2092–2093.

11. Zacharakis G, Koskinaris J, Kotsiou S *et al*. The role of serial measurement of HBV-DNA levels in patients with chronic HBeAg (–) hepatitis B infection: association with liver disease progression. A prospective cohort study. *Hepatology* 2007;46(Suppl 1):636A.

12. European Association for the Study of the Liver. EASL clinical practice guidelines: management of chronic hepatitis B. *Journal of Hepatology* 2009;50:227–242.

13. Hsu YS, Chien RN, Yeh CT *et al*. Long-term outcome after spontaneous HBeAg seroconversion in patients with chronic hepatitis B. *Hepatology* 2002;35:1522–1527.

14. Chu CM, Liaw YF. Incidence and risk factors of progression to cirrhosis in inactive carriers of hepatitis B virus. *American Journal of Gastroenterology* 2009;104:1693–1699. **A large natural history study from Taiwan representing nearly 2000 asymptomatic HbsAg-positive carriers incidentally identified during blood donation. This study demonstrates that a significant risk of reactivation to chronic hepatitis or progression to cirrhosis warrants regular surveillance and monitoring of inactive HBV carriers.** 🔑

15. Fattovich G, Olivari N, Pasino M, D'Onofrio M, Martone E, Donato F. Long-term outcome of chronic hepatitis B in Caucasian patients: mortality after 25 years. *Gut* 2008;57:84–90. **A well-defined Italian cohort study following treatment-naive patients for more than 20 years after spontaneous seroconversion to HBeAg-negative CHB highlights the natural history of the inactive carrier state in a non-endemic population.** 🔑

16. Nguyen MH, Trinh HN, Garcia RT *et al*. High prevalence of significant histologic disease in patients with chronic hepatitis B (CHB) and normal ALT. *Hepatology* 2007;46(Suppl 1):680A.

17. Kumar M, Sarin SK, Hissar S *et al*. Virologic and histologic features of chronic hepatitis B virus infected asymptomatic patients with persistently normal ALT. *Gastroenterology* 2008;134:1376–1384.

18. Bortolotti F, Guido M, Bartolacci S *et al*. Chronic hepatitis B in children after e antigen seroclearance: final report of a 29 year longitudinal study. *Hepatology* 2007;43:556–562.

19. Chu CM, Liaw YF. HbsAg seroclearance in asymptomatic carriers of high endemic areas: appreciable high rates during a long-term follow-up. *Hepatology* 2007;45:1187–1192.

20. Chen CJ, Yang HI, Su J *et al*. Risk of hepatocellular carcinoma across a biological gradient of serum hepatitis B virus DNA level. *Journal of the American Medical Association* 2006;295:65–73. **Seminal work from the REVEAL-HBV Study Group in which more than 3600 HBsAg-positive persons free of cirrhosis or HCC were prospectively followed for more than 12 years. This study demonstrated that the risk of developing cirrhosis or HCC increases in a stepwise fashion with incremental changes in viral load.** 🔑

21. Iloeje U, Yang H, Su J *et al*. HBV viral load less than 104 copies/ml is associated with significant risk of hepatocellular carcinoma in chronic hepatitis B patients: an update

from the REVEAL study. *Hepatology* 2007;46(Suppl 1): 640A.

22. Chu CJ, Hussain M, Lok AS. Hepatitis B virus genotyope is associated with earlier HBeAg seroconversion compared with hepatitis B virus genotype C. *Gastroenterology* 2002;122:1756–1762.

23. Chu CM, Liaw YF. Genotype C hepatitis B virus infection is associated with a higher risk of reactivation of hepatitis B and progression to cirrhosis than genotype B: a longitudinal study of hepatitis B e antigen-positive patients with normal aminotransferase levels at baseline. *Journal of Hepatology* 2005;43:411–417.

24. Tong MJ, Hsien C, Hsu L, Sun HE, Blatt LM. Treatment recommendations for chronic hepatitis B: an evalution of current guidelines based on a natural history study in the Unites States. *Hepatology* 2008;48:1070–1078.

25. Manno M, Camma C, Schepis F *et al*. Natural history of chronic HBV carriers in northern Italy: morbidity and mortality after 30 years. *Gastroenterology* 2004;127:756–763.

HBeAg-negative chronic hepatitis B infection with abnormal transaminases and minimal changes on liver biopsy

Graham R. Foster

Queen Mary's University of London, Blizard Institute of Cell and Molecular Science, London, UK

LEARNING POINTS

- HBeAg-negative chronic hepatitis B infection with minimal histological damage has an uncertain prognosis.

- The benefits of therapy in patients with HBeAg-negative chronic hepatitis B infection and minimal histological damage are uncertain.

- Discussion of the risks and benefits of therapy is required to reach the correct management decision.

- If therapy is not introduced, long-term monitoring with regular review is mandatory.

Introduction

Chronic infection with hepatitis B virus (HBV) is usually associated with different phases of disease that change over time. For patients with HBeAg-negative infection two phases of disease are recognized: (i) 'inactive carriers', individuals with low-level HBV DNA (usually defined as < 2000 IU/mL) and normal liver function tests; and (ii) HBeAg-negative disease, patients with higher levels of HBV DNA (> 2000 IU/mL) and abnormal liver function tests [1]. Since patients with HBeAg-negative disease often have fluctuating disease, it is important to monitor patients with HBeAg infection regularly to avoid diagnostic errors. Management of patients in the 'inactive carrier' phase of infection usually involves periodic review without further

Clinical Dilemmas in Viral Liver Disease, 1st edition. Edited by Graham R. Foster and K. Rajender Reddy. © 2010 Blackwell Publishing.

intervention. For patients with HBeAg-negative disease who have significant liver disease on liver biopsy, management usually involves antiviral therapy with either peg-interferon or oral antiviral agents. However, many patients with HBeAg-negative disease present with moderately high levels of HBV DNA, fluctuating mildly deranged liver function tests and minimal changes on liver biopsy. The most appropriate management of such patients is unclear.

Natural history of HBeAg-negative disease with minimal histological activity and effects of therapy

The natural history of HBeAg-negative disease has been evaluated in a number of studies, chiefly from the Far East [2,3], where cohorts of patients were followed up for many years without therapy. Patients were assessed at the start of the study with virological and serological assays but a liver biopsy was not usually performed. These studies showed that people with relatively low levels of HBV DNA at presentation had an increased risk of developing liver disease in the medium term. However, since these studies did not assess liver histology at enrolment, it is unclear whether the risk of liver disease relates to viral load *per se* or to liver damage, which is most often associated with high levels of viral replication. Although these pivotal studies have often been used to argue for a policy of early therapy in all patients with moderate to high levels of viraemia, it is unclear whether reducing the viral load in patients with minimal histological activity will reduce progression of liver disease. It is clear that antiviral therapy in patients with advanced liver disease reduces the risk of liver decompensation [4] but whether this extends to those with minimal histological lesions is less well defined. Thus the outcome of disease in patients with minimal histological activity remains unclear and the benefits of therapy are unproven.

The case for early therapy

The data from cohort studies indicate that persisting medium- to high-level viraemia in patients with HBeAg-negative HBV is associated with an increased risk of liver disease. Since studies of antiviral therapy have shown that therapy may improve liver histology and reduce the risk of developing complications in patients with severe disease, it seems reasonable to presume that therapy in patients with persisting viraemia and minimal liver damage will confer long-term benefits. These benefits are likely to include a reduction in the lifetime risk of developing severe liver disease. If patients with minimal histological disease are not offered antiviral therapy, the risks of disease progression are such that long-term follow-up with regular monitoring of liver function tests and viral load is required. Most physicians would agree that liver biopsy should be repeated at regular intervals (perhaps every few years) and therefore avoiding therapy requires extensive follow-up with regular histological assessment. Such an approach is often unpopular with patients and retention in long-term follow-up of untreated cohorts has never been assessed but is likely to be low. Furthermore, reduction in viraemia in patients with HBV may reduce the risk of onward transmission, and in countries where universal vaccination is not practised or where uptake of the vaccine is poor it might be argued that early therapy may have public health benefits. Thus it can be argued that early therapy for patients with minimal histological damage reduces the risk of long-term liver damage, avoids repeat liver biopsy assessment and facilitates compliance as well as potentially reducing the risk of inadvertent transmission.

The case for delaying therapy

As noted above the studies completed to date by no means show unequivocal evidence of benefit in treating patients with minimal disease. Therapy in minimal disease requires a long-term commitment by the patient to take medication regularly and undergo frequent monitoring. For patients who choose to take interferon-based therapies, the side effects may be considerable [5]; for patients who choose

oral antiviral agents, regular review with repeated blood tests over many years is required. For patients who choose to take oral antiviral agents there is a risk that in the long term drug-resistant mutations will emerge and reduce the efficacy of therapy. Although the oral drugs that are currently available to treat patients with HBV (e.g. entecavir and tenofovir) have an excellent safety record in the short term [6,7], their long-term safety in patients with HBV has not been determined and their effects on the developing fetus are currently unknown, although the available data does not give rise to any concerns. Thus treating patients with minimal disease exposes them to therapy with no proven benefits and an unknown risk of long-term complications, including viral resistance.

Expert opinion

Two international groups have recently compiled guidelines for the management of chronic HBV infection [1,8]. In view of the lack of high-quality evidence relating to the management of patients with minimal histological disease, it is not surprising to find that the two groups have reached slightly different conclusions. The American guidelines produced on behalf of the American Association for the Study of Liver Diseases (AASLD) [1] suggest that 'These patients generally should not be initiated on treatment but a liver biopsy may be considered in patients with fluctuating or minimally elevated ALT levels, especially in those aged over 40 years of age'. The guidelines suggest that 'treatment may be initiated if there is moderate or severe necroinflammation or significant fibrosis on liver biopsy'. The European guidelines [8] adopt a subtly different approach, recommending that 'patients with slightly elevated ALT (less than 2 times ULN) and mild histological lesions (less than A2F2 with METAVIR scoring) may not require therapy. Follow-up is mandatory'. Thus there is no clear consensus as to the most appropriate management strategy.

Suggestions for management

All clinical decisions require a discussion between the patient and the clinician and this dialogue is of particular importance where the evidence base is weak or equivocal. Patients with minimal histological damage and persistent moderate/high-level viraemia should be advised that therapy is of unproven value but that it is likely to reduce the risk of long-term liver damage. The side effects of therapy and the risks of resistance should be discussed along with the differing advantages and disadvantages of oral therapy and interferon-based treatment regimens. In general, I usually advise young fertile women who are considering starting a family to defer therapy but to continue to undergo regular monitoring. For patients with a family history of liver disease, particularly those with a history of liver cancer, I usually advocate early therapy. For patients who have other risk factors for progressive disease (e.g. men over the age of 40) early therapy is probably the most appropriate option but for patients who have no risk factors that predispose them to advanced liver disease a policy of careful observation is appropriate, provided that the patient is willing to consider regular liver biopsies to monitor disease progression.

The choice of therapy in patients with mild early HBeAg-negative disease is not yet clear. Interferon-based therapies have the advantage of a short fixed course of therapy without the risk of long-term viral resistance. A small proportion of patients will undergo HBsAg seroconversion (effectively a virological cure) and thereby avoid long-term follow-up. However, interferon-based therapies are associated with a wide range of side effects and are often unpopular with patients. Oral therapy is convenient, has few immediate side effects but requires long-term medication with regular clinical review. The optimal therapy is best determined by a careful discussion with the patient.

The future

The management of chronic HBV infection is evolving rapidly. For patients with mild disease it is likely that long-term cohort studies will continue to define the groups at greatest risk of long-term liver damage and, as more sophisticated stratification of risk becomes possible, it is probable that management decisions will be based on the probability of developing liver damage. Studies are currently in progress to determine factors that predict the response to interferon-based therapy in patients with HBeAg-negative disease and it is likely that in the near future it may be possible to identify those patients who are likely to undergo HBsAg seroconversion. Therapy for such patients is likely to be recommended regardless of the histological damage at presentation. Until such studies have been completed and ratified by repetition, clinicians and their patients will continue to balance the risks and benefits of early therapy to maximize the gains.

References

1. Lok AS, McMahon BJ. Chronic hepatitis B. *Hepatology* 2007;45:507–539.
2. Iloeje UH, Yang HI, Su J, Jen CL, You SL, Chen CJ. Predicting cirrhosis risk based on the level of circulating hepatitis B viral load. *Gastroenterology* 2006;130:678–686. **Critical study indicating that liver disease occurs with increased frequency in patients with very low levels of HBV DNA.** 🔑
3. Chen CJ, Yang HI, Su J et al. Risk of hepatocellular carcinoma across a biological gradient of serum hepatitis B virus DNA level. *Journal of the American Medical Association* 2006;295:65–73.
4. Liaw YF, Sung JJ, Chow WC et al. Lamivudine for patients with chronic hepatitis B and advanced liver disease. *New England Journal of Medicine* 2004;351:1521–1531. **Pivotal study illustrating the improvements in mortality in patients receiving effective antiviral therapy.** 🔑
5. Fattovich G, Giustina G, Favarato S, Ruol A. A survey of adverse events in 11 241 patients with chronic viral hepatitis treated with alfa interferon. *Journal of Hepatology* 1996;24:38–47.
6. Yurdaydin C. Entecavir: a step forward in combating hepatitis B disease. *Expert Opinion in Pharmacotherapy* 2008;9:3095–3109.
7. Marcellin P, Heathcote EJ, Buti M et al. Tenofovir disoproxil fumarate versus adefovir dipivoxil for chronic hepatitis B. *New England Journal of Medicine* 2008;359:2442–2455.
8. European Association for the Study of the Liver. EASL Clinical Practice Guidelines: management of chronic hepatitis B. *Journal of Hepatology* 2009;50:227–242.

29 Combination therapy for chronic hepatitis B virus infection: should we use it *ab initio* or sequentially?

William Alazawi[1], Graham R. Foster[2]

[1]Barts and The London School of Medicine, London, UK
[2]Queen Mary's University of London, Blizard Institute of Cell and Molecular Science, London, UK

LEARNING POINTS

- HBV is highly mutable and with drugs that have low genetic barriers to resistance, combination therapy is important to prevent the development of drug resistance.

- For drugs such as entecavir and tenofovir that have high genetic barriers to resistance, it is not clear whether combination therapy is required at the outset or whether treatment initiation followed by careful monitoring and introduction of a second agent in the absence of a virological response is appropriate.

- It is generally agreed that in patients at high risk of resistance, combination therapy should be considered at the initiation of therapy.

Introduction

Combination therapy for the treatment of chronic hepatitis B virus (HBV) monoinfection has been a hotly debated topic since the licensing of lamivudine expanded the HBV formularly from interferon alfa-based treatment. Early studies looking at the combination of peginterferon and lamivudine showed no significant added value of combination therapy over monotherapy [1]. Since then, a further six drugs have become licensed or are in clinical use (adefovir, telbivudine, clevudine, tenofovir, entecavir and emtricitabine), and their utility in combination continues to be

Clinical Dilemmas in Viral Liver Disease, 1st edition. Edited by Graham R. Foster and K. Rajender Reddy. © 2010 Blackwell Publishing.

considered in a range of clinical settings. For example, following the development of resistance to lamivudine, Italian studies demonstrated the superiority of continuing lamivudine in combination with adefovir rather than switching to adefovir alone [2]. This chapter outlines the issues surrounding combination therapy and summarizes the arguments for and against its use *ab initio* versus sequential introduction of antiviral agents. The debate is informed by the biology of viral resistance, the evidence (in particular its paucity), health economic considerations and lessons from the management of other infectious diseases such as tuberculosis and HIV.

Aims of treatment

In chronic HBV infection the ideal outcome from therapy is eradication of HBV, yet surface antigen seroconversion (in so far as it correlates with viral clearance) remains a rare event. Therefore the effective goal of therapy is to control viral replication and to prevent (and, where possible, reverse) the complications of chronic HBV infection, while minimizing side effects of therapy and avoiding the emergence of resistance to antiviral therapy. The emergence of resistant species is associated acutely with hepatitis flares and episodes of decompensation and in the long term with the progression of chronic liver disease and the development of hepatocellular carcinoma [3–5]. Use of the term 'treatment failure' to describe the emergence of resistant species is therefore not unreasonable.

The key to this control is in deciding whom to treat and when to commence treatment. Maximal benefit is gained in patients at risk of progression (male sex, African ethnicity, age, family history, advanced disease) who are in either the immunoactive or immunoescape phases of infection. However, once the decision to treat has been made, the treatment strategy should be designed to minimize the long-term consequences of viral resistance.

Treatment strategy

The lack of proofreading capability of HBV polymerase as well as the very large number of virions produced on a daily basis are important factors in the emergence and propagation of resistance genes. The mantra 'no replication equals no resistance' underpins the strategy that irrespective of whether treatment is with single agents or combinations of drugs, the rapid reduction of HBV DNA levels to undetectable levels is a key goal. Once a treatment has been instigated, regular monitoring is required for early detection of treatment failure.

A rise in alanine aminotransferase (ALT) to greater than twice the upper limit of normal on therapy after normalization is considered biochemical resistance; however, this is preceded by virological breakthrough where viraemia increases, usually by several logs, many weeks before the emergence of overt biochemical resistance. Primary treatment failure is defined as a failure to reduce viral load by 1 log IU/mL after 3 months' therapy and secondary failure as a rebound of greater than 1 log IU/mL from nadir on two occasions at least 1 month apart [6]. The viral mutations associated with resistance to each drug have been studied and can be detected in the clinical setting. Knowledge of so-called genotypic resistance is key to selecting the most appropriate treatment strategy and some advocate HBV DNA sequencing in all cases both before and during therapy, although the value and cost-effectiveness of this approach has not been demonstrated.

Strategies to lessen the risk of resistance include the use of interferon therapy (to which resistance does not develop) or an oral direct-acting antiviral agent that effectively suppresses viral replication and which has a high genetic barrier to resistance. To achieve these two aims many have proposed the use of *ab initio* combination therapy. However, common practice (and national/international society recommendations) has hitherto been to use a single agent and to add a second complementary drug when signs of treatment failure arise.

The logical combination of antiviral agents depends largely on the molecular biology of the resistance that develops to them. A viral mutation that confers resistance to one nucleotide analogue is likely to confer resistance to other drugs in that class, but unlikely to confer resistance to nucleoside analogues [7]. Therefore if resistance arises to a drug in one class, a drug from the other class (hence complementary) should be used and if *ab initio* combination is used, then the drugs should be complementary for the same reasons (see Chapters 33 and 38 for further details on complementary antiviral agents).

Sequential or *ab initio* combination?

The introduction of new direct-acting antiviral agents has been supported by a large body of evidence demonstrating safety and efficacy over existing therapeutic options. Unsurprisingly, most studies have been sponsored by pharmaceutical companies to address regulatory issues and, as such, most trials publish 1-year data with some subsequently extended up to 5 years. These data have informed our therapeutic choices but they do not answer the question as to whether treatment should start with monotherapy or combination therapy. Given the range of pharmaceutical companies involved and the very low rates of resistance with current agents, necessitating very large trials over very long periods of time, the studies needed to evaluate *ab initio* versus sequential combination therapy are unlikely to be conducted. In this era of evidence-based medicine, the absence of large randomized controlled trial data to support a management strategy can sometimes be taken as evidence for its ineffectiveness, although this is clearly not the case.

There are strong virological and economic arguments for initiating therapy with a single antiviral agent and only adding a complementary drug should treatment failure occur. Until the summer of 2007, lamivudine or adefovir were the only oral drugs available, and both are associated with high rates of resistance after 5 years' treatment (approximately 80% and 29%, respectively) [8]. However, sequential addition of adefovir to patients who have shown resistance to lamivudine results in effective suppression of viral load to undetectable in 72% of patients at 2 years [2]. This strategy also results in low rates of acquisition of new adefovir mutations (4% after 42 months) and this approach is the basis for the 'road-map' approach to therapy in which treatment is initiated with one drug and then changed to include additional agents if early virological control is not achieved. This concept is based on the fact that while resistance rates are high, treatment failure is not universal and much evidence demonstrates that the addition of a nucleotide analogue usually rescues virological and biochemical breakthrough. The use of multiple drugs in series rather than in combination decreases the risk of adverse effects and if these do arise then the responsible agent is more readily identified. Although the road-map concept is theoretically attractive, it has never been tested in prospective studies and the definition of treatment failure is unclear.

The argument that supports the use of these drugs in combination *ab initio* is that combination therapy may achieve the goals of treatment more effectively than any single drug alone; in particular, combination therapy may be predicted to reduce the long-term risk from viral resistance. However, no randomized controlled trials have been conducted to test this hypothesis. In the absence of such evidence, many have turned to the lessons learned from HIV medicine over the past 25 years [9] and the management of tuberculosis over the past 50 years [10]. The development of resistance in HIV is rapid and the significant superiority of combination therapy over monotherapy was established very early after the drugs became available. However, HBV resistance occurs at a comparatively slow rate (over months and years versus days and weeks with HIV) and therefore the same rates of resistance have not been observed.

The results of a 2-year study comparing lamivudine monotherapy with lamivudine plus adefovir combination therapy in treatment-naive non-cirrhotic, predominantly Asian, patients demonstrate a degree of superiority of combination therapy over montherapy but are not as emphatic as advocates of combination therapy would have hoped [11]. HBV DNA levels were undetectable after 2 years' therapy in 26% of patients on combination therapy compared with 14% on lamivudine alone, and ALT normalized in 45% and 34% of patients respectively. However, after 52 weeks, more patients had normal liver function tests in the monotherapy arm than in combination (70% vs. 47%). Virological breakthrough was more frequently observed on monotherapy (44%) than on combination treatment (19%). Despite combination therapy, rtM204 mutations were detected in 9% and 15% at 52 and 104 weeks, respectively.

The nucleotide analogue tenofovir and the similarly effective nucleoside analogue entecavir have changed the landscape and expectations of antiviral therapy for HBV. Suppressing HBV DNA to undetectable levels in a minority of patients (such as the 26% in the above study) is no longer considered an adequate level of control and the third-generation drugs have viral suppression rates of greater than 80% for both HBeAg-positive and HBeAg-negative patients. For both of these drugs the medium-term resistance rates are low (well below 5% after several years) [12] and the arguments in favour of combination therapy are much reduced by these highly effective drugs. Nevertheless, the long-term resistance rates (i.e. over a patient's lifetime) with these drugs remains unclear and factors that predict the development of resistance are still unknown.

Consequences of treatment failure

The main advantages of sequential combination therapy – identification of side effects, cost and individualized therapy – are counteracted by the consequences of allowing treatment failure to one drug to develop; in other words, are we storing up problems for the future? The arguments for and against the use of combination therapy are based on the extrapolation of data from studies that report 1-year, 2-year or up to 5-year outcomes on these drugs. The natural history of chronic HBV infection both on and off treatment should be considered in terms of decades rather than years and, as far as we know, so should the intended duration of treatment. Therefore the durability of drugs should be measured over the same period of time.

Viral mutations that result in resistance to one drug will frequently lead to cross-resistance with agents from the same class. Therefore the use of lamivudine effectively precludes subsequent use of telbivudine. Similarly, prior use of adefovir is associated with a decreased response to tenofovir. Interestingly, even though entecavir is a structurally distinct (pentacyclic) nucleoside analogue and the viral mutations associated with resistance to it are not the same as those associated with resistance to lamivudine and telbivudine, prior use of lamivudine adversely affects response to entecavir such that after 4 years' therapy with entecavir 39.5% of lamivudine-resistant patients had also become resistant to entecavir [13]. In lamivudine-experienced patients who already have the rtM240V mutation, emergence of the entecavir-specific mutation rtM250V causes a marked drop in entecavir's effect, while in the absence of the lamivudine-resistance mutation rtM250V alone has minimal effect [14].

The emergence of mutations in suboptimally controlled patients with HBV infection can therefore have significant ramifications to future therapy and the consequences of early treatment decisions can have lifelong consequences for patients. Given that suppression of viral replication is probably the most important determinant of the emergence of resistant strains, the proponents of *de novo* combination therapy argue that the most responsible management strategy is early and effective viral load suppression.

Conclusions

The ongoing debate that this chapter has summarized will continue but for today's patients decisions need to be made regarding their treatment options. Clearly this will be a two-way dialogue and different patients and their physicians will reach different conclusions. Our current approach is to recommend combination therapy with lamivudine and tenofovir in HBeAg-positive patients who either elect not to undertake interferon therapy or who have failed to respond to it. We use this approach as a proportion of patients will not achieve complete suppression of viral replication with montherapy. In patients with HBeAg-negative disease, the same combination therapy is considered although here the arguments for its use are much reduced as most patients achieve undetectable viraemia with monotherapy. For these patients we often employ entecavir or tenofovir unless we are concerned about resistance in which case we use tenofovir plus lamivudine. For patients who are intolerant of combination therapy we use entecavir monotherapy. It remains unclear as to whether this approach will lead to long-term benefits and emerging data over the next few years will decide whether this approach is necessary or is simply overprescribing. It is probable that as long-term resistance data emerges, pretreatment factors that predispose to long-term treatment failure will emerge and it will then become possible to reserve combination therapy for those patients in whom it is clearly indicated.

References

1. Janssen HL, van Zonneveld M, Senturk H *et al.* Pegylated interferon alfa-2b alone or in combination with lamivudine for HBeAg-positive chronic hepatitis B: a randomised trial. *Lancet* 2005;365:123–129.
2. Lampertico P, Vigano M, Manenti E, Iavarone M, Sablon E, Colombo M. Low resistance to adefovir combined with lamivudine: a 3-year study of 145 lamivudine-resistant hepatitis B patients. *Gastroenterology* 2007;133:1445–1451. **Important study of combination therapy in a resistant prone population.** 🔑
3. Dienstag JL, Goldin RD, Heathcote EJ *et al.* Histological outcome during long-term lamivudine therapy. *Gastroenterology* 2003;124:105–117.
4. Liaw YF, Sung JJ, Chow WC *et al.* Lamivudine for patients with chronic hepatitis B and advanced liver disease. *New England Journal of Medicine* 2004;351:1521–1531.
5. Lok AS, Lai CL, Leung N *et al.* Long-term safety of lamivudine treatment in patients with chronic hepatitis B. *Gastroenterology* 2003;125:1714–1722.
6. Lok AS, Zoulim F, Locarnini S *et al.* Antiviral drug-resistant HBV: standardization of nomenclature and assays and recommendations for management. *Hepatology* 2007;46:254–265.
7. Zoulim F, Buti M, Lok AS. Antiviral-resistant hepatitis B virus: can we prevent this monster from growing? *Journal of Viral Hepatitis* 2007;14(Suppl 1):29–36.
8. Hoofnagle JH, Doo E, Liang TJ, Fleischer R, Lok AS. Management of hepatitis B: summary of a clinical research workshop. *Hepatology* 2007;45:1056–1075.
9. De Clercq E. Anti-HIV drugs: 25 compounds approved within 25 years after the discovery of HIV. *International Journal of Antimicrobial Agents* 2009;33:307–320.
10. Guy ES, Mallampalli A. Managing TB in the 21st century: existing and novel drug therapies. *Therapeutic Advances in Respiratory Disease* 2008;2:401–408.
11. Sung JJ, Lai JY, Zeuzem S *et al.* Lamivudine compared with lamivudine and adefovir dipivoxil for the treatment of HBeAg-positive chronic hepatitis B. *Journal of Hepatology* 2008;48:728–735.
12. Alazawi W, Foster GR. Advances in the diagnosis and treatment of hepatitis B. *Current Opinion in Infectious Diseases* 2008;21:508–515.
13. Colonno RJ, Rose RE, Pokornowski K *et al.* Four year assessment of ETV resistance in nucleoside-naive and lamivudine refractory patients. *Journal of Hepatology* 2007;46(Suppl 1):S294. **Important data showing minimal resistance with long-term monotherapy with a highly potent drug.** 🔑
14. Tenney DJ, Levine SM, Rose RE *et al.* Clinical emergence of entecavir-resistant hepatitis B virus requires additional substitutions in virus already resistant to lamivudine. *Antimicrobial Agents and Chemotherapy* 2004;48:3498–3507.

30 Management of hepatitis B virus infection in pregnancy

Eleri S.W. Wilson-Davies, William F. Carman

West of Scotland Specialist Virology Centre, Gartnavel General Hospital, Glasgow, UK

LEARNING POINTS

- The management of a pregnant woman who is HBsAg positive remains based on e-markers.

- There is convincing evidence available that one dose of hepatitis B-specific immunoglobulin as soon as possible after birth, along with a course of HBV vaccination, significantly reduces the chronic carrier rate in infants born to mothers who are HBeAg positive.

- HBeAg-positive women with an HBV DNA level above 10^7 copies/mL before 32 weeks require referral for specialist assessment for consideration of antiviral treatment, as this has been shown to further reduce transmission to their children.

- There is no major evidence to support the use of hepatitis B-specific immunoglobulin in the infants of anti-HBe-positive women. No chronic carriage appears to occur when these infants are treated with an accelerated course of HBV vaccination.

- Women who lack e-markers (i.e. are HBeAg and anti-HBe negative) should be managed in the same way as HBeAg-positive pregnant women.

Introduction

Mother-to-child (vertical) transmission of hepatitis B virus (HBV) accounts for approximately 35–40% of chronic infections worldwide [1]. Vertical transmission can occur in the prenatal period, during delivery or early after birth, although most transmissions occur during labour and delivery. Infections in this period from HBeAg-positive mothers usually result in chronic carriage of HBV.

Clinical Dilemmas in Viral Liver Disease, 1st edition. Edited by Graham R. Foster and K. Rajender Reddy. © 2010 Blackwell Publishing.

Management of the HBsAg-positive pregnant woman

The literature is in agreement that the management of a chronically infected pregnant woman is based on the presence of HBeAg or anti-HBe. As more experience accumulates on the routine use of quantitation of HBV DNA, this recommendation may become modified.

If the mother is HBeAg positive and no immunoprophylaxis is given, more than 85% of offspring will become chronically infected with HBV [2]. If the mother is anti-HBe positive and no immunoprophylaxis is given, less than 5% of offspring become chronically infected with HBV [3]. However, children of anti-HBe-positive mothers are also at risk of acute and fulminant HBV infection which, while rare, has a mortality rate of up to 75% [4].

Passive–active immunization administered to infants of HBeAg-positive women results in vertical transmission being reduced from 90% to between 1.1% [5] and 15% [6–8]. This variation is likely to reflect differing compliance with the recommended follow-up vaccination programme. When an accelerated course of HBV vaccination is started within 24 hours of birth for neonates whose mothers are anti-HBe positive, vertical transmission is reduced to less than 1% [6,8–11] with a significantly reduced risk of acute and fulminant hepatitis.

Immunization with hepatitis B immunoglobulin and HBV vaccine

The effect of passive immunization with hepatitis B immunoglobulin (HBIG) is immediate and lasts between 3 and 6 months [12], but it is expensive and there is limited availability in countries with low prevalence of HBV. As with all human blood derivatives, there is also a potential risk of transmission of pathogens, both known (e.g. new-variant Creutzfeldt–Jakob disease) and those yet to be discovered. For infants born to HBeAg-positive mothers, administration of HBIG in addition to a course of vaccine reduces vertical transmission further than the use of vaccine alone [5,7,8]. However, despite active–passive immunoprophylaxis being employed in a timely manner, not all vertical transmission is prevented.

Of 235 Hong Kong infants of HBeAg-positive mothers, 20% of those in the group who received one dose of HBIG and vaccine were HBsAg positive at 3 years of age [7], and 35% of infants who received accelerated vaccine only were HBsAg positive at 3 years compared with 73% HBsAg positive in the placebo group. While some infections may not have been vertical, the benefit of HBIG at birth in infants of HBeAg-positive mothers is clear. A 10-year (1982–1992) neonatal HBV vaccination program in the Netherlands provides further evidence [5]. Of 705 infants born to HBeAg-positive women, eight (1.1%) became HBsAg positive despite passive–active immunoprophylaxis. No significant difference was found between the groups receiving one or two doses of HBIG. Of 140 infants born to HBeAg-positive mothers in Hong Kong, chronic carriage was 6.8% in children who received passive–active vaccination compared with 21.0% in those who received vaccine alone (with 73.2% chronic carriage in the control group) [8].

HBV DNA level determines consideration of antiviral treatment

In the Netherlands study discussed above (8 of 705 infants from HBeAg-positive mothers became chronic carriers despite passive–active vaccination), the only factor that was found to increase the risk of failure was the maternal HBV DNA level [5]. The protective efficacy rate was 100% if maternal HBV DNA was less than 150 pg/mL, but this was reduced to 68% for those with HBV DNA in excess of 150 pg/mL ($P = 0.009$). In an earlier paper based on the same cohort, median maternal HBV DNA was 314 pg/mL in the group which became chronic carriers in comparison with a median maternal HBV DNA of 4.5 pg/mL in the group which responded to passive–active immunoprophylaxis [13].

In a South Korean study, 17 of 144 (11.8%) children of HBsAg-positive mothers who received HBIG and vaccine suffered immunoprophylaxis failure [6]. Chronic carriage only occurred in children with a detectable maternal HBV DNA level (27% vs. 0% when maternal HBV DNA was undetectable). Chronic infection did not occur in children of HBeAg-positive mothers with undetectable HBV DNA. In one Chinese study, 7 of 95 infants (7.4%) became chronic carriers at 1 year despite passive–active immunization [14]. In mothers who transmitted the infection, mean HBV DNA was significantly increased ($P = 0.04$). In Taiwan, of 52 HBeAg-positive mothers, five had active–passive vaccination failure [15]. The high-infectivity group of 34 mothers with HBV DNA above 0.04 ng/mL contained all five cases of transmission. There was evidence of maternal–fetal haemorrhage in three cases.

Lamivudine taken in the third trimester by mothers with a high viral load reduces vertical transmission further than that achieved by passive–active immunization of the infant alone, but does not prevent all cases [16–18]. In one pilot study, eight women with HBV DNA in excess of 1.2×10^9 copies/mL were treated with lamivudine 150 mg from 34 weeks' gestation [18]. One of the eight (12.5%) children was HBsAg positive at 1 year in the lamivudine treatment group; in a historical control group, 7 of 25 (28%) were HBsAg positive at 1 year. All 33 infants received active–passive immunization. In China, lamivudine was provided throughout pregnancy for 38 women [16]. No complications were observed in the 38 children. Only 12 infants were tested for HBsAg at 1 year, none of whom were positive. Another study compared lamivudine treatment with HBIG administration for the prevention of intrauterine vertical transmission [17]. Both HBIG and lamivudine reduced intrauterine infection compared with the control arm (chronic carrier rate after HBIG prophylaxis 16.3%, chronic carrier rate after maternal lamivudine treatment 16.1%, control group 32.7%). No pregnancy-related complications were observed.

Because of evidence of an increased risk of chronic carriage in infants of HBeAg-positive women with a high HBV DNA level, we recommend that a conservative approach is taken in the rare case of an anti-HBe-positive women, previously known to have HBV DNA in excess of 10^7 copies/mL.

Use of HBIG in infants of anti-HBe-positive women

A Cochrane review did not identify any well-conducted trials which supported the addition of HBIG to vaccine for infants of anti-HBe carrier mothers. It identified no

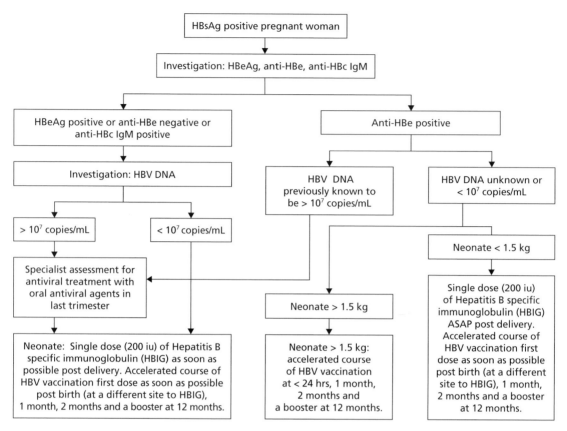

FIG. 30.1 Algorithm for the management of HBsAg-positive women. This algorithm was developed at a consensus meeting of the British Viral Hepatitis Group in summer 2008. It represents one approach to managing women who are HBsAg positive.

evidence for a role of higher viral level in anti-HBe carrier mothers that would support intervention beyond active vaccination [19]. In a study from Taiwan [9], 94 infants received one dose of HBIG and an accelerated course of vaccine; two infants were HBsAg positive at 2 months of age, but both children cleared the infection by 7 months of age. Another group of 122 infants received an accelerated course of vaccine only; one infant was HBsAg positive at 2 months of age, but once again the child cleared the infection by 7 months of age. None of the 122 infants who received vaccine alone became chronic carriers of HBV. In 125 Vietnamese infants born to anti-HBe-positive mothers who received vaccine alone, none became chronic carriers [10]. Of 88 infants born to HBeAg-positive mothers, 12 children became chronically infected despite active vaccination. Finally, in 125 British vaccinated infants born to anti-HBe-positive mothers, none became chronically

infected. In 21 cases born to HBeAg-positive women, six infants became chronic carriers [11]. The use of HBIG in infants weighing less than 1.5 kg whose mothers are anti-HBe positive, while commonly included in guidelines, is not based on evidence.

Management of women who lack e-markers

Some 1% of HBsAg-positive mothers are both HBeAg and anti-HBe negative [8]. Currently, it is recommended to treat them in the same way as mothers who are HBeAg positive.

Conclusion

The approaches outlined above are evidence based. Although it is tempting to offer HBIG to all infants born to

HBsAg-positive mothers, it has to be understood there is little if any evidence to support such a stance. Further studies could be done to investigate the theoretical benefit of lamivudine prophylaxis for anti-HBe-positive mothers. It would be of interest to know if acute and fulminant hepatitis could be reduced by further management of the infant or if the maternal viral load is correlated with this outcome. Figure 30.1 presents a simplified algorithm for the management of women who are infected with HBV.

References

1. Ghendon Y. Perinatal transmission of hepatitis B virus in high-incidence countries. *Journal of Virological Methods* 1987;17:69–79.

2. Okada K, Kamiyama I, Inomata M, Imai M, Miyakawa Y. e antigen and anti-e in the serum of asymptomatic carrier mothers as indicators of positive and negative transmission of hepatitis B virus to their infants. *New England Journal of Medicine* 1976;294:746–749.

3. Stevens CE, Neurath RA, Beasley RP, Szmuness W. HBeAg and anti-HBe detection by radioimmunoassay: correlation of vertical transmission of hepatitis B virus in Taiwan. *Journal of Medical Virology* 1979;3:237–241.

4. Chen HL, Chang CJ, Kong MS *et al*. Pediatric fulminant hepatic failure in endemic areas of hepatitis B infection: 15 years after universal hepatitis B vaccination. *Hepatology* 2004;39:58–63.

5. del Canho R, Grosheide PM, Mazel JA *et al*. Ten-year neonatal hepatitis B vaccination program, The Netherlands, 1982–1992: protective efficacy and long-term immunogenicity. *Vaccine* 1997;15:1624–1630.

6. Song YM, Sung J, Yang S, Choe YH, Chang YS, Park WS. Factors associated with immunoprophylaxis failure against vertical transmission of hepatitis B virus. *European Journal of Pediatrics* 2008;167:489–490.

7. Ip HM, Lelie PN, Wong VC, Kuhns MC, Reesink HW. Prevention of hepatitis B virus carrier state in infants according to maternal serum levels of HBV DNA. *Lancet* 1989;i:406–410.

8. Wong VC, Ip HM, Reesink HW *et al*. Prevention of the HBsAg carrier state in newborn infants of mothers who are chronic carriers of HBsAg and HBeAg by administration of hepatitis-B vaccine and hepatitis-B immunoglobulin. Double-blind randomised placebo-controlled study. *Lancet* 1984;i:921–926.

9. Yang YJ, Liu CC, Chen TJ *et al*. Role of hepatitis B immunoglobulin in infants born to hepatitis B e antigen-negative carrier mothers in Taiwan. *Pediatric Infectious Disease Journal* 2003;22:584–588.

10. Milne A, West DJ, Chinh DV, Moyes CD, Poerschke G. Field evaluation of the efficacy and immunogenicity of recombinant hepatitis B vaccine without HBIG in newborn Vietnamese infants. *Journal of Medical Virology* 2002;67:327–333.

11. Wheeley SM, Jackson PT, Boxall EH *et al*. Prevention of perinatal transmission of hepatitis B virus (HBV): a comparison of two prophylactic schedules. *Journal of Medical Virology* 1991;35:212–215.

12. Previsani N, Lavanchy D, Zuckerman AJ. Hepatitis B. *Perspectives in Medical Virology* 2004;10:31–98.

13. del Canho R, Grosheide PM, Schalm SW, de Vries RR, Heijtink RA. Failure of neonatal hepatitis B vaccination: the role of HBV-DNA levels in hepatitis B carrier mothers and HLA antigens in neonates. *Journal of Hepatology* 1994;20:483–486.

14. Wang Z, Zhang J, Yang H *et al*. Quantitative analysis of HBV DNA level and HBeAg titre in hepatitis B surface antigen positive mothers and their babies: HBeAg passage through the placenta and the rate of decay in babies. *Journal of Medical Virology* 2003;71:360–366.

15. Lin HH, Chang MH, Chen DS *et al*. Early predictor of the efficacy of immunoprophylaxis against perinatal hepatitis B transmission: analysis of prophylaxis failure. *Vaccine* 1991;9:457–460.

16. Su GG, Pan KH, Zhao NF, Fang SH, Yang DH, Zhou Y. Efficacy and safety of lamivudine treatment for chronic hepatitis B in pregnancy. *World Journal of Gastroenterology* 2004;10:910–912.

17. Li XM, Yang YB, Hou HY *et al*. Interruption of HBV intrauterine transmission: a clinical study. *World Journal of Gastroenterology* 2003;9:1501–1503.

18. van Zonneveld M, van Nunen AB, Niesters HG, de Man RA, Schalm SW, Janssen HL. Lamivudine treatment during pregnancy to prevent perinatal transmission of hepatitis B virus infection. *Journal of Viral Hepatitis* 2003;10:294–297.

19. Lee C, Gong Y, Brok J, Boxall EH, Gluud C. Hepatitis B immunisation for newborn infants of hepatitis B surface antigen-positive mothers. *Cochrane Database of Systematic Reviews* 2006;19:CD004790.

Maureen M. Jonas

Children's Hospital Boston, Division of Gastroenterology, Boston, Massachusetts, USA

LEARNING POINTS

- Most individuals with chronic HBV acquired infection either perinatally or during childhood. Chronic HBV acquired during childhood may be associated with significant morbidity later in life, such as cirrhosis and hepatocellular carcinoma.

- Most children with chronic HBV are in the immune-tolerant stage. Treatment is not helpful or indicated during this stage, and indiscriminate use of nucleotide/nucleoside analogues may elicit resistance, with serious negative ramifications for later treatment.

- Some children with chronic HBV infection may be candidates for treatment. This includes those primarily in the immune activation stage, with persistently abnormal ALT values and histological chronic hepatitis.

- Therapeutic options for chronic HBV infection during childhood are limited.

When making treatment decisions, it is important to remember that the natural history of chronic hepatitis B virus (HBV) infection in children is variable, depending on age, mode of acquisition and ethnicity. These differences are likely due to the immune tolerance that is known to develop when infection occurs at an early age, although the exact mechanisms are unknown. Children from endemic countries in whom HBV is acquired perinatally are usually HBeAg positive with high levels of viral replication [1]. Rates of spontaneous seroconversion are less than 2% per year in children younger than 3 years of age, and 4–5% after age 3. In contrast, children in non-endemic countries are

less likely to have acquired the disease perinatally. In this case, they frequently clear HBeAg and HBV DNA from serum during the first two decades of life [2]. In a 29-year longitudinal study of Italian children with chronic HBV who underwent HBeAg seroconversion, 95% of those without cirrhosis had inactive HBV infection at most recent follow-up and 15% cleared HBsAg [3]. Children who seroconvert spontaneously tend to have higher alanine aminotransferase (ALT) levels early in life. Although inflammatory changes are often mild in liver biopsies from children with chronic hepatitis B, fibrosis may be significant. In a recent study of 76 children with chronic HBeAg-positive HBV and elevated ALT (mean age 9.8 years), at least half had moderate to severe fibrosis, with 35% having either bridging fibrosis with lobular distortion or cirrhosis [4]. Cirrhosis is an infrequent complication of HBV infection during childhood, although precise incidence is uncertain. One of the largest studies included 292 consecutive children who were HBsAg positive and had an elevated serum ALT level [5]. Cirrhosis was found in 10 patients (3%) at a mean age of 4.0 ± 3.3 years. No child developed cirrhosis during follow-up (ranging from 1 to 10 years).

There are no data regarding treatment of acute HBV infection in children. Most children infected perinatally are asymptomatic, and the small percentage in whom acute, even fulminant, hepatitis develops rapidly clear HBsAg and viraemia. It has become apparent that some children with chronic HBV infection do require treatment in order to prevent serious sequelae, such as cirrhosis and hepatocellular carcinoma (HCC), in young adult life. Management of children with chronic HBV infection involves education and counselling, surveillance for HCC, and antiviral therapies in some cases.

There are few large trials in children to guide treatment decisions. Treatment is generally considered in patients

Clinical Dilemmas in Viral Liver Disease, 1st edition. Edited by Graham R. Foster and K. Rajender Reddy. © 2010 Blackwell Publishing.

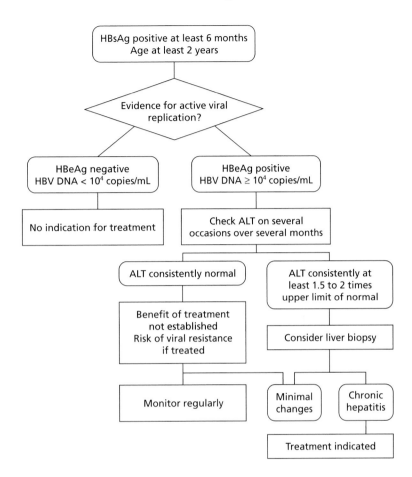

FIG. 31.1 Selection of paediatric patients with chronic hepatitis B for treatment.

who are in the immune active phase, usually defined as ALT more than twice normal and HBV DNA more than 20 000 IU/mL for at least 6 months [6] (Figure 31.1). Almost all children with chronic HBV are HBeAg positive, but therapy can also be considered for the few who are HBeAg negative, provided that viraemia above 10^4 IU/mL is documented and other diseases are excluded. None of the available treatments are highly efficacious. Therefore, the choice of whether to treat depends on patient-specific characteristics that predict the efficacy of treatment, including persistently abnormal ALT levels and active disease on liver biopsy, as well as considerations regarding the likelihood of achieving appropriate therapeutic goals.

The likelihood of response to any of the currently available drugs very much depends on the degree of elevation of serum aminotransferases [7–9]. ALT levels less than 1.5–2 times the upper limit of normal (ULN) generally indicate that the patient is in the immune-tolerant phase of HBV

infection. Such children are not typically candidates for treatment, because treatment with any of the currently available drugs does not result in higher rates of HBeAg seroconversion compared with no treatment. Prolonged treatment with nucleoside or nucleotide analogues at this stage are associated with little benefit, but impose the important risk of viral resistance, both to the agent chosen and similar drugs. An exception may be those immune-tolerant children who will be undergoing immunosuppression, such as those who will have chemotherapy or stem-cell or solid organ transplantation. Just as in adults, HBV suppression should be considered during these critical periods to avoid activation of hepatitis. Children with ALT values greater than 10 times ULN may be in the process of spontaneous HBeAg seroconversion, and should be observed for several months before treatment is begun. There may be several other considerations in deciding on treatment in individual patients, such as co-infection with hepatitis C virus (HCV), hepatitis D virus or HIV, or other comorbidities.

A number of drugs are currently approved for treatment of chronic HBV infection in adults. However, in the USA, only lamivudine and interferon alfa are licensed for use in children, and adefovir dipivoxil is available for use in those over 12 years of age. Interferon alfa leads to a beneficial response in 30–40% of patients. However, it is expensive and may be accompanied by frequent and unpleasant side effects. Success rates of interferon alfa treatment in children have varied significantly in different regions of the world. Response rates have been highest in Western countries, where treatment with interferon alfa results in loss of HBV DNA or HBeAg seroconversion in 20–58% compared with 8–17% in untreated controls. In contrast, only 3–17% of children treated with interferon alfa in Asian countries clear HBV DNA or seroconvert from HBeAg to anti-HBe. However, if aminotransferases are elevated, there may be no difference in response rates between children born in Asian countries (22%) and those from Europe and North America (26%) [10]. Children most likely to respond to interferon alfa, regardless of ethnicity, are of younger age with elevated aminotransferases and low HBV DNA levels. A large, multinational, randomized controlled trial of interferon alfa was performed in 144 children with chronic HBeAg-positive infection and ALT greater than twice ULN [8]. Serum HBeAg and HBV DNA became negative in 26% of treated children compared with 11% of untreated controls. In addition, 10% of treated children lost HBsAg compared with 1% of controls.

Interferon is not a good option in children with an underlying autoimmune disorder, organ transplant or serious neuropsychiatric disease. An advantage of interferon is that it has a finite duration of treatment and is not associated with the development of resistant HBV mutants. For children with HBeAg-positive chronic HBV infection, interferon alfa is given at a dose of 6 MU/m^2 (maximum 10 MU) three times a week for 24 weeks, followed by an observation period of 6–12 months. A year of treatment may be preferable in those with HBeAg-negative chronic HBV infection, based on data in adults. Patients should be monitored regularly for hepatitis flares during the first few months after the drug is discontinued. The efficacy of peginterferon alfa in children with chronic HBV infection has not been investigated. However, based on efficacy in adults and experience in children with HCV, it may be a reasonable choice for children with HBV, using a 48-week course and HCV doses, as recommended for adults.

Lamivudine is the only oral nucleoside analogue approved in the USA for treatment of children younger than 12 years with chronic HBV. In 2002, a multicenter, randomized, double-blind, placebo-controlled trial in HBeAg-positive children with ALT greater than 1.3 times ULN demonstrated clearance of HBeAg and HBV DNA at 52 weeks in 23% of treated children compared with 13% of controls [7]. In children whose baseline ALT was at least twice normal, this response rate increased to 35%. Subsequently, open-label lamivudine given to non-responders showed a cumulative 3-year virological response rate of 35%. HBsAg loss occurred in 3% of patients. HBeAg seroconversion from the first year was durable in 88% of patients at 3 years [11]. However, viral resistance developed in 64% of children who received lamivudine for 3 years. Of the children who participated in this trial, 151 were then followed for two more years [12]. Subjects were divided into two groups for analysis: those who had already achieved virological response by the end of the 3 years of therapy, and those who had not. In those who had achieved virological response, long-term durability of HBeAg seroconversion was 82% and greater than 90% in those who had received lamivudine for 52 weeks and at least 2 years, respectively. This compares with 75% for those who had achieved seroconversion after placebo. In those who had not already achieved virological response, an additional 11% did so during the next 2 years; they had all received lamivudine in the previous trial and none had received further treatment. Eight more children lost HBsAg; all had received lamivudine at some point during the previous trials. Although these findings are consistent with a recent study in Korean children where long-term treatment with lamivudine led to significant improvement in the seroconversion rates of HBeAg and HBsAg [13], results of several other small studies of children receiving long-term lamivudine have reported low rates of HBeAg seroconversion and no clearance of HBsAg.

Lamivudine is safe for children with hepatitis B and is well tolerated. Serious side effects were not reported after 3 years of continuous treatment. In comparison to treatment with interferon alfa, decreased height velocity and weight loss were not observed [11]. Children with higher pretreatment ALT and histological activity index scores on liver biopsy were more likely to respond to lamivudine. Other factors such as HBV DNA levels, age, gender, race, ethnicity, body weight and body mass index did not appear to significantly influence response to lamivudine treatment in children [14]. Initial data suggested that continued treatment of patients who develop resistance might be beneficial in those in whom HBV DNA continues to be suppressed. However, long-term follow-up of such patients suggests that the disease continues to progress. Thus, it may be prudent to discontinue lamivudine in children who develop lamivudine-resistant HBV. Patients should be monitored regularly for hepatitis flares during the first few months after the drug is discontinued. For those who require additional therapy, options are limited at this time.

A double-blind placebo-controlled trial of adefovir dipivoxil (ADV) has been recently reported [15]; 173 children with HBeAg-positive chronic HBV were stratified by age and prior treatment. In the 12–18 year age group, as had been noted in adults, significantly more ADV-treated subjects achieved the primary efficacy end-point (serum HBV DNA < 1000 copies/mL and normal ALT at the end of blinded treatment) compared with placebo-treated subjects (23% vs. 0%; $P = 0.007$). In the younger groups, the differences between ADV and placebo at the end of blinded treatment were not statistically significant. The HBeAg seroconversion rate was 16% compared with 5% in the placebo group. No subject developed an ADV-associated mutation that has been linked to resistance. Each group achieved ADV concentrations in the target range. ADV treatment was well tolerated by all subjects, and no safety issues were identified. An open-label Phase 2 pharmacokinetic and dose-finding study of entecavir in children is underway. A randomized placebo-controlled trial of tenofovir in adolescents is currently enrolling subjects. Telbivudine has not yet been tested in children with chronic HBV.

The only treatments currently approved for chronic HBV infection in children are standard interferon and lamivudine. ADV is available for patients 12 years and older. However, these are less than ideal for the reasons discussed, and some practitioners have begun to use peginterferon in children without contraindications. In my own practice, we use peginterferon in some, and we are enrolling children in the entecavir trial. The adolescent tenofovir trial is in progress. For these reasons, at this time initiation of treatment should be reserved for those children with histological evidence of significant chronic hepatitis or fibrosis. At present, there are no recommendations regarding the best treatment of children co-infected with HCV or HIV, since these co-infections are rare in paediatric patients.

Children with chronic HBV in the immune-tolerant stage (normal ALT, HBeAg positive) need to be monitored carefully for activation. ALT should be determined twice yearly, and HBeAg and anti-HBe yearly. Patients who are in the inactive phase of HBV infection (HBeAg negative, anti-HBe positive, persistently normal ALT, serum HBV DNA < 10^4 copies/mL) should undergo monitoring of ALT every 6–12 months. The infection may reactivate even after years of quiescence; 4–20% of inactive 'carriers' have one or more reversions to HBeAg, and approximately 20–25% will develop HBeAg-negative chronic HBV. Periodic measurement of serum alpha-fetoprotein levels and hepatic ultrasound for HCC surveillance have been recommended in adults based on observational data and expert opinion, even after HBeAg seroconversion, either spontaneous or after treatment. The risk of HCC increases with increasing age, but childhood cases have been well described. Currently, there are no guidelines as to when this surveillance should be initiated, and how often testing should be done.

Children with HBV infection should be allowed to participate in all regular activities of childhood. There is no need to exclude infected children from regular school and sports participation [16]. HBV-infected children should receive hepatitis A vaccine. Household contacts should receive HBV immunization and be tested to ensure vaccine efficacy. They should be counselled not to share items that may be contaminated with blood and to carefully dispose of such items. Adolescents need to be informed of the risks of transmission of HBV by sexual activity and needle sharing.

Optimal treatment for children with chronic HBV infection should be individualized, depending on clinical and histological status, comorbid conditions, ability to take medications, contraindications and family concerns. The goal of treatment should be suppression of HBV DNA and durable HBeAg seroconversion, indicating cessation of active viral replication, to prevent the long-term consequences. Appropriate patient selection and understanding of the strengths and limitations of each of the therapeutic options are key to successful treatment.

References

1. Lok ASF, Lai CL. A longitudinal follow-up of asymptomatic hepatitis B surface antigen-positive Chinese children. *Hepatology* 1988;8:1130–1133.

2. Bortolotti F, Cadrobbi P, Crivellaro C *et al*. Long-term outcome of chronic type B hepatitis in patients who acquire hepatitis B virus infection in childhood. *Gastroenterology* 1990;99:805–810.

3. Bortolotti F, Guido M, Bartolacci S *et al*. Chronic hepatitis B in children after e antigen seroclearance: final report of a 29-year longitudinal study. *Hepatology* 2006;43:556–562.

4. Godra A, Perez-Atayde AR, Jonas MM. Histologic features of chronic hepatitis B in children [Abstract]. *Hepatology* 2005;42(Suppl 1):478A.

5. Bortolotti F, Calzia R, Cadrobbi P *et al*. Liver cirrhosis associated with chronic hepatitis B virus infection in childhood. *Journal of Pediatrics* 1986;108:224–227.

6. Shah U, Kelly D, Chang M-H *et al*. Management of chronic hepatitis B in children. *Journal of Pediatric Gastroenterology and Nutrition* 2009;48:399–404. **This is a recent review of management issues in paediatric hepatitis B infections.**

7. Jonas MM, Kelly DA, Mizerski J *et al*. Clinical trial of lamivudine in children with chronic hepatitis B. *New England Journal of Medicine* 2002;346:1706–1713. **This was the first large trial of a nucleotide analogue for childhood HBV, providing not only indications of safety and efficacy, but features of infection associated with likelihood of response.**

8. Sokal EM, Conjeevaram HS, Roberts EA *et al*. Interferon alfa therapy for chronic hepatitis B in children: a multinational randomized controlled trial. *Gastroenterology* 1998;114:988–995. **This is a major randomized trial of interferon for children with chronic HBV.**

9. Torre D, Tambini R. Interferon-alpha therapy for chronic hepatitis B in children: a meta-analysis. *Clinical Infectious Diseases* 1996;23:131–137.

10. Narkewicz MR, Smith D, Silverman A, Vierling J, Sokol RJ. Clearance of chronic hepatitis B virus infection in young children after alpha interferon treatment. *Journal of Pediatrics* 1995;127:815–818.

11. Sokal EM, Kelly DA, Mizerski J *et al*. Long-term lamivudine therapy for children with HBeAg-positive chronic hepatitis B. *Hepatology* 2006;43:225–232.

12. Jonas MM, Little NR, Gardner SD. Long-term lamivudine treatment of children with chronic hepatitis B: durability of therapeutic responses and safety. *Journal of Viral Hepatitis* 2007;15:20–27.

13. Choe B-H, Lee JY, Jang YC *et al*. Long-term therapeutic efficacy of lamivudine compared with interferon-alfa in children with chronic hepatitis B: the younger the better. *Journal of Pediatric Gastroenterology and Nutrition* 2007;44:92–98.

14. Hom X, Little NR, Gardner SD, Jonas MM. Predictors of virologic response to lamivudine treatment in children with chronic hepatitis B. *Pediatric Infectious Disease Journal* 2004;23:441–445.

15. Jonas MM, Kelly D, Pollack H *et al*. Safety, efficacy, and pharmacokinetics of adefovir dipivoxil in children and adolescents (age 2 to < 18 years) with chronic hepatitis B. *Hepatology* 2008;47:1863–1871.

16. American Academy of Pediatrics. Hepatitis B. In: Pickering LK, Baker CJ, Kimberlin DW, Long SS eds. *Red Book: Report of the Committee on Infectious Diseases.* 28th ed. EIK Grove Village, IL: American Academy of Pediatrics; 2009:337–56.

32   Hepatitis B infection in surgeons and healthcare workers: what should we do to protect patients?

Graham R. Foster

Queen Mary's University of London, Blizard Institute of Cell and Molecular Science, London, UK

LEARNING POINTS

- Healthcare workers with chronic HBV infection can transmit the virus to their patients.

- The risk of transmission is related to viral load, with HBeAg-positive individuals being at greater risk of inadvertent transmission. However, HBeAg-negative patients can transmit HBV to their patients.

- Effective antiviral therapy can reduce the risk of transmission but the optimal treatment regimen and the definition of a 'safe' viral load remains unclear.

Chronic infection with hepatitis B virus (HBV) may be associated with very high levels of circulating viraemia. Transmission of the virus by blood to blood contact is well recognized and infection by contact with other contaminated bodily fluids is established. It is therefore not surprising to find that infected healthcare workers have occasionally and inadvertently infected their patients, sometimes with catastrophic results [1,2]. The risks of transmission are inevitably greater in those who perform prolonged, open surgical procedures but healthcare workers who take part in any invasive procedure may also pose a risk to their patients. The recognition that healthcare workers who are HBeAg positive have high levels of viral replication and pose the greatest risk has led most countries to insist that all those who perform high-risk interventional

procedures should be tested for HBV and those who are HBeAg positive are usually barred from performing such high-risk procedures [1]. The definition of a high-risk procedure is not universally agreed: in the UK the definition of an 'exposure-prone procedure' is one in which the operator's hands are in a body cavity with a sharp instrument. This definition includes surgical operations, dental procedures and obstetric interventions but does not include endoscopic procedures or venesection. In some units concern has been expressed that this definition does not prevent laparoscopic procedures that may escalate rapidly to open surgery and some units have redefined exposure-prone procedures to include 'procedures that may progress to a procedure where the operator's hands are in a body cavity with a sharp instrument'. Similar definitions have been adopted in many other jurisdictions. Unfortunately, excluding healthcare workers at greatest risk of transmitting chronic HBV infection has not completely prevented inadvertent HBV transmission to patients and detailed studies have shown that healthcare workers with HBeAg-negative HBV may also transmit the virus to patients, particularly if the healthcare worker has high-level viraemia [3]. The recognition that some people with HBeAg-negative disease can transmit the virus to other patients led to the introduction of amended guidelines in many countries, whereby patients with HBeAg-negative disease were barred from high-risk procedures if they had high levels of circulating viraemia [4]. The level of viraemia deemed 'safe' varies from country to country but in the UK a value of less than 10^3 genome equivalent per ml is regarded as safe and healthcare workers with viral loads below this level are permitted to operate freely. Other countries have adopted slightly higher viral loads.

Clinical Dilemmas in Viral Liver Disease, 1st edition. Edited by Graham R. Foster and K. Rajender Reddy. © 2010 Blackwell Publishing.

The introduction and widespread use of potent antiviral agents has led to calls for a re-evaluation of the guidelines on infected healthcare workers and many authorities have argued that surgeons and other healthcare workers receiving antiviral therapy should be allowed to operate provided that their viral load is reduced to an acceptable, very low, level [5]. However, a policy whereby surgeons are allowed to operate if their viral load is reduced by antiviral therapy is potentially hazardous: the viral load may rise rapidly if a drug-resistant mutation develops and the prospect of an infected healthcare worker with a drug-resistant viral mutation infecting a patient with a resistant virus led many authorities to impose strict limits on healthcare workers undergoing therapy. The UK has one of the most rigorous policies and current UK policy is to allow infected healthcare workers to perform exposure-prone procedures only if their pretreatment viral load is low ($< 10^5$ genome equivalents per mL) and only if they are undergoing therapy that is carefully monitored by a named physician [4]. In view of the variation in different laboratories testing HBV viral loads, the tests need to be performed in one of two designated laboratories in the UK. The rationale for allowing only healthcare workers with low pretreatment viraemia to operate is based on the assumption that people with low pretreatment viraemia are least likely to develop on-treatment mutations and, in the unlikely event of a resistant mutation developing, it is reasonable to presume that the viral load will not rise rapidly to very high levels, thereby providing an opportunity for early detection of resistance and intervention to prevent transmission from healthcare worker to patient.

The optimal approach to managing healthcare workers with HBV is fraught with difficulty. On the one hand, experienced operators are a scarce resource and are expensive to train and banning healthcare workers from performing exposure-prone procedures may reduce the number of procedures that can be performed. Many HBV-infected healthcare workers have become infected during their work as medical practitioners and preventing them from continuing to work because of a work-related accident seems punitive. This is clearly of particular concern in areas where income is related to the number of procedures performed. On the other hand, patients have a right to expect that they will not be exposed to unnecessary risk while receiving healthcare and placing restrictions on healthcare workers to protect patients from harm is a well-established principle that is widely respected by healthcare professionals. The UK guidelines are among the most restrictive in the world and are generally regarded as reasonable. However, a small number of infected individuals have argued that the restrictions are unnecessary and unduly restrictive.

For healthcare professionals infected with HBV there is an established principle, exemplified by current guidelines, that activity should be restricted when the viral load is very high but there should be few or no restrictions on clinical practice when the viral load is low or when effective therapy is being taken. Some restrictions have been imposed to protect patients from unexpected increases in viraemia caused by viral resistance. Given that the current generation of oral antiviral agents (particularly entecavir and tenofovir) are very potent, have a very low rate of resistance and reduce the viral load in the majority of patients to almost undetectable levels [6,7], it is reasonable to ask whether all infected healthcare workers should be allowed to operate if they are receiving one of these potent antiviral agents. Such a policy has the advantage of restoring experienced professionals to the workplace, of simplifying the management of infected healthcare workers and is highly likely to protect patients because surgeons with viraemia reduced by potent drugs are highly unlikely to transmit virus to their patients. On the other hand, there is a small, but not zero, risk of virological relapse due to either non-compliance or resistance and if a healthcare worker were to infect a patient at a time when his or her viral load was raised it is probable that there would be serious repercussions for all those involved.

Discussion relating to the optimal management of HBV-infected healthcare workers has been led by high-quality studies evaluating the risks of transmission and the effectiveness of antiviral therapies. In many countries the majority of the population are further protected by universal vaccination programmes and hence inadvertent transmission is unlikely. However, policies to protect patients from HBV infection will inevitably establish a precedent that may be used to determine policies for healthcare workers infected with HIV and hepatitis C virus (HCV) and these infections cannot currently be prevented by vaccination and carry a greater stigma than infection with HBV. Thus policies around HBV transmission need to be reviewed in the light of other blood-borne viruses.

The optimal management of healthcare workers with chronic HBV remains controversial. The procedures that carry the highest risk of transmission to patients are well recognized and it seems reasonable to place some restrictions on infected healthcare workers who perform such procedures. At present, most countries prevent those at greatest risk of transmitting virus from performing such procedures but a case could be made for relaxing these restrictions provided that the healthcare worker is taking antiviral medication that can be shown to be effective. Many countries have now introduced complex management algorithms that allow those who have modest levels of viraemia to perform exposure-prone procedures but preclude those with high-level viraemia from performing high-risk procedures. As experience with the new antiviral agents accumulates, it is probable that the current restrictions will be relaxed further and more and more infected healthcare workers will be allowed to return to performing high-risk invasive procedures. It will be important to ensure that all such individuals are very closely monitored to ensure that accidental transmission does not take place: the 'relaxations' in the current restrictions may be rapidly reversed in response to the public pressure that may follow a high-profile inadvertent transmission of viral hepatitis to a patient.

References

1. van der Eijk AA, de Man RA, Niesters HG, Schalm SW, Zaaijer HL. Hepatitis B virus (HBV) DNA levels and the management of HBV-infected health care workers. *Journal of Viral Hepatitis* 2006;13:2–4. **Excellent review of the issues around basing management of healthcare workers on viral load.**

2. Corden S, Ballard AL, Ijaz S *et al.* HBV DNA levels and transmission of hepatitis B by health care workers. *Journal of Clinical Virology* 2003;27:52–58.

3. Public Health Laboratory Service Communicable Disease Surveillance Centre, Incident Investigation Teams and others. Transmission of hepatitis B to patients from four infected surgeons without hepatitis B e antigen. *New England Journal of Medicine* 1997;336:178–184. **The pivotal study demonstrating transmission from HBeAg-negative surgeons.**

4. Department of Health. *Hepatitis B infected health care workers and antiviral therapy*. Available at www.dh.gov.uk/en/ Publications. Published 16 March 2007.

5. Buster EH, van der Eijk AA, de Man RA, Janssen HL, Schalm SW. Prolonged antiviral therapy for hepatitis B virus-infected health care workers: a feasible option to prevent work restriction without jeopardizing patient safety. *Journal of Viral Hepatitis* 2007;14:350–354.

6. Yurdaydin C. Entecavir: a step forward in combating hepatitis B disease. *Expert Opinion in Pharmacotherapy* 2008;9:3095–3109.

7. Marcellin P, Heathcote EJ, Buti M *et al.* Tenofovir disoproxil fumarate versus adefovir dipivoxil for chronic hepatitis B. *New England Journal of Medicine* 2008;359:2442–2455.

33 HBV in the poorly compliant patient: dare we start oral drugs?

Tin Nguyen[1,2], Paul Desmond[1], Stephen Locarnini[2]

[1]Gastroenterology Department, St Vincent's Hospital, Fitzroy, Victoria, Australia

[2]Victorian Infectious Diseases Reference Laboratory, North Melbourne, Victoria, Australia

LEARNING POINTS

- The prevention and treatment of antiviral resistance is a major clinical problem in the management of chronic hepatitis B.

- The emergence of antiviral resistance is dependent on the interplay of viral, host and antiviral drug factors.

- The common pathways of antiviral drug resistance are predictable, and application is advantageous to the treating physician in planning salvage treatment options.

- Non-adherence to therapy is a risk factor for the emergence of antiviral resistance, which can in turn result in virological rebound and clinical progression of disease.

- Ongoing patient counselling and education is a critical component in the management of chronic hepatitis B.

HYPOTHETICAL CLINICAL SCENARIO

Mr T. was a 57-year-old Asian man with HBeAg-negative disease and advanced fibrosis on histology. He was started on lamivudine (LMV) 1 year ago and achieved an on-therapy biochemical and virological response, with normalization of serum alanine aminotransferase (ALT) and an undetectable hepatitis B virus (HBV) load. Unfortunately, Mr T. did not take LMV on a recent 3-month overseas trip, during which he was unwell with a non-specific illness. Upon recommencement of LMV on his return, Mr T. subsequently developed an on-treatment hepatic flare with severe hepatic decompensation. Virological rebound and genotypic resistance to LMV was confirmed, but despite aggressive supportive measures, including attempts at rescue add-on antiviral therapy, Mr T. unfortunately died.

Clinical Dilemmas in Viral Liver Disease, 1st edition. Edited by Graham R. Foster and K. Rajender Reddy. © 2010 Blackwell Publishing.

Introduction

In the past decade, the development of safe and efficacious oral nucleos(t)ide analogue (NA) therapy for chronic HBV has advanced considerably. However, clinical experience with agents such as LMV, adefovir dipivoxil (ADV) and telbivudine highlight the emerging problem of antiviral resistance. The prevention and treatment of antiviral resistance is a major clinical problem in the management of chronic hepatitis B. The clinical impact of antiviral resistance is associated with multiple negative outcomes, including progression of liver disease, an increased risk of hepatocellular carcinoma (HCC), graft failure in post-transplant patients, reduced HBeAg seroconversion rates, and public health concerns including the potential for selection of vaccine escape mutants and transmission of multidrug-resistant virus.

In clinical trials of chronic HBV therapy, medication non-adherence accounts for up to 30% of virological breakthrough [1]. The intensity of monitoring is clearly more rigorous in clinical trials, and there are few published data available on the impact of non-adherence in chronic HBV treatment in everyday clinical practice. Furthermore, although clinical trials often employ an 80% compliance and drug dosing rule as acceptable inclusion in final data analysis (intention to treat versus off-protocol assessment), the applicability of this in the day-to-day post-registration phase of chronic hepatitis B treatment is unclear. While the hypothetical scenario of Mr T. represents the most severe spectrum of potential complications, the increased development of drug-resistant mutants and clinical deterioration in patients non-adherent to therapy is no doubt seen in everyday clinical practice.

This chapter addresses the factors involved in antiviral resistance, specific pathways of resistance to oral NA agents, potential consequences of non-adherence to therapy, and prevention of antiviral resistance.

Antiviral drug resistance

The development of antiviral resistance is dependent on the interplay of multiple factors. These include factors related to the virus (viral replication rate, the error-prone reverse transcriptase/polymerase, replication fitness of viral quasispecies), host (compliance with therapy, prior drug experience, genetic factors such as drug metabolism to active moiety), drug (potency of antiviral agent, genetic barrier of drug to viral resistance, pharmacokinetic properties) and hepatocyte (available replication space). Furthermore, antiviral therapy may not reach potential sequestered sites/sanctuaries of viral replication, and does not eradicate covalently closed circular DNA, which is a crucial HBV replicative intermediate within the hepatocyte.

Specific pathways of resistance to oral NA agents

Antiviral resistance occurs because of the development of adaptive mutations under the selective pressure of antiviral therapy, with the consequence of diminished susceptibility of mutant virus to the inhibitory effect of a drug. The currently available NA agents can be classified according to chemical structure: L-nucleoside analogues such as LMV, telbivudine, emtricitabine and clevudine; acyclic phosphonates such as ADV and tenofovir (TDF); and the cyclopentane

ring group such as entecavir (ETV). This chemical classification of oral NA agents is useful as patterns of antiviral resistance are predictable and generally structure specific (Table 33.1).

L-nucleoside pathway

LMV is the most well-characterized L-nucleoside and is associated with 80% genotypic resistance rates following 5 years of use. Treatment with LMV can lead to the resistant mutation rtM204V/I/S (which is found in the YMDD location in the C domain of HBV polymerase) with or without rtL180M (B domain). Mutations conferring resistance to LMV decrease *in vitro* sensitivity to LMV 100–1000 fold.

Once antiviral resistance to an L-nucleoside occurs, the effect of salvage 'switch' therapy with other agents within the group is attenuated due to cross-resistance, and thus ideally should not be instituted. Furthermore, add-on therapy of drugs within a class is also not recommended, because these drugs may compete for cellular activation mechanisms and viral targets. It should be noted that the rtM204V/I mutation also reduces susceptibility to ETV [2]. In a very small minority of cases, primary LMV resistance can also be observed with the emergence of rtA181T [3].

Acyclic phosphonate pathway

Genotypic resistance rates with ADV occur less frequently than resistance to LMV (Table 33.2). Treatment with ADV can select out rtN236T (D domain) with or without rtA181T/V (B domain). TDF is a nucleotide analogue that is structurally similar to ADV. TDF has much higher potency than ADV, in part because it can be given at a

TABLE 33.1 Pathways of antiviral resistance in chronic HBV infection.

Pathway	Mutation	Associated resistance
L-nucleoside	rtM204V/I/S ± rtL180M rtA181T	Lamivudine Emtricitabine Telbivudine
Acyclic phosphonate	rtN236T rtA181T/V	Adefovir Tenofovir
'Shared'	rtA181T/V	L-nucleosides (see above) Acyclic phosphonates (see above)
Naive entecavir resistance	rt180M + rtM204V with changes at one of rtT184, rtS202 or rtM250 codons	Entecavir
Multidrug resistance	Complex patterns, e.g. rtA181T + rtN236T + rtM250L	Multidrug

TABLE 33.2 Annual resistance rates for oral antiviral agents in chronic HBV infection.

Drug	Cumulative resistance rate (%)				
	1 year	2 years	3 years	4 years	5 years
Treatment naive					
Lamivudine [8,9]	23	46	55	71	80
Adefovir dipivoxil (HBeAg negative) [10]	0	3	11	18	29
Entecavir [11]	0.2	0.5	1.2	1.2	1.2
Emtricitabine [12,13]	13	18	–	–	–
Telbivudine [14]					
HBeAg positive	4.4	21.6	–	–	–
HBeAg negative	2.7	8.6			
Tenofovir fumarate [15]	0	–	–	–	–
Previous lamivudine resistance					
Adefovir dipivoxil (LMV resistant) [16]	0–18	38.3	–	–	–
Adefovir/LMV (LMV resistant) [17]	1	2	4	4	–
Entecavir (LMV resistant) [18]	6	15	35	43	51

much higher dosage because of less nephrotoxicity [1]. Cross-resistance exists between ADV and TDF *in vitro*, and longer-term studies with TDF are required to determine other mutations that may arise in the clinical situation.

Shared pathway

Most patients with antiviral resistance to LMV have rtM204V/I, and thus a salvage option is to add on ADV therapy. However, the shared pathway which selects out rtA181T/V confers resistance to acyclic phosphonates (e.g. ADV), and partial cross-resistance to LMV. rtA181T/V is seen in 40% of ADV treatment failures and 5% of LMV treatment failures [4]. The development of rtA181T/V has also been shown to have a dominant inhibitory effect on wild-type virion secretion, and could challenge the traditional case definition of virological breakthrough ($\geq 1.0 \log_{10}$ IU/mL increase from nadir) [5].

Naive entecavir resistance pathway

ETV is the most potent oral antiviral agent, with *in vitro* studies demonstrating 100–300 times greater potency than LMV [6]. Resistance to ETV was first noted in patients with pre-existing LMV resistance (Table 33.2). Virological breakthrough to entecavir requires at least three substitutions, including two lamivudine-resistant mutations (rtM204V and rtL180M), and an additional substitution at either rtS202I, rtT184G and/or rtM250V [7]. Thus, in treatment-naive patients, ETV has a high genetic barrier to resistance, and the 5-year cumulative genotypic resistance rate is only 1.2% (Table 33.2).

Clinical consequences of non-adherence and antiviral resistance

The impact of non-adherence to therapy in chronic HBV infection on healthcare is difficult to quantify. However, it is likely a significant cause of additional usage of healthcare resources, including repeated visits to clinic, requirement for additional investigations and changes to therapeutic regimens. Furthermore, non-adherence can hasten the emergence of antiviral resistance. The development of antiviral resistance can in turn result in virological breakthrough, reduced HBeAg seroconversion rates (in HBeAg-positive HBV), on/off treatment hepatic flares, histological progression of disease, and hepatic decompensation [1].

Prevention of antiviral resistance

There are multiple factors involved in the prevention of antiviral resistance to oral antiviral therapy. Patient counselling and education regarding the natural history of HBV infection, potential complications, and indications for antiviral therapy are essential (refer to published AASLD, EASL and APASL guidelines) [1,19,20]. Furthermore, given that treatment may be long term, and possibly indefinite in the setting of HBeAg-negative disease and cirrhosis, it is imperative that adherence to therapy is encouraged to minimize the emergence of antiviral resistance.

In chronic hepatitis B, it is not possible to directly measure adherence to therapy by measurement of serum or urinary drug levels. Furthermore, such measures would be both problematic and costly. Thus, general measures that may improve adherence include involvement of a dedicated liver nurse, regular education of both patient and family, provision of written information, empowerment of patients to take ownership of their treatment, monitoring of pill counts, and the development of a strong therapeutic relationship between the treating physician and patient/family.

Once therapy is indicated in treatment-naive patients, careful selection of initial antiviral agent is required. Highly potent drugs with low rates of resistance should be used where possible. Much interest has surrounded the concept of combination therapy for HBV, similar to the highly active antiretroviral therapy used in HIV medicine. Ideally, combination therapy with synergistic drugs with different mechanisms or sites of action should be employed. However, the drugs that comprise the current oral therapeutic arsenal against HBV all have similar mechanisms of action. Furthermore, the combination of immunomodulators such as interferon with oral agents has not shown definitive superiority over monotherapy. As of 2008, there are still insufficient data to recommended initial combination therapy for the management of chronic HBV infection if starting with the newer, more potent NA agents such as ETV or TDF.

On-therapy monitoring includes 3-monthly quantitative serum HBV and ALT measurements. Regular 3-monthly testing facilitates the assessment of antiviral efficacy as indicated by response, durability and development of virological breakthrough. If viral load rises on therapy, compliance needs to be assessed, and in patients adherent to therapy virological breakthrough usually equates with antiviral resistance. At this juncture, genotype testing should ideally be performed to confirm resistance and identify known mutations associated with antiviral resistance (Table 33.1). This in turn allows the appropriate initiation of add-on salvage therapy, which can be determined by understanding the aforementioned pathways of resistance. Clinical experience thus far has shown add-on therapy to be more efficacious than sequential monotherapy. It is emphasized that for optimal suppression of viral replication, salvage therapy should be commenced as soon as resistance is detected. Clearly, it is too late to wait for clinical signs of antiviral resistance such as hepatic flare or hepatic decompensation, particularly in patients with already compromised hepatic reserve.

A critical question is whether a target viral load threshold exists below which the emergence of antiviral resistance does not occur. Ideally, complete suppression to undetectable levels by polymerase chain reaction is preferable, although this may not always be achievable in clinical practice. In clinical practice, consistent and durable suppression of viral replication to less than 3 $\log_{10}$ copies/mL (equivalent to approximately 2.2 $\log_{10}$ IU/mL) may be a reasonable viral threshold target to minimize emergence of resistance, providing a highly potent drug with a high genetic barrier to resistance is used.

Conclusion

The emergence of antiviral resistance in the treatment of chronic HBV infection not only results in virological and biochemical breakthrough, but can lead to histological progression, hepatic decompensation and even death. The combination of a limited spectrum of available drugs and often long-term treatment means that the problem of antiviral resistance will continue to pose a major clinical challenge. Adherence to drug therapy is a critical component in the prevention of antiviral resistance. Strategies for minimizing antiviral resistance include patient education and support from both the physician and liver nurse, careful timing and selection of initial therapy, regular viral load monitoring, and understanding of current pathways for antiviral resistance to determine salvage options.

References

1. Lok AS, McMahon BJ. Chronic hepatitis B. *Hepatology* 2007;45:507–539.
2. Tenney DJ, Levine SM, Rose RE *et al.* Clinical emergence of entecavir-resistant hepatitis B virus requires additional substitutions in virus already resistant to lamivudine. *Antimicrobial Agents and Chemotherapy* 2004;48:3498–3507.
3. Yeh CT, Chien RN, Chu CM, Liaw YF. Clearance of the original hepatitis B virus YMDD-motif mutants with emergence of distinct lamivudine-resistant mutants during prolonged lamivudine therapy. *Hepatology* 2000;31:1318–1326.
4. Locarnini S. Primary resistance, multidrug resistance, and cross-resistance pathways in HBV as a consequence of treatment failure. *Hepatology International* 2008;2:147–151. **Summary of resistance pathways.** ☞

5. Warner N, Locarnini S. The antirviral drug selected HBV rtA181T/sW172* mutant has a dominant negative secretion defect and alters the typical profile of viral rebound. *Hepatology* 2008;48:88–98.

6. Levine S, Hernandez D, Yamanaka G *et al.* Efficacies of entecavir against lamivudine-resistant hepatitis B virus replication and recombinant polymerases in vitro. *Antimicrobial Agents and Chemotherapy* 2002;46:2525–2532.

7. Tenney DJ, Rose RE, Baldick CJ *et al.* Two-year assessment of entecavir resistance in lamivudine-refractory hepatitis B virus patients reveals different clinical outcomes depending on the resistance substitutions present. *Antimicrobial Agents and Chemotherapy* 2007;51:902–911.

8. Lai CL, Dienstag J, Schiff E *et al.* Prevalence and clinical correlates of YMDD variants during lamivudine therapy for patients with chronic hepatitis B. *Clinical Infectious Diseases* 2003;36:687–696.

9. Leung NW, Lai CL, Chang TT *et al.* Extended lamivudine treatment in patients with chronic hepatitis B enhances hepatitis B e antigen seroconversion rates: results after 3 years of therapy. *Hepatology* 2001;33:1527–1532.

10. Hadziyannis SJ, Tassopoulos NC, Heathcote EJ *et al.* Long-term therapy with adefovir dipivoxil for HBeAg-negative chronic hepatitis B. *New England Journal of Medicine* 2005;352:2673–2681.

11. Gish RG, Lok AS, Chang TT *et al.* Entecavir therapy for up to 96 weeks in patients with HBeAg-positive chronic hepatitis B. *Gastroenterology* 2007;133:1437–1444.

12. Lim SG, Ng TM, Kung N *et al.* A double-blind placebo-controlled study of emtricitabine in chronic hepatitis B. *Archives of Internal Medicine* 2006;166:49–56.

13. Gish RG, Trinh H, Leung N *et al.* Safety and antiviral activity of emtricitabine (FTC) for the treatment of chronic hepatitis B infection: a two-year study. *Journal of Hepatology* 2005;43:60–66.

14. Leung N. Recent data on treatment of chronic hepatitis B with nucleos(t)ide analogues. *Hepatology International* 2008;2:163–178.

15. Marcellin P, Buti M, Krastev Z *et al.* A randomized, double-blind, comparison of tenofovir DF (TDF) for the treatment of HBeAg-negative chronic hepatitis B (CHB): study GS-US-174-0102. *Hepatology* 2007;46(Suppl 1):80A.

16. Chen CH, Wang JH, Lee CM *et al.* Virological response and incidence of adefovir resistance in lamivudine-resistant patients treated with adefovir dipivoxil. *Antiviral Therapy* 2006;11:771–778.

17. Lampertico P, Vigano M, Manenti E, Iavarone M, Sablon E, Colombo M. Low resistance to adefovir combined with lamivudine: a 3-year study of 145 lamivudine-resistant hepatitis B patients. *Gastroenterology* 2007;133:1445–1451. **Demonstration of the beneficial effects of combination therapy in patients who are lamivudine resistant.** ⚷

18. Colonno R, Rose R, Pokornowski K *et al.* Four year assessment of entecavir resistance in nucleoside naive and lamivudine refractory patients. *Journal of Hepatology* 2007;46(Suppl 1):S294.

19. Liaw YF, Leung N, Kao JH *et al.* Asian-Pacific consensus statement of the management of chronic hepatitis B: a 2008 update. *Hepatology International* 2008;2:263–283.

20. Keeffe EB, Dieterich DT, Han SH *et al.* A treatment algorithm for the management of chronic hepatitis B virus infection in the United States: an update. *Clinical Gastroenterology and Hepatology* 2006;4:936–962.

34 Acute liver failure and HBV: is there a role for HBV therapy?

Hank S. Wang, Tram T. Tran

Geffen UCLA School of Medicine, Cedars Sinai Medical Center, Los Angeles, California, USA

LEARNING POINTS

- Acute liver failure secondary to HBV infection remains a significant problem worldwide.

- Most patients with acute HBV will recover spontaneously.

- Treatment with oral nucleoside/nucleotide analogues may be initiated in cases of severe acute HBV infection with severe jaundice, coagulopathy and/or encephalopathy, but definitive data are lacking that it improves clinical outcomes.

- Further studies on viral genotypes, host immune factors and more potent therapies are needed to determine the true indication of treatment.

The aetiology of acute liver failure (ALF), characterized by coagulopathy and encephalopathy in a patient without pre-existing cirrhosis [1], varies by geography. In the USA and the UK, paracetamol toxicity remains the leading cause of ALF, while acute hepatitis B virus (HBV) infection constitutes 7–19% of all cases [2]. In Asia, HBV remains an important cause of ALF, accounting for 21–38% of all cases based on various studies from different countries [3].

The clinical spectrum of acute HBV infection varies from subclinical asymptomatic hepatitis to fulminant hepatic failure. Age at the time of infection, as well as host immune status, are key determinants of the clinical outcome of acute infection. Perinatally acquired HBV is usually associated with a more benign asymptomatic hepatitis but leads to high rates of chronicity. This is in contradistinction to

adult-acquired HBV, which has a more symptomatic clinical presentation with a constitutional prodrome and icterus in approximately 30% of adults, but a more benign course as ultimate clearance of HBsAg occurs in approximately 95% of infected individuals [4].

The natural history of patients with ALF due to acute HBV who do not undergo liver transplantation is poor, with a published survival rate thought to range between 19 and 33% [5]. Moreover, ALF due to acute HBV is generally considered to have a worse prognosis than ALF due to most other aetiologies as reported in a large study involving 17 tertiary care centres in the USA [2]. Liver transplantation, the only therapeutic treatment shown to prevent death, is associated with a greater than 80% survival in patients with ALF due to acute HBV [6]. However, its use is exceedingly limited by timely availability of donor organs within a short interval from diagnosis to death. In patients who do undergo transplantation, the recurrence rate of HBV infection is estimated to be 20% [6]. In general, studies on the prevalence of acute HBV as a cause of ALF have been limited by a lack of consistency in the serological diagnosis of acute HBV.

While no randomized controlled trials have evaluated the efficacy of medical treatment in patients specifically with ALF due to acute HBV, studies in acute HBV infection suggest that antiviral therapy may be beneficial in the treatment of ALF due to HBV. Importantly, nucleoside analogue antiviral therapy has been shown to be extremely well tolerated and to have an excellent safety profile in both patients with chronic HBV [7] and in patients with decompensated liver disease [8]. Moreover, the use of antiviral therapy in ALF due to acute HBV also reduces the risk of HBV recurrence should the patient undergo liver transplantation. In contrast to the oral therapies, interferon therapy may actually accelerate the course of liver disease in

Clinical Dilemmas in Viral Liver Disease, 1st edition. Edited by Graham R. Foster and K. Rajender Reddy. © 2010 Blackwell Publishing.

TABLE 34.1 Summary of available studies evaluating nucleoside analogue therapy for HBV-induced acute liver failure.

Reference	Methods and inclusion criteria	Drug	Serological status prior to therapy	Serological response	Clinical response
Schmilovitz-Weiss et al. [10]	Prospective study 15 patients with HBV ALF defined by two of the following: (i) HE; (ii) serum bilirubin ≥ 10.0 mg/dL; (iii) INR ≥ 1.6	Lamivudine 100 mg daily for 3–6 months	15/15 HBsAg positive 13/15 HBeAg positive 15/15 IgM HBcAb positive	11/11 HBsAg negative 11/13 HBeAg negative 9/13 HBeAb positive within 6 months of follow-up	13/15 survived without transplant 2/15 required liver transplantation
Tillman et al. [11]	Prospective study 17 patients with HBV ALF defined by INR > 2.0 or HE	Lamivudine 100 or 150 mg daily until HBsAg cleared	17/17 HBsAg positive 5/17 HBeAg positive 17/17 IgM HBcAb positive	17/17 HBsAg negative within 6 months of follow-up	14/17 survived without transplant 2/17 required liver transplantation 1/17 died from herniation
Kumar et al. [12]	Randomized controlled trial 71 patients randomized to treatment (31) or placebo (40) with HBV ALF defined by two of the following: (i) HE; (ii) serum bilirubin ≥ 10.0 mg/dL; (iii) INR ≥ 1.6	Lamivudine 100 mg or placebo daily for 3 months	31/31 HBsAg positive 26/31 HBeAg positive 31/31 IgM HBcAb positive	30/31 HBsAg negative 26/26 HBeAg negative 22/31 HBeAb positive within 18 months of follow-up	31/31 survived without transplant No significant biochemical or clinical improvement seen between placebo and treatment groups
Seremba et al. [13]	Retrospective study 57 patients with HBV ALF of whom 32 received a nucleoside analogue	Lamivudine (N = 29) Adefovir/lamivudine (N = 1) Entecavir (N = 2) Median use 9 days	Not available	Not available	20/32 who received a nucleoside analogue survived (14 were transplanted) 20/25 who did not receive a nucleoside analogue survived (9 were transplanted)

HBsAg, hepatitis B surface antigen; HBeAg, hepatitis B e antigen; IgM HBcAb, immunoglobulin M antibody to hepatitis B core antigen; HBeAb, hepatitis B e antigen antibody; HE, hepatic encephalopathy; INR, International Normalized Ratio.

ALF because of its immunomodulatory effect [9] and is not recommended in the setting of acute disease.

In 2004, Schmilovitz-Weiss et al. [10] published the first pilot study evaluating lamivudine treatment (100 mg daily for 3–6 months) for severe acute HBV infection (Table 34.1). They enrolled 15 patients who fulfilled at least two of the following criteria for severe acute HBV: hepatic encephalopathy, serum bilirubin 10.0 mg/dL or greater, or INR 1.6 or greater. Thirteen patients (86.7%) responded to treatment with resolution of hepatic encephalopathy within 3 days and coagulopathy within 1 week. Serum HBV

DNA was undetectable within 4 weeks and serum liver enzymes normalized within 8 weeks. Two patients in whom lamivudine administration was delayed by 6 weeks developed fulminant hepatitis and underwent urgent liver transplantation. No adverse events were reported [10].

Based on this initial study, and on case reports of successful lamivudine use in patients with fulminant reactivation of chronic HBV after chemotherapy for hepatocellular carcinoma, Tillman et al. [11] sought to evaluate lamivudine therapy (100 or 150 mg daily) in patients with acute (INR > 2.0) or fulminant (hepatic encephalopathy) HBV in an attempt to prevent HBV reinfection following potential liver transplantation. Instead, they found that 14 of 17 (82.4%) lamivudine-treated patients survived without liver transplantation at all. All these 14 patients cleared HBsAg on lamivudine therapy within less than 6 months. In addition, prothrombin time normalized and bilirubin decreased in 12 of these 14 patients within a week of therapy, while the other two patients had normalization of prothrombin time and a decline in bilirubin after 2 weeks of therapy. No drug-related adverse events were recorded. Furthermore, of the three patients who progressed to transplant despite lamivudine therapy, one became HBsAg negative after 3 days of therapy allowing transplantation without hepatitis B immunoglobulin therapy after transplantation. These three patients included patients with the most severe liver disease (as indicated by severe coagulopathy) or concomitant paracetamol ingestion (> 5 g). In contrast, only 4 of 20 historical control patients not receiving lamivudine antiviral therapy survived without transplantation. The study also included 20 other patients with ALF treated with lamivudine referred to the authors for inclusion; only 5 of 20 (25%) required transplantation in this subgroup [11].

In contrast to these non-randomized studies, Kumar et al. [12] recently reported results of a randomized controlled trial comparing lamivudine 100 mg daily for 3 months versus placebo in the treatment of acute HBV infection and found no differences in clinical or biochemical improvement between the two groups. While the study included all patients with acute HBV, the majority of patients in both the lamivudine-treated group (22 of 31 patients, 71%) and in the placebo group (25 of 40 patients, 62.5%) had severe acute viral hepatitis as defined by the presence of any two of three criteria: hepatic encephalopathy, serum bilirubin 10.0 mg/dL or greater, and INR 1.6 or greater. Two patients in the lamivudine-treated group and one patient in the placebo-treated group had encephalopathy, thus suggesting ALF. While HBV DNA levels were significantly lower in the lamivudine group compared with placebo at week 4, thereafter no differences in HBV DNA levels were seen between the two groups. Furthermore, no differences in clinical or biochemical tests, including serum bilirubin, alanine aminotransferase (ALT) and INR, were seen up to 1 year after therapy. Interestingly, the rate of development of protective anti-HBs in the lamivudine-treated group after 1 year was lower than in the placebo-treated group (67.7% vs. 85%; $P = 0.096$) [12].

Additionally, a retrospective study (reported as an abstract) examined whether use of nucleoside analogues favourably influenced outcomes in HBV-induced ALF using the ALF Study Group registry [13]. In total, the authors identified 57 patients with HBV ALF, 32 (56.1%) of whom received a nucleoside analogue (29 lamivudine, one adefovir/lamivudine and two entecavir). The median duration of nucleoside analogue use was 9 days (range 1–36). The group that received a nucleoside analogue was older (51 vs. 38 years; $P = 0.03$), had greater bilirubin levels (23.4 vs. 15.2 mg/dL; $P = 0.01$) and lower ALT (1234 vs. 2416 IU/L; $P = 0.06$) and aspartate aminotransferase (AST) levels (676 vs. 1347 IU/L; $P = 0.03$). Overall survival was 20 of 32 (62.5%) for the nucleoside analogue treatment group and 20 of 25 for the non-treatment group ($P = 0.15$). From this retrospective non-randomized study, no benefit for therapy was identified in HBV ALF though selection bias and differences in treatment duration likely confounded presented results [13]. Indeed, in a study published by Wai et al. [14] evaluating the clinical features and prognostic factors in patients with HBV ALF, the authors found that advanced age was the only independent factor associated with a poor outcome while no laboratory test predicted outcome.

Virological factors have not been shown to affect overall survival or the rate of recovery among patients with ALF due to acute HBV; however, a number of viral factors are thought to increase the likelihood of development of ALF [14]. From several Asian studies, the presence of precore stop codon (G1896A) and core promoter dual (T1762A, A1764T) variants is associated with a greater rate of HBV ALF, suggesting that these factors may portend a worsened prognosis [14]. In addition, HBV genotype D has also been found to have a greater association with HBV ALF compared with chronic HBV infection, suggesting that this genotype may also be associated with a more aggressive disease course. Further studies are needed to determine the effect of antiviral therapy in acute HBV ALF in these subgroups of patients with possible markers of a more aggressive disease course.

Based on the above clinical information weighing the risks of therapy with nucleoside/nucleotide treatment (few) with the potential benefit of initiating therapy in a patient with severe acute HBV presenting with signs of liver failure (many), most clinicians and guidelines, despite a lack of robust randomized controlled studies showing efficacy, will initiate therapy on presentation, and we agree with this strategy [15]. Future studies should be aimed at evaluating more potent antiviral drugs, including entecavir and tenofovir in patients with ALF due to HBV, host immune responses to HBV, and viral predictors of liver failure.

References

1. Polson J, Lee WM. AASLD position paper: the management of acute liver failure. *Hepatology* 2005;41:1179–1197.
2. Ostapowicz G, Fontana RJ, Schiodt FV *et al.* Results of a prospective study of acute liver failure at 17 tertiary care centers in the United States. *Annals of Internal Medicine* 2002;137:947–954.
3. Lee H. Acute liver failure related to hepatitis B virus. *Hepatology Research* 2008;38:S9–S13.
4. McMahon BJ, Alward WL, Hall DB *et al.* Acute hepatitis B virus infection: relation of age to the clinical expression of disease and subsequent development of the carrier state. *Journal of Infectious Diseases* 1985;151:599–603.
5. Shakil AO, Kramer D, Mazariegos GV *et al.* Acute liver failure: clinical features, outcome analysis, and applicability of prognostic criteria. *Liver Transplantation* 2000;6:163–169.
6. Steinmuller T, Seehofer D, Rayes N *et al.* Increasing applicability of liver transplantation for patients with hepatitis B-related liver disease. *Hepatology* 2002;35:1528–1535.
7. Lai CL, Chien RN, Leung NWY *et al.* A one year trial of lamivudine for chronic hepatitis B. *New England Journal of Medicine* 1999;329:61–68.
8. Fontanta RJ. Management of patients with decompensated HBV cirrhosis. *Seminars in Liver Disease* 2003;23:89–100.
9. Leifeled L, Cheng S, Ramakers J *et al.* Imbalanced intrahepatic expression of interleukin 12, interferon gamma, and interleukin 10 in fulminant hepatitis B. *Hepatology* 2002;36:1001–1008.
10. Schmilovitz-Weiss H, Ben-Ari Z, Sikuler E *et al.* Lamivudine treatment for acute severe hepatitis B: a pilot study. *Liver International* 2004;24:547–551.
11. Tillman HL, Hadem J, Leifeld L *et al.* Safety and efficacy of lamivudine in patients with severe acute or fulminant hepatitis B, a multicenter experience. *Journal of Viral Hepatitis* 2006;13:256–263.
12. Kumar M, Satapathy S, Monga R. A randomized controlled trial of lamivudine to treat acute hepatitis B. *Hepatology* 2007;45:97–101. **The only randomized controlled trial assessing the efficacy of treatment versus placebo in acute hepatitis B showing no clinically significant difference between the two groups. A small study, but the only randomized trial.** ⚬━━
13. Seremba E, Sanders CM, Jain MK *et al.* Use of nucleoside analogues in HBV related acute liver failure. *Hepatology* 2007;46(Suppl):276a. **The US experience in the NIH Acute Liver Failure Study on the use of oral therapies essentially reflecting clinician decision-making regarding treatment in those with more severe disease. Again, no difference between those treated and those not treated for acute HBV.** ⚬━━
14. Wai CT, Fontana RJ, Polson J *et al.* Clinical outcome and virological characteristics of hepatitis B-related acute liver failure in the United States. *Journal of Viral Hepatitis* 2005;12:192–198.
15. Degertekin B, Lok A. Indications for therapy in hepatitis B. *Hepatology* 2009;49:S129–S137.

35 High-risk needle exposure in hepatitis B vaccine failures: what are the options?

Pari Shah[1,2], Kimberly A. Forde[1,2]

[1]Division of Gastroenterology, Department of Medicine, University of Pennsylvania, Philadelphia, Pennsylvania, USA
[2]Center for Clinical Epidemiology and Biostatistics, School of Medicine, University of Pennsylvania, Philadelphia, Pennsylvania, USA

LEARNING POINTS

- Protective immunity after completion of the HBV vaccination schedule is defined as an anti-HBs titre of ≥ 10 mIU/mL.

- Protective immunity is achieved in 90–95% of healthy individuals after completion of the HBV vaccination series. However, up to 50% of people with chronic medical conditions and/or specific HLA haplotypes fail to respond to the vaccination series.

- Predictors of non-response include age, male gender, obesity, tobacco use, alcoholism, chronic medical conditions, immunocompromised states and genetic predisposition.

- The algorithm for post-exposure prophylaxis must take into account the adequacy of the host's vaccination response.

Background

Infection with hepatitis B virus (HBV) has long been regarded as an occupational hazard for those employed as healthcare workers (HCWs). While HBV may be transmitted through a myriad of routes, parenteral or mucosal exposure to hepatitis B surface antigen (HBsAg)-positive blood or body fluids is clearly the largest threat to HCWs [1]. Prior to the discovery and formulation of a vaccine against HBV, HCWs exposed to HBsAg-positive/hepatitis

Clinical Dilemmas in Viral Liver Disease, 1st edition. Edited by Graham R. Foster and K. Rajender Reddy. © 2010 Blackwell Publishing.

Be antigen (HBeAg)-positive blood had a 37–62% chance of developing serological markers of infection. A 20–40% seroconversion rate was observed if the exposure in question was to HBsAg-positive/HBeAg-negative blood [2].

The first vaccine against HBV became commercially available in 1982 [1]. This vaccination, a series of three intramuscular injections administered at baseline, 30 days and 180 days, is highly effective at preventing chronic HBV infection [3]. Since the advent of clinical guidelines mandating vaccination for HCWs, the incidence of HBV seroconversion has declined by 95% [4].

As appropriate vaccine administration for HCWs has been undertaken, other high-risk groups have emerged whose seroconversion rates surpass that of HCWs. Currently, despite the continued targeting of high-risk groups for HBV vaccination, there are still instances where vaccination fails to provide protective immunity. Vaccination failure in those exposed to HBV may result in chronic HBV infection, with its inherent risk of cirrhosis, liver failure, hepatocellular carcinoma and even death. This chapter discusses strategies for the post-exposure management of high-risk exposures in the setting of HBV vaccination failures.

Identification of high-risk populations for vaccination

The Centers for Disease Control and Prevention (CDC) recommend that in addition to the vaccination of all infants and children previously not vaccinated, all adults at high risk for HBV infection should undergo vaccination. The high-risk groups targeted for vaccination include HCWs, inmates of long-term correctional facilities, injection drug users, men who have sex with men, those with high-risk heterosexual practices, household contacts of HBV-positive patients, haemodialysis patients, recipients of clotting factor concentrates, and long-term international travellers. Estimates obtained by the CDC from the 2004 National Health Interview Survey indicate that only 45.4% of these high-risk populations are actually vaccinated against HBV [5]. Although vaccination is required of HCWs, surveys show that only about 75% complete the full vaccination series [6].

HBV vaccination and characteristics of failure

Current anti-HBV vaccines consist of single-antigen formulations of recombinant HBsAg. The two commercially available vaccine preparations, Recombivax HB and Engerix-B, are administered in typical doses that contain 10–40 μg/mL of the HBsAg protein. With administration of the three-aliquot series, the accepted protective serum antibody level is defined as a detectable titre of 10 mIU/mL (or 10 IU/L) or greater. Seroconversion with protective serum titres of anti-HBs is achieved in 90–95% of healthy individuals after completion of the vaccination series [1,7].

Non-response is defined as an anti-hepatitis B surface antigen (anti-HBs) titre below 10 mIU/mL, typically measured 1–6 months after the last dose of a full immunization schedule. Hyporesponse is defined as an anti-HBs titre greater than 10 and less than 99 mIU/mL. Predictors of non-response include age 30 years, male gender, obesity, tobacco use, alcoholism, diabetes, chronic renal disease, chronic liver disease and immunocompromised states (such as HIV or medication-induced immunomodulation) (Table 35.1) [3,7]. Additionally, studies have demonstrated that genetics may play a role in the degree of response to vaccination. Data have shown that individuals who are homozygous for two extended major histocompatibility complexes (MHCs) of HLA haplotypes (HLA-B8, DR3, SC01 and HLA-B44, DR7, FC31) are likely to be non-responders while heterozygous individuals tend to be hyporesponders [8].

The true non-responder is not protected against HBV infection if exposure occurs. Several strategies have been employed to address those who, after a full vaccination schedule, are deemed non-responders. The CDC recommends revaccination of non-responders with one or more

TABLE 35.1 Predictors of non-response to HBV vaccination.

Vaccine administration
Site of injection (gluteal >> deltoid)
Length of needle
Depth of injection (intradermal >> intramuscular)
Incomplete vaccination series

Host characteristics
Male gender
Age > 30 years
Obesity
Genetic predisposition

Habits
Tobacco
Alcohol

Disease states
HIV/AIDS
Chronic liver disease
Chronic renal disease

additional vaccine doses. In the case of three or more additional booster injections, as many as 30–50% of recipients respond with appropriate production [3]. For individuals with risk factors for non-response, some clinicians also advocate using higher doses of vaccine, specifically 40-μg dosing for the initial three injections instead of the standard adult dosing of 10–20 μg.

Along with changing the dose and/or dosing schedule of the HBV vaccine, the use of adjuvant therapy with vaccination has been explored. This has included the use of various antigen delivery systems and immunomodulators intending to increase the rate of immune response (Table 35.2). For instance, various cytokines, including interferon alfa, have been studied in HBV vaccine non-responders and hyporesponders. Unfortunately, these agents have been unsuccessful in decreasing vaccine failure rates [9]. Hence there are no current recommendations for the use of adjuvant delivery systems.

Although the use of adjuvant delivery system for HBV vaccines has been disappointing, newer more immunogenic vaccines have shown promising results in increasing vaccine response rates. Most recently, a third-generation HBV vaccine containing PreS1, PreS2 and S antigens, surface proteins of HBV that play a role in immunogenicity, has shown an increase in antibody titres when used in non-responders compared with conventional vaccination (S antigen alone). Several studies have examined use of this vaccine in high-risk populations [10].

TABLE 35.2 Adjuvant strategies for HBV vaccination in healthy non-responders/hyporesponders.

Immunization strategy	Intervention group response rate[*]	Control group response rate[*]	P-value
Rendi-Wagner et al. [10] PreS/S vaccination, non-responders	81.7%	49.1%	< 0.001
Goldwater et al. [9] Interferon alfa			
Non-responders	53.0%	41.0%	NS
Hyporesponders	87.5%	70.0%	NS
Kim et al. [12] GM-CSF[†], non-responders	55.2%	53.3%	0.60
Goldwater et al. [13] SRL 172, non-responders	41.7%	45.4%	NS

* Response is defined as anti-HBs titres > 10 mIU/mL after vaccination.
† Studies in haemodialysis and HIV-infected patients have established efficacy of GM-CSF [7,14].

In addition, there is a growing body of evidence that the use of granulocyte/macrophage colony-stimulating factor (GM-CSF) may enhance the immune response to HBV vaccination. However, the exact mechanism by which GM-CSF may improve the response in HBV vaccination remains unclear. Proposed mechanisms for the action of GM-CSF have included macrophage activation, an increase in MHC class II antigen expression, enhancement of cell maturation, migration, T- and B-cell activation, and induction of localized inflammation. A recent meta-analysis published in 2007 reviewed 13 randomized studies evaluating GM-CSF as an adjuvant to HBV vaccination and found a more favorable rate of response compared to conventional vaccination (RR 1.54, 95% CI 1.04–2.27) [7]. GM-CSF has been found to be beneficial for inducing seroconversion in both healthy non-responders and groups of high-risk non-responders such as haemodialysis patients [7]. Because additional research into the role of GM-CSF needs to be explored, there are no current recommendations for its clinical use at this time.

High-risk exposure in non-responders

High-risk exposures for HCWs include blood splashes to mucous membranes or open cuts/abrasions, needle or sharps injury with hollow-bore needles contaminated with blood, or direct introduction of blood or body fluids into an open cut. In these settings, the addition of inadequate vaccination or hyporesponse or non-response to a full vaccination schedule results in a high risk of infection, ranging from 4 to 30% in those with inadequate vaccination and up to 100% in non-responders [11]. Further complicating the matter is that at the time of their exposure, HCWs are unlikely to know that they may have had an inadequate response to vaccination.

Algorithm for management of high-risk needle exposures in HBV vaccination failures

Hepatitis B immunoglobulin (HBIG) is a human immune globulin extracted from the plasma of healthy donors with high levels of HBsAb. In addition to an exhaustive process to eliminate donors who have serological markers of other viral infections (e.g. HIV, hepatitis C virus), the multistep process utilized for its preparation also targets such viruses for deactivation.

HBIG provides passive immunity against HBV. After an intramuscular injection of 0.06 mL/kg, the mean half-life of the immune globulin is 17.5–25 days. Given the long half-life of this antibody in the blood, we recommend that all known non-responders and hyporesponders to the full HBV vaccination series receive HBIG after a high risk HBV exposure. The initiation of a revaccination series in this group may also be performed if this has not already been undertaken. If the quality of the prior anti-HBs response is unknown in an individual with a

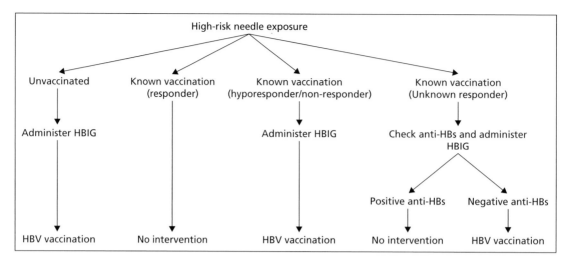

FIG. 35.1 Algorithm for post-exposure prophylaxis in high-risk needle exposures.

reported history of HBV vaccination, anti-HBs titres should be assessed and HBIG administered. If anti-HBs titres are inadequate, revaccination may be attempted although the yield may be low. If intermediate anti-Hbs titres are found, a booster injection is not required given a documented amnestic immune response.

Revaccination may certainly play a role in boosting the immunity of hyporesponders, although this role may be limited in those individuals who are truly non-responders. Regardless, revaccination has been suggested in the algorithm of the post-prophylaxis therapy for high-risk exposures in non-responders and hyporesponders as noted above (Figure 35.1).

Conclusion

HCWs remain at high risk for the acquisition of HBV in the setting of high-risk needle or sharps exposures. Although vaccination against HBV has decreased the transmission rate of HBV in healthcare settings, vaccination non-adherence or hyporesponse/non-response may still leave providers and patients cared for by those providers at risk. While some risk factors for non-response are modifiable, such as obesity, tobacco use and alcoholism, some are non-modifiable host factors or comorbidities. In this case, aggressive post-exposure prophylaxis with HBIG and potentially HBV revaccination are of the utmost importance. In the future, immune response primers such as

GM-CSF may be added to traditional HBV vaccination in order to boost the immune response in traditional non-responders or hyporesponders.

References

1. Quaglio G, Lugoboni F, Mezzelani P *et al.* Hepatitis vaccination among drug users. *Vaccine* 2006;24:2702–2709.
2. Werner BG, Grady GF. Accidental hepatitis-B-surface-antigen-positive inoculations. Use of e antigen to estimate infectivity. *Annals of Internal Medicine* 1982;97:367–369.
3. Sjogren MH. Prevention of hepatitis B in nonresponders to initial hepatitis B virus vaccination. *American Journal of Medicine* 2005;118(Suppl 10A):34S–39S.
4. Mahoney FJ, Stewart K, Hu H *et al.* Progress toward the elimination of hepatitis B virus transmission among health care workers in the United States. *Archives of Internal Medicine* 1997;157:2601–2605.
5. Hepatitis B vaccination coverage among adults: United States, 2004. *Morbidity and Mortality Weekly Report* 2006;55:509–511.
6. Simard EP, Miller JT, George PA *et al.* Hepatitis B vaccination coverage levels among healthcare workers in the United States, 2002–2003. *Infection Control and Hospital Epidemiology* 2007;28:783–790.
7. Cruciani M, Mengoli C, Serpelloni G *et al.* Granulocyte macrophage colony-stimulating factor as an adjuvant for hepatitis B vaccination: a meta-analysis. *Vaccine* 2007;25:709–718.

8. Craven DE, Awdeh ZL, Kunches LM *et al.* Nonresponsiveness to hepatitis B vaccine in health care workers. Results of revaccination and genetic typings. *Annals of Internal Medicine* 1986;105:356–360.

9. Goldwater PN. Randomized comparative trial of interferon-alpha versus placebo in hepatitis B vaccine non-responders and hyporesponders. *Vaccine* 1994;12:410–414.

10. Rendi-Wagner P, Shouval D, Genton B *et al.* Comparative immunogenicity of a PreS/S hepatitis B vaccine in non- and low responders to conventional vaccine. *Vaccine* 2006;24:2781–2789.

11. Puro V, De Carli G, Scognamiglio P *et al.* Risk of HIV and other blood-borne infections in the cardiac setting: patient-to-provider and provider-to-patient transmission. *Annals of the New York Academy of Sciences* 2001;946:291–309.

12. Kim MJ, Nafziger AN, Harro CD *et al.* Revaccination of healthy nonresponders with hepatitis B vaccine and prediction of seroprotection response. *Vaccine* 2003;21:1174–1179.

13. Goldwater PN. A pilot study of SRL 172 (killed *Mycobacterium vaccae*) in healthy chronic hepatitis B carriers and hepatitis B vaccine non-responders. *Human Vaccines* 2006;2:8–13.

14. Yu AS, Cheung RC, Keeffe EB. Hepatitis B vaccines. *Infectious Disease Clinics of North America* 2006;20:27–45. **This is a comprehensive review of the evolution of hepatitis B vaccine development and the guidelines for its use for primary prevention and post-exposure prophylaxis.** ⚷

36 Antiviral prophylactic treatment of chronic hepatitis B to prevent viral reactivation during cytotoxic chemotherapy

Mohsin Ali[1], K. Rajender Reddy[2]

[1]Thomas Jefferson University, Philadelphia, Pennsylvania, USA
[2]University of Pennsylvania, Philadelphia, Pennsylvania, USA

LEARNING POINTS

- HBV reactivation, characterized by an increase in serum HBV DNA levels in individuals with chronic or resolved HBV infection, occurs at increased rates in patients undergoing cytotoxic chemotherapy.

- Although few have been definitively authenticated, numerous risk factors for reactivation have been suggested. These include, but are not limited to, HBsAg seropositivity, detectable pre-chemotherapy HBV DNA levels, male gender, younger age, and treatment with glucocorticoids, anthracyclines or rituximab.

- Lamivudine prophylaxis has been shown to effectively reduce the risk of HBV reactivation, with the only noteworthy drawback being the selection for lamivudine-resistant mutant HBV strains.

- Newer and more potent antivirals with better resistance profiles are likely to be successful as prophylactic strategies, although specific data are lacking and clinical trials are needed.

Chronic hepatitis B virus (HBV) infection, a disease defined by the presence of hepatitis B surface antigen (HBsAg) in the circulation for longer than 6 months, afflicts approximately 350 million individuals worldwide. The prevalence of the infection varies from highly endemic regions such as sub-Saharan Africa and East Asia ($\geq$ 8%) to areas of relatively low prevalence such as North America

and northern Europe (< 2%) [1]. HBV is transmitted both vertically or perinatally, and horizontally, often as a result of sexual exposure or intravenous drug use. The development of chronic infection is closely associated with the mode of transmission, such that vertical transmission leads to chronicity in up to 90% of infected patients whereas horizontal transmission during adulthood does not progress beyond the acute stage in 95% of infected patients [2]. It is estimated that 15–40% of HBV carriers will develop liver failure, cirrhosis or hepatocellular carcinoma during their lifetimes [1].

One of the current clinical dilemmas encountered in the management of chronic HBV individuals with resolved or inactive infection revolves around the increased risk of viral reactivation during or following cytotoxic chemotherapy. HBV reactivation has been somewhat vaguely defined as an increase in HBV viral replication in individuals with chronic or resolved HBV infection. Although there are no standardized diagnostic criteria for this condition, a recent study proposes the following: an increase in serum HBV DNA level to above 1 log higher than baseline, an absolute increase greater than 6 $\log_{10}$ copies/mL, or transition from negative to positive serum HBV DNA [3]. Reactivation may occur in an average of up to 50% of chronic HBV cases undergoing cytotoxic chemotherapy while not on antiviral prophylaxis. Such a development may pose a significant health challenge by impairing overall survival and obligating delays and interruptions in chemotherapeutic treatment regimens as a result of associated liver complications such as icteric hepatitis flares [4]. Studies have reported delays as long as 100 days and direct mortality rates between 4 and 60% due to HBV reactivation [5].

It is believed that the risk of viral reactivation is subject to variance depending on the aggressiveness and duration of the chemotherapy, the types of drugs administered, the type of malignancy, and a patient's gender, age and serological profile. Important surveys of the literature by Kohrt *et al.* [5], Lalazar *et al.* [6] and Yeo and Johnson [7] inform much of the following summary of the suspected key risk factors involved in HBV reactivation. However, it is important to note that small sample sizes and heterogeneity in factors such as malignancies studied, treatment regimens and baseline serological status prevent definitive elucidation of risk stratification for HBV reactivation.

Univariate analysis in a study of 78 HBsAg-positive cases with various malignancies has shown an increased risk of viral reactivation associated with male gender and younger age. Use of corticosteroids, due perhaps to their interaction with a glucocorticoid response element in HBV DNA that may lead to increased viral replication, and of anthracyclines, which have been shown to increase viral DNA secretion *in vitro*, have also been identified as risk factors in a multivariate analysis of 138 HBsAg-positive individuals with various malignancies. It is important to note here that although corticosteroids confer a greater risk of reactivation, steroid-free chemotherapy should not necessarily be considered a better alternative given that studies have shown a significantly decreased rate of remission and overall survival as a result of this potentially weaker treatment regimen. Use of CD20 monoclonal antibody therapy with rituximab has also been suggested in multiple reports to be a risk factor. In a recent study of a homogeneous population of 46 HBsAg-negative/anti-HBc-positive patients with diffuse large B-cell lymphoma undergoing chemotherapy (CHOP therapy) with or without rituximab, it was found that rituximab was significantly associated with HBV reactivation [8]. Univariate analysis in a study of 46 HBsAg-positive patients with lymphoma also suggested that treatment using second- or third-line chemotherapy led to an increased incidence of reactivation.

In terms of risk factors related to the patient's serological profile, it has been determined that the greatest risk of reactivation exists in patients positive for HBsAg and the lowest risk in patients with hepatitis B surface antibody (anti-HBs) levels above 10 IU/L. Detectable anti-HBc in the absence of positive HBsAg or anti-HBs has also been suggested to confer a risk, though lower, for reactivation. Seropositivity for HBeAg has been identified as a risk factor, but the absence of HBeAg does not preclude the possibility of reactivation

given the existence of HBeAg-negative precore and core promoter mutations preventing production of HBeAg. A recent multivariate analysis that examined predictors of viral reactivation in 133 patients who had undergone HBeAg seroconversion found that genotype C (compared with genotype B), male gender and alanine aminotransferase (ALT) levels above five times upper limit of normal during the HBeAg-positive phase, and age older than 40 years at the time of HBeAg seroconversion were all significantly associated with greater incidence of reactivation [9].

A detectable pre-chemotherapy HBV DNA level has been associated with increased risk in a univariate analysis of 41 breast cancer patients (viral load $> 3 \times 10^5$ copies/mL) and a multivariate analysis of 138 patients with various malignancies (viral load $> 2.9 \times 10^5$ copies/mL). Kohrt and colleagues suggest that this may be the strongest indicator of reactivation risk.

The highest reported risk of reactivation (67%) was found in patients undergoing glucocorticoid-containing therapy for haematological malignancies. The lowest overall risk ($\leq 40\%$) was observed in patients undergoing glucocorticoid-free chemotherapy for solid tumours. It is not yet clear whether differences in reactivation risks in varying malignancy types are due to variation in tumour histology or variation in the form and drugs used in their respective chemotherapy treatments. A summary of many of the above-mentioned risk factors is provided in Table 36.1.

Given the significant risk of viral reactivation and the chances of life-threatening sequelae occurring, prophylactic treatment of HBV has been suggested for preventing reactivation of HBV during and after chemotherapeutic

TABLE 36.1 Risk factors associated with an increased risk of HBV reactivation in patients undergoing cytotoxic chemotherapy.

Detectable pre-chemotherapy HBV DNA level

HBsAg seropositivity

HBeAg seropositivity

Male gender

Younger age

Corticosteroid and anthracycline use

Rituximab/CD20 monoclonal antibody therapy

Second- or third-line chemotherapy

TABLE 36.2 Summary of the meta-analyses by Loomba *et al.* and Ziakas *et al.*.*

Study	Patients	Serological profile	Malignancy	Chemotherapy regimen	Prophylactic strategy	HBV reactivation risk reduction	HBV-related mortality risk reduction
Loomba *et al.* [10]	275 treatment 485 control	HBsAg positive	Various	Varied	Lamivudine	9/240 vs. 156/424 RR 0.00–0.21	4/208 vs. 27/394 RR[†] 0.00–0.20
Ziakas *et al.* [11]	127 treatment 269 control	HBsAg positive	Lymphomas	Varied	Lamivudine	11/127 vs. 136/269 RR 0.21	2/117 vs. 15/254 RR 0.68

* Loomba *et al.* studied patients with a variety of malignancies including lymphomas, hepatocellular carcinoma, breast cancer, leukaemia, nasopharyngeal carcinoma and solid tumours, whereas Ziakas *et al.* studied only lymphoma patients. Lamivudine administration was highly variable in both studies, ranging widely from 28 days to 1 day before and from 1 to 12 months after chemotherapy.
† For simplicity, this RR range does not include the one conflicting study, published only as an abstract, from the Loomba survey that showed three deaths in the treated group and none in the control group.

treatment. Although hepatitis B is relatively uncommon in developed Western countries, except within subsets of immigrant communities from highly endemic regions, there is an increasingly large number of individuals expected to develop cancer and subsequently undergo chemotherapy. This calls for serious consideration of prevention of chemotherapy-induced HBV reactivation, in both hypoendemic and hyperendemic regions, given the important clinical and public health implications [10]. Most studies of antiviral prophylaxis have focused exclusively on the use of lamivudine, a nucleoside analogue used in conventional treatment of chronic hepatitis B to curtail HBV replication, reduce viral loads and improve liver injury while maintaining a highly favourable side-effect profile [10]. A variety of different studies with small datasets have analysed the efficacy of lamivudine prophylaxis, leading to the recent publication of several meta-analyses. Table 36.2 summarizes the relevant findings of the two recent meta-analyses discussed below.

Loomba *et al.* [10] reviewed published literature until June 2007 and conducted a meta-analysis of two randomized controlled trials, eight prospective controlled studies and four retrospective studies in order to assess the risk of HBV reactivation, HBV-related morbidity and HBV-related mortality in HBsAg-positive patients receiving chemotherapy with or without lamivudine prophylaxis. The authors did not pool the data of these smaller studies due to inconsistencies in their experimental designs and patient populations and instead reported their results as

patterns based on study-specific estimates. A total of 485 control patients were administered deferred or no lamivudine treatment while 275 patients were administered lamivudine prophylactically. All studies showed a relative risk ratio (RR) in favour of prophylactic lamivudine ranging from 0.00 to 0.21 in assessments of both viral reactivation and HBV-related hepatitis. No patient undergoing prophylactic lamivudine suffered HBV-related hepatic failure in the seven studies reporting this outcome as opposed to a total of 21 patients from the control groups (RR 0.00). Nine of ten studies reporting HBV-related death showed decreased numbers of this outcome associated with prophylaxis (RR 0.00–0.20) while the remaining study, published only as an abstract, cited three deaths among the 26-patient prophylactic group and no deaths in the 25-patient control group. No harmful side effect was seen as a result of lamivudine prophylaxis and a smaller percentage of prophylaxis patients experienced chemotherapy interruptions (27 of 156 patients, 17.3%) relative to the control group (127 of 322 patients, 39.4%) in the six studies reporting this outcome. Cancer-related mortality (34.9% or 15/43 vs. 26.2% or 11/42) and all-cause mortality (36.3% or 57/157 vs. 17.8% or 21/118) were also reduced in the group receiving lamivudine prophylaxis. In summary, this meta-analysis determined that lamivudine prophylaxis for HBsAg-positive patients undergoing chemotherapy results in fewer interruptions, confers a 79% or greater risk reduction for viral reactivation and HBV-related hepatitis, and reduces the risk of HBV-related death and HBV-related hepatic failure. The limitations of this meta-analysis include the heterogeneity of the patient populations, treatment regimens and cancer type as well as the overall weak experimental methodology of the incorporated studies. These limitations may potentially have resulted in some bias.

Identifying the failure of previous meta-analyses to distinguish between antiviral prophylactic effect on lymphoma versus solid tumours, Ziakas *et al.* [11] conducted a meta-analysis focusing solely on HBsAg-positive lymphoma patients undergoing chemotherapy or immunotherapy. They reviewed published literature until December 2008 and selected one randomized controlled trial, three prospective cohorts and five retrospective cohorts comprising a total of 396 participants, 269 in the control group and 127 in the lamivudine prophylaxis group. The RR was pooled and calculated according to the fixed effects method and statistical heterogeneity between studies was evaluated using the chi-squared Q test and the I^2 statistic. The authors found no evidence of statistical heterogeneity and identified a significant reduction in the risk of HBV reactivation (RR 0.21, 95% CI 0.13–0.35) in the prophylaxis group (11 of 127, 8.6%) compared with the control group (136 of 269, 50.6%). There was also a trend, though not statistically significant (RR 0.68, 95% CI 0.19–2.49), for reduced risk of HBV-related mortality in the prophylaxis group (2 of 117, 1.7%) compared with the control group (15 of 254, 5.9%).

An economic analysis of prophylactic lamivudine use demonstrates that prophylaxis used until 6 months after chemotherapy cessation is a cost-effective strategy (incremental cost-effective ratio $33 514) compared with use of lamivudine after hepatitis is evident [12]. Despite the evidence of HBV reactivation risk reduction using antiviral prophylaxis, quite alarmingly a recent survey of oncologists in Washington, DC showed that only 56% knew of the existence of prophylactic therapy and 48% were doubtful of which antiviral agent to use [13].

One drawback to lamivudine therapy is that extended use of lamivudine allows the selection of lamivudine-resistant HBV strains with mutations in the YMDD (tyrosine-methionine-aspartate-aparate) motif. A cohort study of 58 patients undergoing conventional (non-prophylactic) lamivudine treatment of chronic HBV infection showed that 12–20% of patients developed mutations after 1 year and 67% developed mutations after 4 years [5]. The risk of viral resistance with prophylactic lamivudine

is not well established, nor is the clinical significance of such an occurrence. Given the possibility of this complication, more trials investigating the efficacy of non-lamivudine antiviral prophylaxis are greatly needed, as data are currently very limited.

In a recent case report, three HBsAg-positive patients undergoing cytotoxic chemotherapy with steroids for solid tumours were given entecavir prophylaxis until 6 months after completion of chemotherapy [14]. None of the patients developed HBV reactivation. Another case report mentioned an HBsAg-positive lymphoma patient who received adefovir prophylaxis while undergoing chemotherapy with rituximab but who developed HBV reactivation after 3 months of treatment [15]. Despite the limited data on prophylactic use of non-lamivudine drugs, their success in conventional treatment of chronic HBV makes them reasonable candidates for prophylaxis as well. As a result, the 2007 AASLD guidelines propose that newer antiviral drugs such as adefovir and entecavir should be considered for prophylaxis that is expected to be maintained over a long duration (> 12 months) rather than lamivudine [16]. The more recently approved drug tenofovir may also be considered for prophylactic therapy. Although these newer antiviral drugs may prove efficacious, their use may be limited in certain parts of the world by their higher costs.

Summary

It is suggested that clinicians administer prophylactic treatment with lamivudine or other antiviral agents prior to chemotherapy to reduce the risk of viral reactivation in HBV carriers. For this purpose, a therapeutic model adapted from Kohrt and colleagues is proposed in Figure 36.1. A full serological work-up for HBV markers is recommended for all at-risk patients prior to chemotherapy, especially those from highly endemic regions. Prophylactic treatment is recommended for those testing positive for HBsAg and risk assessment should be performed on HBsAg-negative patients. The duration of treatment is not yet clearly established but reasonable guidelines are as follows: a minimum of 6 months after cessation of conventional chemotherapy and 12 months or longer for patients with high pre-chemotherapy HBV DNA levels or immunosuppression regimens involving monoclonal antibodies such as rituximab [3].

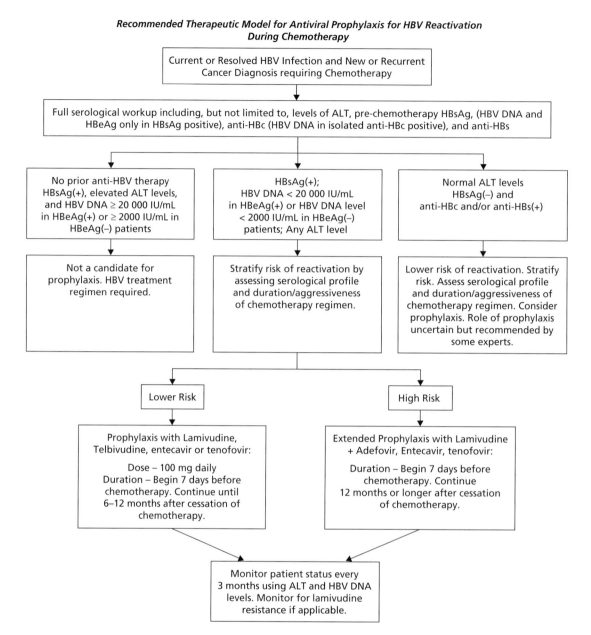

Recommended Therapeutic Model for Antiviral Prophylaxis for HBV Reactivation During Chemotherapy

Current or Resolved HBV Infection and New or Recurrent Cancer Diagnosis requiring Chemotherapy

Full serological workup including, but not limited to, levels of ALT, pre-chemotherapy HBsAg, (HBV DNA and HBeAg only in HBsAg positive), anti-HBc (HBV DNA in isolated anti-HBc positive), and anti-HBs

No prior anti-HBV therapy HBsAg(+), elevated ALT levels, and HBV DNA ≥ 20 000 IU/mL in HBeAg(+) or ≥ 2000 IU/mL in HBeAg(–) patients

HBsAg(+); HBV DNA < 20 000 IU/mL in HBeAg(+) or HBV DNA level < 2000 IU/mL in HBeAg(–) patients; Any ALT level

Normal ALT levels HBsAg(–) and anti-HBc and/or anti-HBs(+)

Not a candidate for prophylaxis. HBV treatment regimen required.

Stratify risk of reactivation by assessing serological profile and duration/aggressiveness of chemotherapy regimen.

Lower risk of reactivation. Stratify risk. Assess serological profile and duration/aggressiveness of chemotherapy regimen. Consider prophylaxis. Role of prophylaxis uncertain but recommended by some experts.

Lower Risk

High Risk

Prophylaxis with Lamivudine, Telbivudine, entecavir or tenofovir:

Dose – 100 mg daily
Duration – Begin 7 days before chemotherapy. Continue until 6–12 months after cessation of chemotherapy.

Extended Prophylaxis with Lamivudine + Adefovir, Entecavir, tenofovir:

Duration – Begin 7 days before chemotherapy. Continue 12 months or longer after cessation of chemotherapy.

Monitor patient status every 3 months using ALT and HBV DNA levels. Monitor for lamivudine resistance if applicable.

FIG. 36.1 A model adapted from the work of Kohrt *et al*. [5] that summarizes the treatment strategies to be employed in the management of chemotherapy patients with resolved or current HBV infection. Note that although most data exists with the use of lamivudine, other antiviral HBV drugs (entecavir and tenofovir) can be considered because of a better resistance profile. However, the cost-effectiveness of lamivudine versus other strategies has not been studied.

References

1. Lavanchy D. Hepatitis B virus epidemiology, disease burden, treatment, and current and emerging prevention and control measures. *Journal of Viral Hepatitis* 2004;11: 97–107.

2. Post A, Nagendra S. Reactivation of hepatitis B: pathogenesis and clinical implications. *Current Infectious Disease Reports* 2009;11:113–119.

3. Liang R. How I treat and monitor viral hepatitis B infection in patients receiving intensive immunosuppressive therapies or undergoing hematopoietic stem cell transplantation. *Blood* 2009;113:3147–3153.

4. Hoofnagle JH. Reactivation of hepatitis B. *Hepatology* 2009;49(5 Suppl):S156–S165. **A nice overview on HBV reactivation and the consequences related to it.** ☞

5. Kohrt HE, Ouyang DL, Keeffe EB. Antiviral prophylaxis for chemotherapy-induced reactivation of chronic hepatitis B virus infection. *Clinics in Liver Disease* 2007;11:965–991.

6. Lalazar G, Rund D, Shouval D. Screening, prevention and treatment of viral hepatitis B reactivation in patients with haematological malignancies. *British Journal of Haematology* 2007;136:699–712.

7. Yeo W, Johnson PJ. Diagnosis, prevention and management of hepatitis B virus reactivation during anticancer therapy. *Hepatology* 2006;43:209–220.

8. Yeo W, Chan TC, Leung NWY *et al.* Hepatitis B virus reactivation in lymphoma patients with prior resolved hepatitis B undergoing anticancer therapy with or without rituximab. *Journal of Clinical Oncology* 2009;27:605–611.

9. Chu C, Liaw Y. Predictive factors for reactivation of hepatitis B following hepatitis B e antigen seroconversion in chronic hepatitis B. *Gastroenterology* 2007;133:1458–1465.

10. Loomba R, Rowley A, Wesley R *et al.* Systematic review: the effect of preventive lamivudine on hepatitis B reactivation during chemotherapy. *Annals of Internal Medicine* 2008;148: 519–528. **A systematic review on the published literature on HBV prophylaxis during chemotherapy.** ☞

11. Ziakas PD, Karsaliakos P, Mylonakis E. Effect of prophylactic lamivudine for chemotherapy-associated hepatitis B reactivation in lymphoma: a meta-analysis of published clinical trials and a decision tree addressing prolonged prophylaxis and maintenance. *Haematologica* 2009;94:998–1005.

12. Saab S, Dong MH, Joseph TA, Tong MJ. Hepatitis B prophylaxis in patients undergoing chemotherapy for lymphoma: a decision analysis model. *Hepatology* 2007;46:1049–1056.

13. Khokhar OS, Farhadi A, McGrail L, Lewis JH. Oncologists and hepatitis B: a survey to determine current level of awareness and practice of antiviral prophylaxis to prevent reactivation. *Chemotherapy* 2009;55:69–75.

14. Okita R, Takahashi M, Narahara H *et al.* Use of entecavir to prevent hepatitis B virus reactivation during cytotoxic chemotherapy for solid malignancy. *Clinical Journal of Gastroenterology* 2009;2:214–217.

15. Khaled Y, Hanbali A. Hepatitis B virus reactivation in a case of Waldenstrom's macroglobulinemia treated with chemotherapy and rituximab despite adefovir prophylaxis. *American Journal of Hematology* 2007;82:688.

16. Lok ASF, McMahon BJ. Chronic hepatitis B. *Hepatology* 2007;45:507–539.

Management of hepatitis B in HIV-infected and other immunosuppressed patients

Kaiser Raja, Douglas T. Dieterich

Division of Liver Diseases, Mount Sinai School of Medicine, New York, New York, USA

LEARNING POINTS

- Hepatitis B has an aggressive course in patients co-infected with HIV, with increased risk of development of chronicity after acute HBV infection, persistence of HBeAg with high levels of HBV viraemia, and accelerated progression to cirrhosis.

- Therapy for HBV in HIV/HBV co-infected patients should preferably be administered as part of HAART to prevent emergence of drug-resistant HIV strains. In those co-infected with HIV, drugs with antiretroviral activity (lamivudine, tenofovir, entecavir) should be avoided as monotherapy for HBV in the absence of HAART is likely to lead to HIV resistance.

- Immunosuppression administered after renal or other organ transplantation in patients with chronic HBV infection leads to enhanced HBV replication and progressive liver disease that can be effectively prevented by nucleos(t)ide analogues.

- Patients with rheumatological diseases and inflammatory bowel disease being considered for treatment with biological agents should be screened for HBV and administered antiviral prophylaxis if HBsAg positive.

Introduction

Hepatitis B virus (HBV) is widely prevalent and it is not uncommon to encounter patients who have active or inactive HBV infection and develop immunosuppression because of a disease state (i.e. HIV) or who require immunosuppressive therapy for management of an unrelated disorder (i.e. chemotherapy for haematological or

Clinical Dilemmas in Viral Liver Disease, 1st edition. Edited by Graham R. Foster and K. Rajender Reddy. © 2010 Blackwell Publishing.

other malignancy, immunosuppression after organ transplantation). Patients with chronic kidney disease on dialysis are also intrinsically immunosuppressed and a significant proportion have associated HBV infection. Another group of patients recently recognized are those receiving biological agents for rheumatic disorders or inflammatory bowel disease. Patients with chronic HBV infection, under these conditions, have a substantial risk of reactivation of HBV that may lead to liver-related morbidity, liver failure and death. In this chapter we discuss the natural history, clinical presentation and diagnosis of chronic HBV infection in the above patient subgroups, followed by the essential role of antiviral therapy to suppress viral replication and prevent progressive liver disease.

HIV/HBV co-infection

Co-infection with HBV is common in HIV-infected individuals since both viruses are transmitted predominantly by percutaneous and sexual routes. In areas of low HBV endemicity, about 5–7% of HIV-positive individuals are co-infected with HBV, whereas this figure is 10–20% in areas of high HBV prevalence [1]. Men who have sex with men have higher co-infection prevalence rates (9–17%) than heterosexual individuals and intravenous drug users [2]. Although the effects of HBV on the natural history of treated and untreated HIV infection is debatable, there is well-documented evidence that HIV adversely affects all phases of the natural history of HBV. Following acute HBV infection, HIV-infected individuals are more likely to progress to chronic HBV infection rather than clear the virus. The risk of progression to chronic HBV is higher in patients with low CD4 T-cell counts [2]. Chronic co-infected patients who are HBeAg positive are less likely to have HBeAg seroclearance. HBV DNA levels are higher in co-infected patients compared with HBV monoinfected patients. Alanine aminotransferase (ALT) levels tend to remain normal in co-infected patients and thus do not reflect ongoing hepatic inflammation [3]. HIV-positive patients who have evidence of resolved past HBV infection (anti-HBc positive with or without anti-HBs positivity), although not shown to be at risk for progressive liver disease, are at risk for subsequent reactivation of HBV when CD4 T-cell count decreases or when administered chemotherapy for malignancies, especially lymphoma [4]. Although hepatocyte injury is immune mediated in HBV, there is accelerated progression of chronic hepatitis to cirrhosis in co-infected patients, despite the existence of an immunosuppressed state. The rate of progression is in fact faster in patients with low CD4 T-cell counts [5]. With regard to hepatocellular carcinoma (HCC), it is unclear whether HIV/HBV co-infected patients have an increased risk compared with HBV monoinfected patients. Recent studies suggest that the incidence of HCC is higher than the population average in HIV-positive patients co-infected with HBV or hepatitis C virus (HCV) and receiving highly active antiretroviral therapy (HAART). Underlying cirrhosis and increased longevity has been suggested as the principal reason for this phenomenon [6]. Overall, HIV/HBV co-infected individuals are more likely to die of liver-related causes than those infected with HBV alone. An eightfold risk of liver-related mortality has been shown in the Multicentre AIDS Cohort Study among HBV/HIV co-infected individuals compared with HIV monoinfected individuals, particularly in patients with low CD4 nadir counts [7]. Similarly, a large European study (EuroSIDA) has also reported a 3.6-fold higher risk of liver-related deaths in co-infected patients [8]. However, there are reports that effective suppression of HBV with potent antiviral agents, particularly tenofovir, may halt progression of liver fibrosis and prevent development of decompensated liver disease [9].

Diagnosis of HBV infection in HIV/HBV co-infected patients

Diagnosis of HBV in HIV-infected patients is similar to individuals not infected with HIV. Screening should be performed in all patients, with tests for HBsAg, anti-HBs and anti-HBc. Standard HBV vaccination is recommended for those who are negative for HBsAg and anti-HBs. Adequate antibody titres are achieved in only 17–56% of

HIV patients; vaccine failures are therefore common and periodic testing is necessary in patients who continue to show high-risk behaviour [9]. Those who are diagnosed with chronic hepatitis B (evident by presence of HBsAg for at least 6 months) should have further evaluation with liver chemistries, imaging and testing for HBeAg, anti-HBe and HBV DNA. Liver biopsy is often necessary to stage the disease and occasionally to differentiate from other causes of hepatitis. The significance of isolated anti-HBc positivity in patients with HIV infection is not known. It may represent either resolved past infection or an occult HBV infection. The latter may be diagnosed by performing a sensitive assay for HBV DNA (lower limit of detection 10–20 IU/mL). Positive HBV DNA by such assays has been variably reported (2–89%) [2]. Although liver disease has not been associated with occult HBV infection, such patients may be at risk for reactivation during periods of further immunosuppression such as administration of chemotherapy for haematological malignancies. Reactivation with spontaneous disappearance of anti-HBs and reappearance of HBsAg can also occur, especially if CD4 T-cell counts are less than 200×10^6/L [2]. Therefore, even in HBsAg-negative patients with prior positive anti-HBs and/or anti-HBc, extended evaluation with all HBV-related serologies and HBV DNA should be performed in the presence of unexplained liver disease.

Management of chronic HBV in HIV/HBV co-infected patients (Figure 37.1)

The goal of antiviral therapy in HIV/HBV co-infected patients is suppression of HBV replication to prevent development of end-stage liver disease. Drug regimens should be carefully designed, since including agents effective against both HIV and HBV can promote drug resistance if either virus is inadequately suppressed. Most patients require therapy for both viruses and usually patients are initiated on HAART containing tenofovir in combination with either emtricitabine or lamivudine as the nucleoside backbone [2,9,10]. In co-infected patients it has been shown that using two drugs effective against HBV (including tenofovir) is more effective in reducing HBV DNA levels to less than 100 IU/mL than tenofovir, emtricitabine or lamivudine therapy alone [2]. Most importantly, a combination of two drugs effective against HBV prevents development of drug resistance. Patients with prior lamivudine-resistant HBV can also be adequately suppressed with tenofovir and

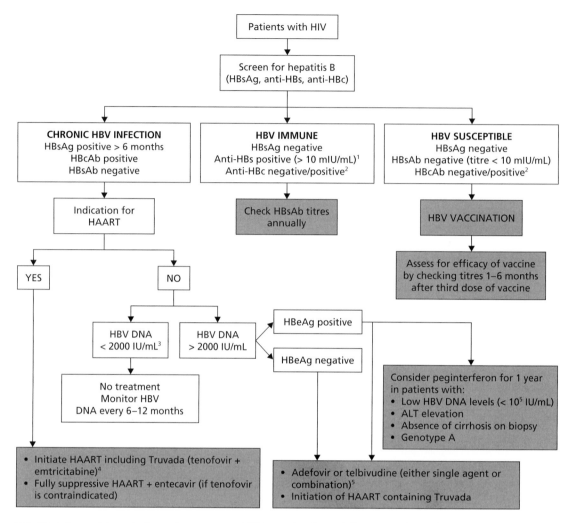

FIG. 37.1 Approach to evaluation and management of HBV infection in HIV-infected patients. 1, Anti-HBs titres must be checked annually; titres may fall with progression of HIV disease. 2, Anti-HBc-positive patients (with or without anti-HBs positivity) are at risk for HBV reactivation especially during periods of severe immunosuppression (organ transplantation, treatment of lymphoma, fall in CD4 T-cell counts). 3, Patients with cirrhosis and any level of detectable HBV DNA need nucleos(t)ide therapy. 4, Patients with lamivudine-resistant HBV also respond well to Truvada. 5, Patients who do not reach undetectable serum HBV DNA at week 24 of single-agent therapy should have add-on therapy with the other nucleos(t)ide.

emtricitabine combination. If tenofovir cannot be used as part of the initial regimen in patients with or without lamivudine resistance, alternatives include adefovir and entecavir. Compared with adefovir, entecavir is more potent and has a high genetic barrier to resistance. However, even though entecavir is effective in lamivudine-resistant HBV, resistance develops more rapidly. Moreover, since entecavir inhibits HIV replication, it should be used only with a fully suppressive HAART.

If there is no indication to treat HIV, use of nucleos(t)ide analogues for HBV treatment alone may result in development of HIV drug resistance mutations. Therefore it is important to assess the replication status of HBV as well as the stage of liver disease to guide treatment decisions. There are no established cut-off values of HBV DNA for initiation of treatment in co-infected patients. Patients with levels of 2000 IU/mL or more should preferably be treated [9,10,11]. Biopsy is ideal for assessing inflammatory activity and fibrosis stage since aminotransferase levels tend to be low in patients with HIV. The presence of more than mild inflammation should be a consideration for therapy. Patients with advanced fibrosis and established cirrhosis should be treated in the presence of any detectable HBV DNA. Patients who need treatment for HBV without therapy for HIV should ideally be treated with agents that have no activity against HIV [10]; adefovir and telbivudine are two such drugs. Adefovir is unable to achieve complete HBV suppression due to its low potency, while telbivudine has been shown to manifest rapid development of resistance in HBV monoinfected individuals when used alone. Peginterferon can be considered for HBeAg-positive patients, although data are limited. Ideal patients for peginterferon treatment are those with low HBV DNA levels, elevated transaminases, genotype A and absence of significant fibrosis/cirrhosis on biopsy. A 1-year course of peginterferon can be expected to lead to HBeAg seroconversion in 20–30% patients [9,11]. Another option is to initiate HAART earlier than recommended by HIV treatment guidelines. Many clinicians prefer this approach, since this allows treatment of HBV with more potent drugs, allowing complete suppression of HBV replication and preventing long-term consequences of progressive liver disease.

It is important to monitor both HIV and HBV infections during therapy. HBV DNA and ALT levels should be monitored every 3 months to detect emergence of drug-resistant virus. Patients who are HBeAg positive should be monitored every 6 months for HBeAg loss and anti-HBe seroconversion. Patients who do not meet criteria for HIV therapy and who have low HBV viral load (< 2000 IU/mL) with no or minimal inflammation and absence of fibrosis on biopsy do not need treatment [11]. However, they need monitoring with HBV DNA and ALT levels every 6 months. If a HAART regimen containing anti-HBV agents needs to be discontinued, there is a risk of HBV reactivation in up to one-third of patients [12]. This is manifested by elevation in ALT and HBV DNA levels. Reactivation hepatitis can occasionally lead to severe hepatitis and liver failure, especially in patients with underlying cirrhosis [12]. Reactivation can be prevented by treating with an agent effective only against HBV (and not HIV) when HAART is discontinued.

HAART can lead to a rapid decline in HIV RNA levels and rise in CD4 T-cell counts. Reconstitution of the immune system is usually seen within the first 4–8 weeks of initiating HAART. This may lead to immune-mediated damage of HBV-infected hepatocytes that may cause worsening of the liver disease and occasionally hepatic decompensation and liver failure. Since HIV suppression occurs earlier than HBV suppression, it may be logical to initiate anti-HBV therapy before HAART therapy especially in patients with high HBV DNA levels. Such an approach is not universal and has not been studied to prove its effectiveness in preventing immune reconstitution hepatitis.

HBV in chronic kidney disease and renal transplantation

Universal screening, vaccination and strict infection control measures have reduced the prevalence of HBV in chronic kidney disease patients on long-term haemodialysis to between 0 and 7% in the developed world, although the prevalence may be higher in developing countries (5–20%) [13,14]. The course of HBV infection in patients on long-term dialysis is variable with only a few studies reporting excess liver-related morbidity and mortality. Patients usually have normal ALT levels and stable low levels of HBV DNA. Studies documenting histological evolution of liver disease are lacking in this patient population. However, HBV does have a detrimental effect on outcome after renal transplantation [15]. HBV DNA levels rise after renal transplantation and this may be related to immunosuppression and use of corticosteroids. A study evaluating serial liver biopsies after renal transplantation has shown histological deterioration in more than 80% of patients [16]. Accelerated progression to cirrhosis occurs in one-quarter of patients and survival is markedly reduced in patients who develop cirrhosis. Annual risk of development of HCC is 2.5–5% [13].

In patients with chronic kidney disease, antiviral therapy is indicated in chronically infected HBsAg-positive patients with detectable serum HBV DNA. Although controversial, even patients with low HBV DNA levels (< 2000 IU/mL) are being treated at many centres. Patients with undetectable HBV DNA (< 100 IU/mL) do not usually warrant treatment, unless they receive immunosuppression or chemotherapy [13]. Reports of interferon treatment are anecdotal and the mainstay of therapy has been the nucleoside analogue lamivudine. The dose of lamivudine has to be adjusted according to creatinine clearance and doses of 50–100 mg after each dialysis session or 10–20 mg daily have been used [14]. Although there are no published data on the use of entecavir and tenofovir in patients with

TABLE 37.1 Modification of entecavir dose in patients with renal impairment and in those on haemodialysis.

Creatinine clearance (mL/min)	Lamivudine-sensitive HBV	Lamivudine-resistant HBV
> 50	0.5 mg once daily	1.0 mg once daily
30–49	0.25 mg once daily or 0.5 mg every 48 hours	0.5 mg once daily
10–29	0.15 mg once daily or 0.5 mg every 72 hours	0.30 mg once daily or 0.5 mg every 48 hours
< 10	0.05 mg once daily or 0.5 mg every 7–10 days (administer after haemodialysis)	0.10 mg once daily or 0.5 mg every 72 hours

Oral solution (0.05 mg/mL) is recommended for doses less than 0.5 mg.
No dose adjustment is recommended based on age or for patients with hepatic dysfunction.

chronic kidney disease, these drugs are being preferred for the treatment of chronic HBV infection considering their favourable resistance profile. Patients with creatinine clearance below 50 mL/min as well as those on haemodialysis need reduced doses of entecavir and tenofovir (Tables 37.1 and 37.2). All patients, irrespective of HBV DNA levels require ongoing surveillance for HCC as well as serial ALT and HBV DNA to monitor for spontaneous HBV reactivation. Biopsy is desirable especially in patients being evaluated for renal transplantation to stage fibrosis and detect cirrhosis, since the presence of cirrhosis adversely affects post-transplant outcome. Presence of decompensated cirrhosis necessitates assessment for combined liver and kidney transplantation. Isolated renal transplantation in patients with well-compensated cirrhosis is controversial. With the availability of several nucleos(t)ide analogues that are quite potent at suppressing HBV replication and thereby preventing progression of cirrhosis, patients with stable well-compensated cirrhosis who have undetectable HBV DNA on treatment may be considered for isolated renal transplantation [13]. For renal transplant patients, nucleos(t)ide analogues should be started at least 4–6 weeks prior to transplantation in those with detectable HBV DNA. Patients with undetectable HBV DNA may be started on treatment at the time of transplantation. Choice of nucleos(t)ide analogue should consider long-term risk of resistance since treatment is required for prolonged periods. Entecavir or tenofovir may be preferred over lamivudine, although published experience on these drugs in post-transplant settings is limited. Regular monitoring of ALT and HBV DNA should be done every 3 months to detect reactivation. HCC surveillance should be continued especially in patients with cirrhosis. Risk of reactivation in HBsAg-negative HBcAb-positive patients is negligible and

TABLE 37.2 Modification of tenofovir dose in patients with renal impairment and in those on haemodialysis.

Creatinine clearance (mL/min)	Tenofovir dose
> 50	300 mg once daily
30–49	300 mg every 48 hours
10–29	300 mg twice weekly
< 10, or patients on haemodialysis	300 mg once a week (administer after three dialysis sessions)

prophylaxis is not recommended routinely. HBV vaccination has been suggested prior to transplantation in the subgroup of HBsAg-negative HBcAb-positive patients with a low titre of HBsAb (< 100 IU/mL) who are at a higher risk for reactivation [13].

HBV in rheumatic diseases

Although most of the published literature on HBV reactivation is from the fields of oncology and transplantation, an increasing number of cases are being reported in patients with rheumatic diseases on immunosuppressants. Not uncommonly, patients with rheumatic diseases receive long-term low-dose immunosuppression (with or without corticosteroids). Corticosteroids specifically enhance HBV replication and this is related to the presence of a glucocorticoid responsive element in the HBV genome. HBV reactivation has been reported after brief interruption of immunosuppression as well as during chronic therapy [17]. There have been several recent reports of patients developing HBV reactivation while on therapy with biological agents such as tumour necrosis factor (TNF)-α inhibitors and anti-B-cell therapy (rituximab) [18]. All patients developing HBV reactivation were HBsAg positive prior to initiation of treatment with infliximab. Prophylaxis with lamivudine has been shown to prevent HBV reactivation in HBsAg-positive patients on infliximab in a few case reports [18]. Although there are no guidelines for HBV screening in rheumatology patients, those being considered for corticosteroids, TNF-α inhibitors or rituximab therapy should be screened for HBV. HBV prophylaxis should be given to patients who are HBsAg positive irrespective of HBV DNA levels. Currently, HBsAg-negative and anti-HBc-positive patients may not receive preventive treatment, although periodic monitoring of HBV status is desirable.

HBV in inflammatory bowel disease

There have been reports of HBV reactivation following infliximab therapy for Crohn's disease. Death from HBV reactivation-induced liver failure has also been reported [18]. Similar to rheumatic diseases, it may be prudent to screen patients prior to initiation of infliximab and offer lamivudine prophylaxis to all HBsAg-positive individuals. Since infliximab is administered intermittently, lamivudine should be given continuously and at least until 6 months after the last infusion. There have been no reports of HBV reactivation with other TNF-α inhibitors (adalimumab, etanercept), although this is likely to occur in these patients as well and therefore prophylaxis appears prudent.

Conclusion

Approximately 10% of HIV-infected individuals have chronic hepatitis B. Liver disease is a leading cause of morbidity and mortality in patients with HIV infection, despite adequate control of HIV with HAART. HIV affects both the natural history and treatment of chronic HBV infection. HIV/HBV co-infected patients have higher HBV DNA levels, lower rates of spontaneous HBeAg loss, increased risk of progression to cirrhosis and possibly an increased risk of HCC. The management of hepatitis B in HIV infection is complicated by the dual activity of several nucleos(t)ide analogues against both HIV and HBV, which can lead to rapid development of drug resistance of either virus if single agents are used and viral suppression is incomplete. Patients with other forms of immunosuppression such as after renal transplantation, where the prevalence of chronic

HBV is higher, are also at risk of HBV reactivation and progressive liver disease. More recently, patients with chronic HBV infection and rheumatological disease or inflammatory bowel disease receiving immunosuppression with high-dose steroids, infliximab or rituximab have also been reported to manifest HBV reactivation. Screening of all immunosuppressed patient groups followed by antiviral prophylaxis with nucleos(t)ide analogues in HBsAg-positive patients can effectively prevent HBV reactivation and associated liver-related morbidity.

References

1. Alter MJ. Epidemiology of viral hepatitis and HIV co-infection. *Journal of Hepatology* 2006;44(1 Suppl):S6–S9.
2. Thio CL. Hepatitis B and human immunodeficiency virus coinfection. *Hepatology* 2009;49:S138–S145. **Excellent review on epidemiology, pathogenesis and approach to management of HIV/HBV co-infected patients.** ⚷
3. Colin JF, Cazals-Hatem D, Loriot MA *et al*. Influence of human immunodeficiency virus infection on chronic hepatitis B in homosexual men. *Hepatology* 1999;29:1306–1310.
4. Sheng WH, Kao JH, Chen PJ *et al*. Evolution of hepatitis B serological markers in HIV-infected patients receiving highly active antiretroviral therapy. *Clinical Infectious Diseases* 2007;45:1221–1229.
5. Di Martino V, Thevenot T, Colin JF *et al*. Influence of HIV infection on the response to interferon therapy and the long-term outcome of chronic hepatitis B. *Gastroenterology* 2002;123:1812–1822.
6. Macdonald DC, Nelson M, Bower M, Powles T. Hepatocellular carcinoma, human immunodeficiency virus and viral hepatitis in the HAART era. *World Journal of Gastroenterology* 2008;14:1657–1663.
7. Thio C, Seaberg E, Skolasky R. HIV-1, hepatitis B virus, and risk of liver-related mortality in the Multicenter AIDS Cohort Study (MACS). *Lancet* 2002;360:1921–1926.
8. Konopnicki D, Mocroft A, de Wit S. Hepatitis B and HIV: prevalence, AIDS progression, response to HAART and increased mortality in the EuroSIDA cohort. *AIDS* 2005;19:2117–2125.
9. Soriano V, Puoti M, Peters M *et al*. Care of HIV patients with chronic hepatitis B: updated recommendations from the HIV-Hepatitis B Virus International Panel. *AIDS* 2008;22:1399–1410.
10. Dieterich DT. Special considerations and treatment of patients with HBV-HIV co-infection. *Antiviral Therapy* 2007;12(Suppl 3):H43–H51. **Review on practical approach to management of HIV/HBV co-infected patients.** ⚷

11. Keeffe EB, Dieterich DT, Han SH *et al*. A treatment algorithm for the management of chronic hepatitis B virus infection in the United States: 2008 update. *Clinical Gastroenterology and Hepatology* 2008;12:1315–1341.

12. Bellini C, Keiser O, Chave JP *et al*. Liver enzyme elevation after lamivudine withdrawal in HIV-hepatitis B virus co-infected patients: the Swiss HIV Cohort Study. *HIV Medicine* 2009;10:12–18.

13. Barclay S, Pol S, Mutimer D *et al*. The management of chronic hepatitis B in the immunocompromised patient: recommendations from a single topic meeting. *Journal of Clinical Virology* 2008;41:243–54. **Good overall review with recommendations from a consensus meeting on management of chronic HBV infection in different immuno-suppressed groups.** ⊙━

14. Fabrizi F, Messa P, Martin P. Hepatitis B virus infection and the dialysis patient. *Seminars in Dialysis* 2008;21:440–446.

15. Mathurin P, Mouquet C, Poynard T *et al*. Impact of hepatitis B and C virus on kidney transplantation outcome. *Hepatology* 1999;29:257–263.

16. Fornairon S, Pol S, Legendre C *et al*. The long-term virologic and pathologic impact of renal transplantation on chronic hepatitis B virus infection. *Transplantation* 1996;62:297–299.

17. Calabrese LH, Zein NN, Vassilopoulos D. Hepatitis B virus (HBV) reactivation with immunosuppressive therapy in rheumatic diseases: assessment and preventive strategies. *Annals of the Rheumatic Diseases* 2006;65:983–989.

18. Carroll MB, Bond MI. Use of tumor necrosis factor-alpha inhibitors in patients with chronic hepatitis B infection. *Seminars in Arthritis and Rheumatism* 2007;38:208–217.

38 Lamivudine and adefovir resistance: what should we do?

Geoff M. Dusheiko

UCL Centre for Hepatology and Royal Free Hospital, London, UK

LEARNING POINTS

- Resistance to the original oral antiviral agents (lamivudine and adefovir) is common but appropriate use of targeted 'rescue' therapies allows resistance to be managed.

- For patients with lamivudine resistance it is important to add on adefovir because resistance to adefovir is common if the drug is substituted for lamivudine in patients with lamivudine resistance.

- For patients with adefovir resistance add-on strategies are probably appropriate and consideration should be given to using the third-generation antiviral agents.

- In the future the newer more potent antiviral agents (such as tenofovir and entecavir) may reduce resistance rates appreciably.

Introduction

Considerable progress has been made in the development of potent and safe inhibitors of hepatitis B virus (HBV). However, nucleoside analogues may lead to the development of antiviral resistance, diminishing their efficacy. Thus choices of therapy depend on a number of factors predictive of treatment response, including clinical circumstances and stage of disease, potency of different agents, and the likelihood and consequences of resistance to treatment. HBeAg-positive disease is typically associated with high levels of HBV replication for a prolonged period of time. In anti-HBe-positive chronic hepatitis B, HBV DNA concentrations are typically in excess of 10^5 copies/mL but less than 10^8 copies/mL.

Clinical Dilemmas in Viral Liver Disease, 1st edition. Edited by Graham R. Foster and K. Rajender Reddy. © 2010 Blackwell Publishing.

Lamivudine and adefovir in HBV infection

Lamivudine (2',3'-dideoxy-3'-thiacytidine or 3TC) is a cytidine analogue. Lamivudine competes with cytosine in the synthesis of viral DNA. It is a (−)enantiomer and a phosphorylation step is required for transformation to active drug. The drug has a strong safety record, and reliably reduces HBV DNA concentrations in serum by $2-4 \log_{10}$. Elevated serum alanine aminotransferase (ALT) levels have likewise been shown to predict a higher likelihood of HBeAg loss in patients with chronic HBV treated with lamivudine. Lamivudine is a relatively inexpensive drug, and the lack of side effects in patients with advanced disease is attractive. As a result, lamivudine has become a widely used first-line drug for the treatment of HBeAg-positive and anti-HBe-positive disease. The major disadvantage of lamivudine treatment is the high rate of resistance observed in both HBeAg-positive and anti-HBe-positive patients.

Adefovir dipivoxil is a phosphonate acyclic nucleoside analogue of adenosine monophosphate [1]. Adefovir diphosphate acts by selectively inhibiting the reverse transcriptase/DNA polymerase of HBV by directly competing with the binding of the endogenous substrate deoxyadenosine 5'-triphosphate (dATP) [2]. A variable proportion of patients, particularly HBeAg-positive patients with higher body mass index (BMI) and high viral load, have slower and poorer primary responses; in one analysis, 25% of patients had less than $2.2 \log_{10}$ reduction. These effects may be seen in routine clinical practice where worse compliance and a higher BMI may affect susceptibility to adefovir, resulting in poor primary responses. In anti-HBe-positive patients [3], adefovir-treated group show significant improvement when compared with placebo. Thus adefovir is an agent that has low rates of resistance and good long-term viral suppression, which is of particular benefit in HBeAg-negative HBV infection.

Lamivudine

What are the characteristics of lamivudine-resistant HBV?

Lamivudine resistance is conferred through acquired selection of HBV with mutations of the YMDD motif of the HBV DNA polymerase gene [4,5]. The incidence of lamivudine resistance is 15–20% per year, with 70% of patients becoming resistant after 5 years of treatment. Variants emerging during lamivudine therapy display mutations in the viral polymerase, within the catalytic domain (C domain), which includes the YMDD motif (e.g. M204V or M204I), and within the B domain (e.g. L180M or V173L). These mutants have a reduced replicative capacity compared with wild-type virus. The commonest mutation is the substitution of methionine to isoleucine or valine (rtM204V/I) at the highly conserved YMDD motif of the reverse transcriptase. Four major patterns have been observed: L180M + M204V; M204I; L180M + M204I; V173L + L180M + M204V; and occasionally L180M + M204V/I. Although viral 'fitness' may be reduced, as lower levels of HBV DNA occur, recent studies have suggested that the disease may progress [6]. Resistance to lamivudine emerges at higher rates in HIV/HBV co-infection [7] and more rapidly in patients with HBV genotype A than in those with genotype D. Lamivudine resistance is accompanied by breakthrough of HBV DNA levels and a subsequent rise in ALT, but this is variable. In patients with decompensated cirrhosis undergoing lamivudine monotherapy, early detection of viral breakthrough is critical.

How should lamivudine resistance be managed?

Adefovir and tenofovir (and to a degree entecavir) are active against lamivudine-resistant HBV, but it is advisable to continue lamivudine in combination in these patients rather than replacing lamivudine with adefovir. Nonetheless, the clinical course after the development of resistance is complex and variable. Hepatitis is common, but is not always severe. Most patients generally experience worsening of liver disease [6]. Adefovir has been an important drug for the treatment of lamivudine-resistant HBV infection. There are a number of reports of successful treatment of lamivudine-resistant patients with adefovir, particularly

for recurrence of HBV before or after transplantation [8–11]. The wisdom of discontinuing lamivudine has been challenged, given the rates of resistance or non-response observed with adefovir monotherapy in some centres [12]. A 1 $\log_{10}$ rise in previously undetectable HBV DNA levels is taken as indicative of phenotypic resistance; adding a rescue therapy before waiting for an increase in ALT levels is advisable for these patients (see below). Thus the early addition of adefovir at the time of detection of a log rise in HBV DNA is advocated, as subsequent resistance (and adverse clinical events) are reduced if adefovir is added at lower concentrations of HBV DNA [13,14]. In the future, tenofovir will replace adefovir for the treatment of lamivudine resistance. In our current state of knowledge it is reasonable to suggest that tenofovir should be added to therapy for patients with lamivudine resistance.

Entecavir shows some efficacy against lamivudine-resistant HBV, but the effect is partial and higher doses of entecavir (1.0 mg) are required. Virological rebound and resistance have been reported in 43% of lamivudine-resistant patients after 4 years of switching treatment to entecavir. Lower rates of HBV suppression were reported in this group when using 1.0 mg of entecavir. Entecavir resistance is thus common in lamivudine-resistant patients and is not the preferred therapy.

Telbivudine cannot be used for the treatment of lamivudine-resistant patients. The magnitude of early HBV suppression (24 weeks) is linked to clinical efficacy and resistance at 1 year.

How should lamivudine be used?

The efficacy of lamivudine monotherapy is offset by the development of resistance, restricting its use as a first-line monotherapy, although monotherapy will suffice for 3–5 years in about 15–20% of anti-HBe-positive patients with low levels of replication. After emergence of resistance, the clinical benefit of continuing lamivudine is doubtful, and resistance can be taken to imply treatment failure.

The value of lamivudine monotherapy is being questioned because of the likelihood of subsequent resistance to a lineage of drugs including entecavir, telbivudine and possibly adefovir. Lamivudine resistance has typically been managed by sequential treatment with adefovir, and more recently tenofovir, but the disadvantage of sequential treatment strategies has been highlighted. If forced to use lamivudine, it is ideal to restrict it to patients likely to benefit, i.e. those with high ALT concentrations and low

HBV DNA concentrations. Early viral suppression, in particular HBV DNA levels below 200 copies/mL or less than 3 $\log_{10}$ after 6 months of treatment, predicts a lower risk of resistance after 1 year of treatment [15,16]. Long-term lamivudine therapy can prevent the complications of HBV-related liver disease as long as viral suppression is maintained [17]. Thus progression of liver disease can be prevented with a prolonged viral response, but this response is attenuated in those with virological break-through (i.e. resistance). In summary, lamivudine is not recommended as a single agent but could form the back-bone of maintenance combination therapies.

Recurrent HBV infection in the transplanted liver has previously been a major problem. Lamivudine for pre-transplant prophylaxis, in combination with hepatitis B immunoglobulin (HBIG), reduces the risk of graft infection to less than 10%, as long as HBV is suppressed before transplantation. With the advent of lamivudine and ade-fovir, outcomes have improved further [18,19]. Currently, both HBIG and lamivudine and/or adefovir are used prophylactically and recurrent HBV is now rare. Other licensed and more potent nucleosides could also be considered. For patients with high levels of replication, or with cirrhosis, many experts would consider initiating treatment concurrently with lamivudine and adefovir, or preferably using drugs with high genetic barriers to resistance (i.e. tenofovir or entecavir).

Adefovir

What are the characteristics of adefovir resistance?

Sequencing of the RT domain of the HBV polymerase has suggested that mutations rtA181V/T in the B domain and rtN236T in the D domain confer resistance to adefovir [20]. The reported mutations correlate with HBV DNA rebounds of more than 1 log above nadir, suggesting phenotypic resistance. Life-table analysis has suggested a cumulative incidence of 3.9–5.9% (in naive patients) after 3 years of treatment. A figure of 18% at 4 years of therapy has been reported. However, in clinical practice, higher rates than this are being reported [21]. Patients with prior lamivudine resistance are at greater risk of adefovir resistance [22]. HBV DNA levels at week 48 predict rate of resistance. Suppression to less than 3 $\log_{10}$ was associated with a 4% rate of adefovir resistance at week 144, but an HBV DNA concentration of greater than 6 $\log_{10}$ was associated

with 67% resistance at week 144. Adefovir resistance is apparently uncommon in treatment-naive patients treated with adefovir and emtricitabine or adefovir and lamivudine in combination.

How should adefovir resistance be treated?

Adefovir mutants remain sensitive to lamivudine, emtric-itabine, telbivudine and entecavir [23,24]. The A181V mutation has a greater effect on subsequent sensitivity to lamivudine than N236T; this compares with observed *in vitro* effects on fold sensitivity.

How should adefovir be used?

It is important to identify patients with high levels of repli-cation, or host factors, for whom adefovir monotherapy will not suffice. Anti-HBe-positive patients could be treated with adefovir monotherapy, as first-line treatment is effective in this group. Long-term therapy is required, and resistance has been reported but at lower rates than with lamivudine therapy. In other groups such as HBeAg-positive patients or anti-HBe-positive patients with decompensated cirrho-sis or high viral loads, rapid suppression of HBV DNA replication with a low risk of primary non-response or resistance is important, and combination therapies could be advantageous. Tenofovir will supplant adefovir shortly.

What about newer agents for the treatment of HBV?

Tenofovir

Tenofovir and adefovir are related molecules with a similar mechanism of action. Tenofovir disoproxil fumarate is the prodrug of tenofovir. Tenofovir diphosphate inhibits the activity of HIV-1 reverse transcriptase by competing with the natural substrate dATP and, after incorporation into DNA, causing DNA chain termination. There is strong clinical evidence of the efficacy of tenofovir in chronic hep-atitis B, with less nephrotoxicity. The drug is active against wild-type and precore mutant HBV, as well as lamivudine-resistant HBV *in vitro* [25–31].

Thus tenofovir is a far more consistent and potent sup-pressor of HBV replication than adefovir. Levels of sup-pression in both HBeAg-positive and anti-HBe-positive patients are similar to those observed with other newer potent nucleosides such as entecavir, although these two drugs have not been compared. Tenofovir is effective against lamivudine-resistant strains of HBV as well as the

A181T strain of adefovir-resistant HBV. Tenofovir shows intermediate activity against the N236T variant associated with adefovir resistance and is effective against entecavir-resistant HBV. Tenofovir will also be more useful than adefovir for the treatment of lamivudine resistance. Tenofovir has proven useful for the management of delayed or suboptimal responses to adefovir. A rapid switch to tenofovir or entecavir for these latter patients is recommended.

Entecavir

Entecavir is a cyclopentyl guanosine analogue. Early studies in animals and humans indicated that entecavir is a potent inhibitor of viral replication. Entecavir has been licensed for the treatment of chronic hepatitis B. Entecavir inhibits all three activities of the HBV polymerase/reverse transcriptase: base priming, reverse transcription of the negative strand from the pregenomic mRNA and synthesis of the positive strand of HBV DNA. Phase III trials have been completed.

In Phase III trials in HBeAg-positive patients, HBV DNA was suppressed to less than 300 copies/mL in 67% and 36% of entecavir- and lamivudine-treated patients, respectively [32]. The mean change from baseline was −6.9 log and −5.4 log respectively. HBeAg seroconversion occurred in 21% and 18% of entecavir- and lamivudine-treated patients, respectively. In HBeAg-negative patients, HBV DNA suppression to less than 300 copies/mL occurred on treatment in 90% of entecavir-treated and 72% of lamivudine-treated patients. The mean change of HBV DNA from baseline was −5.0 log and −4.5 log. ALT normalized in 78% and 71% respectively. Rebound to levels detectable by polymerase chain reaction (PCR) occurs in the majority of patients after cessation of treatment [33].

Entecavir resistance

A complex picture of entecavir resistance is emerging, suggesting a requirement for new reverse transcriptase changes in combination with those conferring lamivudine resistance to reduce susceptibility to entecavir. Entecavir resistance requires M204V/I plus L180M mutations and T184, S202 or M250 mutations [34]. After 4 years of follow-up, a cumulative resistance rate of approximately 1.2% of a subset of naive treated and monitored patients has been reported. At 5 years, resistance rates remain low in virological responders on continued treatment; entecavir thus confers a high genetic barrier to resistance in naive patients.

How can resistance be avoided?

Avoiding resistance should take into account the appropriate indications for treatment and the optimization of therapy to avoid resistance. This is particularly applicable to therapy with agents such as lamivudine and adefovir, which can lead to high rates of resistance. The disadvantages of using a single drug with high-frequency resistance are:

- treatment failure is likely;
- failure is frequently associated with exacerbation of disease;
- an increase in the population with resistant strains will result;
- resistance to lamivudine may increase precedent for resistance or deleterious mutations with other agents;
- resistance represents and the drug may become unusable.

Newer potent agents capable of suppressing HBV in most patients to levels undetectable by current PCR assays (< 10–15 IU/mL) are preferred.

Resistance can be prevented by adhering to the following recommendations.

- There should be a clear indication for starting therapy.
- Encourage patient compliance.
- Maximize antiviral activity.
- Suppress HBV DNA to the lowest possible level.
- Maximize genetic barriers.
- Avoid sequential treatment.
- Avoid treatment interruptions.
- Increase pharmacological barriers.

Table 38.1 shows the cross-resistance data for the most frequently resistant HBV variants and Table 38.2 shows the appropriate management strategy when resistance is encountered.

Who should be treated?

The European Association for the Study of the Liver (EASL) has recently published guidelines for therapy [35]. Serum aminotransferase levels, serum HBV DNA levels and histological grade and stage are taken into account. Thus these guidelines suggest that patients should be considered for treatment when serum ALT levels are above the upper limit of normal for the laboratory and/or HBV DNA levels are above 2000 IU/mL (~ 10 000 copies/mL), and liver biopsy shows moderate to severe active

TABLE 38.1 Cross-resistance data for the most frequently resistant HBV variants.

HBV variant	Lamivudine	Telbivudine	Entecavir	Adefovir	Tenofovir
Wild type	Sensitive	Sensitive	Sensitive	Sensitive	Sensitive
M204I	Resistant	Resistant	Intermediate	Sensitive	Sensitive
L180M + M204V	Resistant	Resistant	Intermediate	Sensitive	Sensitive
A181T/V	Intermediate	Sensitive	Sensitive	Resistant	Sensitive
N236T	Sensitive	Sensitive	Sensitive	Resistant	Intermediate
L180M + M204V/I ± I169T ± V173L ± M250V	Resistant	Resistant	Resistant	Sensitive	Sensitive
L180M + M204V/I ± T184G ± S202I/G	Resistant	Resistant	Resistant	Sensitive	Sensitive

Source: European Association for the Study of the Liver [35].

TABLE 38.2 Appropriate management strategy when resistance is encountered. The safety of some combinations in the long term is unknown.

Drug resistance	Second drug addition
Lamivudine resistance	Add tenofovir
Adefovir resistance	If N236T substitution, add lamivudine, entecavir or telbivudine or switch to tenofovir plus emtricitabine If A181T/V substitution, add entecavir or switch to tenofovir plus emtricitabine
Telbivudine resistance	Add tenofovir
Entecavir resistance	Add tenofovir
Tenofovir resistance (not yet described)	Entecavir, telbivudine, lamivudine or emtricitabine could be added

necroinflammation and/or fibrosis using a standardized scoring system (e.g. at least grade A2 or stage F2 by Metavir scoring). Patients with mild disease and normal ALT levels may not require immediate treatment and should be monitored carefully at appropriate intervals.

The guidelines suggest that therapy with nucleosides should aim to reduce HBV DNA concentrations in serum to as low a level as possible, ideally below the lower limit of detection of real-time PCR assays (10–15 IU/mL), to ensure virological suppression that will then lead to biochemical remission, histological improvement and prevention of complications and reduce the risk of resistance [35]. Prolonged continuous HBV DNA reduction to undetectable levels is necessary to reduce the risk of resistance

to nucleosides. It also increases the chance of HBeAg seroconversion in HBeAg-positive patients and the possibility of HBsAg loss in the mid to long term in HBeAg-positive and HBeAg-negative patients.

The recently formulated EASL guidelines suggest that because entecavir and tenofovir are potent HBV inhibitors and have a high barrier to resistance, they can be confidently used as first-line monotherapy. The role of monotherapy with entecavir or tenofovir could be modified if higher rates of resistance become apparent with longer treatment duration. In a compliant patient with a primary non-response, identification of possible HBV resistance mutations can help formulate a rescue strategy that must reasonably be based on an early change to a more potent drug that is active against the resistant HBV variant. Although there are no data that any combinations tested to date are synergistic, proof of principle exists to suggest that, for example, resistance to lamivudine and adefovir are reduced when used in combination.

There is some urgency to establish the efficacy of potent and appropriate combination therapies, but these will need necessarily large and hence expensive trials. Thus we may need to glean the efficacy of potent monotherapies and combination therapies from direct clinical experience and learning in the next few years.

References

1. Kramata P, Votruba I, Otova B, Holy A. Different inhibitory potencies of acyclic phosphonomethoxyalkyl nucleotide analogs toward DNA polymerases alpha, delta and epsilon. *Molecular Pharmacology* 1996;49:1005–1011.

2. Heijtink RA, De Wilde GA, Kruining J *et al.* Inhibitory effect of 9-(2-phosphonylmethoxyethyl)-adenine (PMEA) on human and duck hepatitis B virus infection. *Antiviral Research* 1993;21:141–153.

3. Hadziyannis SJ, Tassopoulos NC, Heathcote EJ *et al.* Adefovir dipivoxil for the treatment of hepatitis B e antigen-negative chronic hepatitis B. *New England Journal of Medicine* 2003;348:800–807.

4. Ling R, Mutimer D, Ahmed N *et al.* Selection of mutations in the hepatitis B virus polymerase during therapy of transplant recipients with lamivudine. *Hepatology* 1996;24:711–713.

5. Zollner B, Petersen J, Schafer P *et al.* Subtype-dependent response of hepatitis B virus during the early phase of lamivudine treatment. *Clinical Infectious Diseases* 2002;34:1273–1277.

6. Dienstag JL, Goldin RD, Heathcote EJ *et al.* Histological outcome during long-term lamivudine therapy. *Gastroenterology* 2003;124:105–117.

7. Locarnini S, Hatzakis A, Heathcote J *et al.* Management of antiviral resistance in patients with chronic hepatitis B. *Antiviral Therapy* 2004;9:679–693.

8. Perrillo R, Schiff E, Yoshida E *et al.* Adefovir dipivoxil for the treatment of lamivudine-resistant hepatitis B mutants. *Hepatology* 2000;32:129–134.

9. Walsh KM, Woodall T, Lamy P, Wight DGD, Bloor S, Alexander GJM. Successful treatment with adefovir dipivoxil in a patient with fibrosing cholestatic hepatitis and lamivudine resistant hepatitis B virus. *Gut* 2001;49:436–440.

10. Mutimer D, Feraz-Neto BH, Harrison R *et al.* Acute liver graft failure due to emergence of lamivudine resistant hepatitis B virus: rapid resolution during treatment with adefovir. *Gut* 2001;49:860–863.

11. Tillmann HL, Bock CT, Bleck JS *et al.* Successful treatment of fibrosing cholestatic hepatitis using adefovir dipivoxil in a patient with cirrhosis and renal insufficiency. *Liver Transplantation* 2003;9:191–196.

12. Peters MG, Hann HH, Martin P *et al.* Adefovir dipivoxil alone or in combination with lamivudine in patients with lamivudine-resistant chronic hepatitis B. *Gastroenterology* 2004;126:91–101.

13. Lampertico P, Vigano M, Manenti E, Iavarone M, Lunghi G, Colombo M. Adefovir rapidly suppresses hepatitis B in HBeAg-negative patients developing genotypic resistance to lamivudine. *Hepatology* 2005;42:1414–1419.

14. Rapti I, Dimou E, Mitsoula P, Hadziyannis SJ. Adding-on versus switching-to adefovir therapy in lamivudine-resistant HBeAg-negative chronic hepatitis B. *Hepatology* 2007;45:307–313. **Key paper clarifying the importance of add-on versus substitution therapy.** ✑

15. Lai CL, Leung N, Teo EK *et al.* A 1-year trial of telbivudine, lamivudine, and the combination in patients with hepatitis B e antigen-positive chronic hepatitis B. *Gastroenterology* 2005;129:528–536.

16. Yuen MF, Sablon E, Hui CK, Yuan HJ, Decraemer H, Lai CL. Factors associated with hepatitis B virus DNA breakthrough in patients receiving prolonged lamivudine therapy. *Hepatology* 2001;34:785–791.

17. Liaw YF, Sung JJ, Chow WC *et al.* Lamivudine for patients with chronic hepatitis B and advanced liver disease. *New England Journal of Medicine* 2004;351:1521–1531.

18. Grellier L, Mutimer D, Ahmed M *et al.* Lamivudine prophylaxis against reinfection in liver transplantation for hepatitis B cirrhosis. *Lancet* 1996;348:1212–1215.

19. Mutimer D, Dusheiko G, Barrett C *et al.* Lamivudine without HBIg for prevention of graft reinfection by hepatitis B: long-term follow-up. *Transplantation* 2000;70:809–815.

20. Angus P, Vaughan R, Xiong S *et al.* Resistance to adefovir dipivoxil therapy associated with the selection of a novel mutation in the HBV polymerase. *Gastroenterology* 2003;125:292–297.

21. Yeon JE, Yoo W, Hong SP *et al.* Resistance to adefovir dipivoxil in lamivudine resistant chronic hepatitis B patients treated with adefovir dipivoxil. *Gut* 2006;55:1488–1495.

22. Lee YS, Suh DJ, Lim YS *et al.* Increased risk of adefovir resistance in patients with lamivudine-resistant chronic hepatitis B after 48 weeks of adefovir dipivoxil monotherapy. *Hepatology* 2006;43:1385–1391.

23. Villeneuve JP, Durantel D, Durantel S *et al.* Selection of a hepatitis B virus strain resistant to adefovir in a liver transplantation patient. *Journal of Hepatology* 2003;39:1085–1089.

24. Westland CE, Yang H, Delaney WE *et al.* Week 48 resistance surveillance in two phase 3 clinical studies of adefovir dipivoxil for chronic hepatitis B. *Hepatology* 2003;38:96–103.

25. Dore GJ, Cooper DA, Pozniak AL *et al.* Efficacy of tenofovir disoproxil fumarate in antiretroviral therapy-naive and -experienced patients coinfected with HIV-1 and hepatitis B virus. *Journal of Infectious Diseases* 2004;189:1185–1192.

26. Lacombe K, Gozlan J, Boelle PY *et al.* Long-term hepatitis B virus dynamics in HIV-hepatitis B virus-co-infected patients treated with tenofovir disoproxil fumarate. *AIDS* 2005;19:907–915.

27. Nelson M, Portsmouth S, Stebbing J *et al.* An open-label study of tenofovir in HIV-1 and hepatitis B virus co-infected individuals. *AIDS* 2003;17:F7–F10.

28. Benhamou Y, Tubiana R, Thibault V. Tenofovir disoproxil fumarate in patients with HIV and lamivudine-resistant hepatitis B virus. *New England Journal of Medicine* 2003;348:177–178.

29. Bruno R, Sacchi P, Zocchetti C, Ciappina V, Puoti M, Filice G. Rapid hepatitis B virus-DNA decay in co-infected HIV-hepatitis B virus 'e-minus' patients with YMDD mutations after 4 weeks of tenofovir therapy. *AIDS* 2003;17:783–784.

30. Kuo A, Dienstag JL, Chung RT. Tenofovir disoproxil fumarate for the treatment of lamivudine-resistant hepatitis B. *Clinical Gastroenterology and Hepatology* 2004;2:266–272.

31. Van Bommel F, Zollner B, Sarrazin C *et al.* Tenofovir for patients with lamivudine-resistant hepatitis B virus (HBV) infection and high HBV DNA level during adefovir therapy. *Hepatology* 2006;44:318–325.

32. Chang TT, Gish RG, De Man R *et al.* A comparison of entecavir and lamivudine for HBeAg-positive chronic hepatitis B. *New England Journal of Medicine* 2006;354:1001–1010.

33. Lai CL, Shouval D, Lok AS *et al.* Entecavir versus lamivudine for patients with HBeAg-negative chronic hepatitis B. *New England Journal of Medicine* 2006;354:1011–1020.

34. Tenney DJ, Levine SM, Rose RE *et al.* Clinical emergence of entecavir-resistant hepatitis B virus requires additional substitutions in virus already resistant to lamivudine. *Antimicrobial Agents and Chemotherapy* 2004;48:3498–3507.

35. European Association for the Study of the Liver. EASL Clinical Practice Guidelines: management of chronic hepatitis B. *Journal of Hepatology* 2009;50:227–242. **Excellent summary of up-to-date treatment recommendations.**

39 HBV therapy following unsuccessful interferon therapy: how do you see the role for oral therapies?

Grace M. Chee, Fred F. Poordad

Cedars-Sinai Medical Center, Los Angeles, California, USA

LEARNING POINTS

- Interferon is a well-accepted therapy for chronic HBV, particularly HBV genotypes A and B.

- Combination therapy with interferon and an oral nucleos(t)ide analogue has not been shown to be superior to interferon alone.

- In interferon non-responders, oral therapy appears to be the best option.

- Strategies of sequential therapy or single or multiple combination therapies in interferon non-responders need to be evaluated.

Introduction

The two broad treatment options for chronic hepatitis B virus (HBV) infection are the interferon alfas (conventional and pegylated) and oral antivirals (nucleotide and nucleoside analogues). Interferon has a dual mechanism of action involving both immunomodulatory and antiviral actions. Compared with the conventional or standard interferons, pegylated interferons have lower potency *in vitro* but a more favourable pharmacokinetic profile with a half-life that allows weekly dosing. Findings from a Phase II dose-finding study showed that in HBeAg-positive patients, peginterferon alfa-2a had better outcomes than interferon alfa-2a and was more convenient with weekly dosing [1]. Interferon was the first therapy approved for

Clinical Dilemmas in Viral Liver Disease, 1st edition. Edited by Graham R. Foster and K. Rajender Reddy. © 2010 Blackwell Publishing.

chronic HBV in 1992, with peginterferon approved in 2005. Advantages of interferon therapy are a finite duration of treatment, absence of resistance, and immune-mediated viral suppression even after the dosing period. The side-effect profile and subcutaneous administration have limited its use in this era of oral antiviral therapies. Furthermore, the majority of patients treated with interferon do not achieve a response and will require further therapy. This chapter discusses the initial and subsequent efficacy of interferon therapy and treatment options for those who fail.

Interferon efficacy

HBV treatment end-points include HBV DNA suppression, HBeAg seroconversion, and HBsAg loss with or without seroconversion to anti-HBs. Pretreatment factors that are predictors of seroconversion with interferon therapy are low viral load, high serum alanine aminotransferase (ALT) levels and high activity scores on liver biopsy [2,3]. When treated with conventional interferon for 16–24 weeks or peginterferon for 48 weeks, roughly one-third of patients respond with HBeAg seroconversion. The results of two large multicentre trials with peginterferon therapy are summarized in Table 39.1. In HBeAg-positive patients, 25% and 14% of patients achieved HBV DNA below 400 copies/mL at the end of 48 weeks of peginterferon alfa-2a (week 48) and after 24 weeks of follow-up (week 72), respectively. Because of the immunomodulatory effects of interferon, HBeAg seroconversion continues to occur weeks to months after the end of therapy. HBeAg seroconversion occurred in 27% of patients at week 48 and in 32% at week 72 while HBsAg seroconversion occurred in 3% of

TABLE 39.1 Outcomes of studies comparing peginterferon with lamivudine.

	End of treatment (week 48)		End of follow-up (week 72)	
	Peginterferon alfa-2a (%)	Lamivudine (%)	Peginterferon alfa-2a (%)	Lamivudine (%)
HBeAg-positive patients				
Normalization of ALT	39	62	41	28
HBeAg seroconversion	27	20	32	19
HBV DNA < 400 copies/mL	25	40	14	5
HBsAg seroconversion	–	–	3	0
HBeAg-negative patients				
Normalization of ALT	38	73	59	44
HBV DNA < 400 copies/mL	63	73	19	7
HBsAg loss	–	–	4	0
HBsAg seroconversion	–	–	3	0

patients [4]. The results of the study confirmed the efficacy of peginterferon in HBV DNA suppression and seroconversion of HBsAg and HBeAg. In HBeAg-negative patients, 63% and 19% of patients achieved HBV DNA below 400 copies/mL at week 48 and week 72, respectively. HBsAg loss and seroconversion occurred in 4% and 3% of patients [5].

There are few studies with long-term follow-up of patients treated with interferon. Lau *et al.* [6] reviewed the long-term outcomes in both conventional interferon responders and non-responders. Response was defined as HBeAg seroconversion. Interestingly, even beyond the dosing period, seroconversion continued to occur, as did HBsAg loss, particularly in those with initial response. After a mean follow-up of 6.2 years, 100% of initial responders and 65% of non-responders became HBeAg negative while 86% of responders and 11% of non-responders lost HBsAg. In a study by Moucari *et al.* [7], 14 years of follow-up in 97 HBeAg-positive patients treated with interferon revealed continued yearly loss of HBsAg up to 29% by the end of follow-up. Similarly, in HBeAg-negative patients treated with peginterferon, HBsAg loss occurred after the dosing period, reaching 8.7% by 3 years [8]. These studies suggest that there are potential benefits even beyond the dosing period when patients are treated with interferon, especially if they show an initial response.

Not all genotypes of HBV respond well to interferon. Higher responses to interferon have been reported for genotype A than D and for genotype B than C. A study conducted by Hou *et al.* [9] reported response to interferon in 33% of genotype A patients and 11% of genotype D

patients, a difference that was statistically significant. Flink *et al.* [10] found that loss of HBsAg occurred in 14% of genotype A and 2% of genotype D patients. Kao *et al.* [11] found that interferon was more efficacious in genotype B than C, with 41% and 15% responding, respectively. Difference in response by genotype may be explained by the differences in molecular characteristics of each genotype. Given that these differences in outcome based on genotype have been noted in several studies, most recommend considering interferon therapy for genotype A and perhaps B.

Retreatment of interferon non-responders

Therapy options for interferon non-responders are limited to retreatment with interferon, oral antivirals or a combination of both. The role of interferon retreatment in interferon non-responders is limited. In a small pilot study conducted by Janssen *et al.* [12], 18 patients who had failed prior interferon therapy were retreated with 16 weeks of dose-escalating interferon. Although all patients experienced a decrease in their HBV DNA level by 80%, only two of the 18 patients (11%) became HBV DNA negative and had HBeAg seroconversion. None of the patients experienced HBsAg loss. Combination therapy with interferon and an oral antiviral has also not been proven to be of benefit [13].

Because of the lack of efficacy in retreating interferon non-responders with another course of interferon or a combination regimen, monotherapy with oral antivirals appears to be the preferred treatment option. In a small

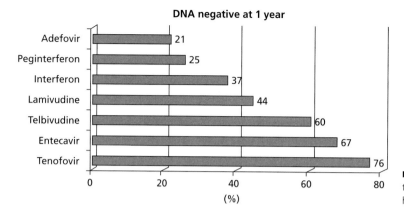

FIG. 39.1 Efficacy of approved therapies for chronic HBeAg-positive hepatitis B.

dose-finding study, Dienstag et al. [14] treated 32 chronic HBeAg-positive patients with lamivudine (25, 100 or 300 mg) or placebo for 12 weeks. Of this group, 17 had previously failed interferon. While the majority had viral suppression, only six maintained suppression and five of them were the interferon non-responders, four of whom seroconverted. In a larger study conducted by Schiff et al. [13], interferon non-responders were treated for 52 weeks with lamivudine or placebo. Although the study failed to show a significant difference in HBeAg seroconversion, more patients experienced HBeAg loss at week 52 with lamivudine compared with placebo (33% vs. 13%; $P = 0.013$). Comparison of liver biopsies at baseline and at week 52 did not show significant changes in fibrosis but did show greater improvement in necroinflammatory activity in the lamivudine group compared with the placebo group.

Oral antivirals

No large datasets have compared nucleoside/nucleotide treatment of interferon non-responders and interferon-naive patients. However, there is little to suggest that efficacy would be lower in the interferon-experienced patients. Indeed, as the apparent benefits of interferon therapy appear to extend beyond the treatment period, oral therapy may further enhance this benefit. This requires further study. As for the choice of oral antiviral, the two preferred compounds are the two most potent with the lowest barriers to resistance, namely entecavir and tenofovir. Further study comparing the two in a post-interferon setting is required before any firm recommendations can be made. Figure 39.1 shows the relative potency of the

compounds with 48–52 weeks of therapy (12–24 weeks with conventional interferon) [15]. These data are not from head-to-head comparisons and patient demographics and trial designs varied considerably. Lamivudine has the largest breadth of data and is well characterized. It does have a weak barrier to resistance and, like telbivudine, the resistance profile has limited its usefulness. Adefovir is a weak antiviral and although there is little early resistance, its lack of efficacy leads to high rates of late resistance.

Conclusions

Interferon remains a viable first-line therapeutic option for genotypes A and B, with potential benefits extending beyond the dosing period. Nevertheless, the majority of these patients will fail therapy and will need an oral agent. At that point, they should be treated in the same way a treatment-naive patient would be. Future studies need to further explore the utility of interferon and antivirals in various schemata in the treatment of chronic HBV infection. Now that there are five oral compounds, conventional interferon and two peginterferons, many permutations exist that can be explored in an effort to optimize therapy. Sequential therapy, priming with one agent followed by another, combination therapies and even alternating therapies can all be explored. One must remain cautious, however, as novel adverse events may occur when drugs are combined. The combination of peginterferon alfa-2a and telbivudine led to several cases of peripheral neuropathy in a clinical trial setting. It is best to study all potential combinations in a rigorous systematic way to minimize toxicity while addressing the aim of the study.

References

1. Cooksley WG, Piratvisuth T, Lee S *et al.* Peginterferon alfa-2a (40 kDa): an advance in the treatment of hepatitis B e antigen-positive chronic hepatitis B. *Journal of Viral Hepatitis* 2003;10:298–305.

2. Wong DK, Cheung AM, O'Rourke K *et al.* Effect of alpha-interferon treatment in patients with hepatitis B e antigen-positive chronic hepatitis B. A meta-analysis. *Annals of Internal Medicine* 1993;119:312–323.

3. Zoulim F, Perrillo R. Hepatitis B: reflections on the current approach to antiviral therapy. *Journal of Hepatology* 2008;48(Suppl 1):S2–S19.

4. Lau GK, Piratvisuth T, Luo KX *et al.* Peginterferon alfa-2a, lamivudine, and the combination for HBeAg-positive chronic hepatitis B. *New England Journal of Medicine* 2005;352:2682–2695.

5. Marcellin P, Lau GK, Bonino F *et al.* Peginterferon alfa-2a alone, lamivudine alone and the two in combination in patients with HBeAg-negative chronic hepatitis B. *New England Journal of Medicine* 2004;350:1206–1217.

6. Lau DT, Everhart J, Kleiner DE *et al.* Long-term follow-up of patients with chronic hepatitis B treatment with interferon alfa. *Gastroenterology* 1997;113:1660–1667.

7. Moucari R, Korevaar A, Lada O *et al.* High rates of HBsAg seroconversion in HBeAg-positive chronic hepatitis B patients responding to interferon: a long-term follow-up study. *Journal of Hepatology* 2009;50:1084–1092.

8. Marcellin P, Bonino F, Lau GK *et al.* Sustained response of hepatitis B e antigen-negative patients 3 years after treatment with peginterferon alpha-2a. *Gastroenterology* 2009;136:2169–2179.

9. Hou J, Schilling R, Janssen HLA *et al.* Molecular characteristics of hepatitis B virus genotype A confer a higher response rate to interferon treatment [Abstract]. *Journal of Hepatology* 2001;34(Suppl 1):15.

10. Flink HJ, van Zonneveld M, Hansen BE *et al.* Treatment with peg-interferon alfa-2b for HbeAg-positive chronic hepatitis B: HBsAg loss is associated with HBV genotype. *American Journal of Gastroenterology* 2006;101:297–303. **A paper that discusses the rate of HBsAg loss, according to genotype, following interferon therapy.** 🔑

11. Kao JH, Wu NH, Chen PJ *et al.* Hepatitis B genotypes and the response to interferon therapy. *Journal of Hepatology* 2000;33:998–1002.

12. Janssen HL, Schalm SW, Berk L *et al.* Repeated courses of alpha-interferon for treatment of chronic hepatitis type B. *Journal of Hepatology* 1993;17:S47–S51.

13. Schiff ER, Dienstag JL, Karayalcin S *et al.* Lamivudine and 24 weeks of lamivudine/interferon combination therapy for hepatitis B e antigen-positive chronic hepatitis B in interferon nonresponders. *Journal of Hepatology* 2003;38:818–826.

14. Dienstag JL, Perrillo RP, Schiff ER *et al.* A preliminary trial of lamivudine for chronic hepatitis B infection. *New England Journal of Medicine* 1995;333:1657–1661.

15. Keeffe EB, Dieterich DT, Han SH *et al.* A treatment algorithm for the management of chronic hepatitis B virus infection in the United States: 2008 update. *Clinical Gastroenterology and Hepatology* 2008;6:1315–1341. **A comprehensive summary of currently available therapies and recommendations for the various HBV clinical situations.** 🔑

40 Hepatitis B and hepatitis C co-infection

Quentin M. Anstee, Belinda C. Smith, Howard C. Thomas

Department of Academic Medicine, St Mary's Hospital Campus, Imperial College London, London, UK

LEARNING POINTS

- HBV/HCV co-infection is a common phenomenon, particularly in areas where both infections are endemic.

- Viral interaction may result in fluctuating HBV/HCV dominance and frequently leads to apparent suppression of HBV replication.

- Peginterferon and ribavirin combination therapy for HCV is as efficacious and safe in HBV/HCV co-infection as in monoinfection.

- Few data are available to guide therapy in patients with dually active co-infection, although addition of a nucleos(t)ide may be appropriate.

- Antiviral therapy may alter the viral dynamics and reverse the suppression of HBV replication. This should be actively sought and nucleos(t)ide therapy instituted as appropriate.

Introduction

The globally high prevalence of hepatitis B virus (HBV) and hepatitis C virus (HCV), in association with the shared routes of transmission of these viruses, explains the inevitable common finding of HBV/HCV co-infection. Such interactions were first described when HCV infection was known as non-A, non-B hepatitis [1]. It is difficult to accurately determine the number of HBV/HCV co-infected individuals and there is considerable geographical variation; it is estimated that 3–22% of chronic HBV-infected patients are HCV antibody positive and that 2–10% of anti-HCV-positive patients are HBsAg positive

Clinical Dilemmas in Viral Liver Disease, 1st edition. Edited by Graham R. Foster and K. Rajender Reddy. © 2010 Blackwell Publishing.

[2]. Outside endemic areas, HBV/HCV co-infection most frequently occurs in specific high-risk populations, particularly intravenous drug users, HIV-positive individuals and patients on haemodialysis [2]. Reports of occult HBV infection (HBsAg negative, HBV DNA positive) suggest it is likely we underestimate the true prevalence of co-infection and implies that co-infection should be actively sought by HBV DNA testing, particularly in anti-HBcAb-positive individuals [2,3]. Dual viral infection may occur rarely by simultaneous acute infection with both viruses or more commonly by a second acute infection in an individual already chronically infected with one hepatitis virus (super-infection). Typically, particularly in areas with high HBV prevalence, acute HCV will be superimposed on chronic HBV [4]. Acute superinfection may provoke a fulminant hepatitis [5] or may lead to a chronic dual hepatitis with sequelae including cirrhosis and hepatocellular carcinoma (HCC). Rarely, superinfection with HCV may result in clearance of HBV [6]. Despite the relatively large disease burden, knowledge regarding the virological interactions, clinical consequences of co-infection and optimum therapy remains incomplete.

Viral interaction in HBV/HCV co-infection

Laboratory and clinical studies demonstrate that HBV and HCV may interact with each other and affect the host immune response. Typically, HBV/HCV co-infection is associated with both lower HBV viraemia *and* lower HCV viraemia than control monoinfected subjects [7]. Cross-sectional studies suggest that many co-infected cases have detectable HCV viraemia but significantly reduced levels of HBV DNA, possibly indicating a dominance of HCV over HBV [2]. In chronic infection, HBsAg/anti-HBs serocon-version occurs at a higher rate in co-infected individuals

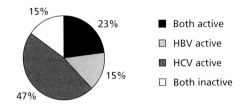

15%

23%

15%

47%

■ Both active

▢ HBV active

■ HCV active

☐ Both inactive

FIG. 40.1 Pattern of viral activity among HBV/HCV co-infected patients (*N* = 103). (Based on data from Raimondo *et al.* [12].)

(2.08% per annum) than monoinfected individuals (0.43%), which may contribute to the development of so-called occult HBV co-infection [4]. This is despite evidence that proliferative responses in peripheral blood mononuclear cells are more reactive against HCV than HBV [8]. This relative lack of immune selective pressure on HBV may result in the observed reduced prevalence of HBV precore mutations in co-infected HBV patients [9].

In vitro evidence indicates that HCV core protein is able to directly interact with HBV X-protein, pol protein and pregenomic RNA and that it may also indirectly affect Enh1 and Enh2/basal core promoter to suppress HBV transcription [10,11]. However, the primacy of HCV over HBV remains controversial, with a number of observational studies reporting the opposite effect. This apparent discrepancy may be explained by the findings of an Italian longitudinal study in a cohort of HBV/HCV co-infected patients which shows that while HCV is the dominant viral infection in the majority, a more complex spectrum of virological profiles with evidence of a dynamic relationship and fluctuating co-dominance occurs in up to one-third of patients [12] (Figure 40.1).

Fibrosis progression and HCC in HBV/HCV co-infection

Cross-sectional studies report that HBsAg-positive patients with active HCV infection show more severe hepatic fibrosis and faster progression to cirrhosis than patients with sole HCV infection [13]. A multicentre Italian study of 59 co-infected patients demonstrates that coexisting HBV and HCV infection is associated with a higher cirrhosis prevalence than in HBV monoinfection (28.8% vs. 15.1%) [14].

Epidemiological data from a large meta-analysis indicates that there may be a synergistic carcinogenic effect between the two viruses, with an odds ratio for HCC of 35.7

(95% CI 26.2–48.5) in individuals with active co-infection compared with 14.1 (95% CI 10.6–18.8) in HBV monoinfection and 4.6 (95% CI 3.6–5.9) in HCV monoinfection [15]. Even when HBV is inactive (HBsAg negative, anti-HBc positive) and apparently does not contribute to inflammation, it still increases the risk of developing HCC by 2–2.5 fold [11].

Treatment of HBV/HCV co-infection

Established guidelines for the treatment of HBV/HCV co-infected patients have been hampered by the lack of high-quality evidence of treatment efficacy as co-infection has been an exclusion criterion in the majority of large clinical trials. In addition, many patients with HCV/HBV co-infection in Western countries have not been suitable for clinical trials, either because of additional HIV infection or due to chaotic lifestyles associated with injecting drug use in some patients with recent acquisition of hepatitis. Based largely on evidence of HCV dominance over HBV infection, recent European guidelines suggest that initial treatment should be targeted at HCV [16]. As HCV is cleared, there is a risk of reactivation of latent HBV that may necessitate subsequent treatment with nucleos(t)ide analogues [16].

Two randomized trials have examined the efficacy of standard HCV treatment (peginterferon alfa-2a/2b and ribavirin) in HCV/HBV co-infection [17,18]. HCV-infected patients (serum alanine aminotransferase > 1.5 times upper limit of normal, RNA > 10^5 copies/mL) with (*N* = 161) or without (*N* = 160) detectable HBsAg were studied in Taiwan. Patients received standard 24/48 weeks therapy according to genotype with peginterferon alfa-2a 180 mg/week plus ribavirin 800–1200 mg daily. Follow-up 6 months after completion of therapy showed that sustained virological response (SVR) rates were no different in those with co-infection compared with HCV alone: 72.2% in co-infected genotype 1 patients compared with 77.3% in genotype 1 monoinfected patients, and 82.8% versus 84% in genotype 2 and 3 patients. Of patients with HBV DNA above 1000 IU/mL at the start of treatment, 45% achieved an HBV virological response at 24 weeks; 19 patients with previously undetectable HBV DNA experienced an increase in HBV DNA load.

The smaller European HEP-NET prospective multi-centre trial of peginterferon alfa-2b and ribavirin that enrolled 19 patients (10 genotype 1, 9 genotype 2/3) has been published in full [17]. A total of 15 patients completed treatment and 24 weeks' post-treatment follow-up. At 24 weeks after therapy, SVR was observed in 86% of genotype 1 and 100% of genotype 2/3 patients. Two of six patients who initially had detectable HBV DNA were cleared of detectable HBV virus and four patients with initially undetectable HBV load experienced a reactivation of HBV replication. The frequency of serious adverse events was in line with previous monoinfection trials.

Both studies demonstrate that standard HCV therapeutic protocols may be applied to HBV/HCV co-infected individuals; however, close monitoring of HBV viral load is advised, even in patients with undetectable HBV DNA at the start of treatment. Similar conclusions were made after treatment with non-pegylated interferon and ribavirin in 42 co-infected patients in a study by Chuang et al. [19]. Only 1 of 42 had simultaneous clearance of HCV and HBV with interferon and ribavirin, although five (11.9%) developed HBsAg seroconversion during follow-up (to 72 weeks). HBV clearance correlated negatively with HCV SVR. Potthoff et al. [20] reported a case of HBV/HCV co-infection treated with peginterferon and ribavirin where the combination of antiviral therapy and active HBV immunization achieved successful clearance of both viruses with development of high-titre anti-HBs.

None of these studies examined the role of nucleos(t)ides in the treatment of co-infection. Data in this area are particularly limited, being confined to a single study of eight patients given standard interferon plus lamivudine; HCV SVR was achieved in 50% and HBeAg clearance was observed in three patients [21]. There have been no studies examining the use of more potent nucleos(t)ides in co-infection.

Summary

HBV/HCV co-infection is a common but insufficiently studied condition, particularly in endemic areas. Interactions occur between the two viruses both at a virological level and, importantly, at a pathogenic level, where co-infection appears to promote accelerated disease progression and increased risk of HCC. HCV treatment response to peginterferon and ribavirin appears to be similar in co-infection to monoinfection, although the possibility of rebound activation of suppressed HBV mandates surveillance. Studies examining the use of combination therapy with interferon, ribavirin and potent nucleos(t)ides are urgently needed.

References

1. Lee CA, Kernoff PB, Karayiannis P, Farci P, Thomas HC. Interactions between hepatotropic viruses in patients with haemophilia. *Journal of Hepatology* 1985;1:379–384.

2. Chu CJ, Lee SD. Hepatitis B virus/hepatitis C virus coinfection: epidemiology, clinical features, viral interactions and treatment. *Journal of Gastroenterology and Hepatology* 2008;23:512–520.

3. Cacciola I, Pollicino T, Squadrito G, Cerenzia G, Orlando ME, Raimondo G. Occult hepatitis B virus infection in patients with chronic hepatitis C liver disease. *New England Journal of Medicine* 1999;341:22–26.

4. Crockett SD, Keeffe EB. Natural history and treatment of hepatitis B virus and hepatitis C virus coinfection. *Annals of Clinical Microbiology and Antimicrobials* 2005;4:13.

5. Wu JC, Chen CL, Hou MC, Chen TZ, Lee SD, Lo KJ. Multiple viral infection as the most common cause of fulminant and subfulminant viral hepatitis in an area endemic for hepatitis B: application and limitations of the polymerase chain reaction. *Hepatology* 1994;19:836–840.

6. Sheen IS, Liaw YF, Chu CM, Pao CC. Role of hepatitis C virus infection in spontaneous hepatitis B surface antigen clearance during chronic hepatitis B virus infection. *Journal of Infectious Diseases* 1992;165:831–834.

7. Pontisso P, Ruvoletto MG, Fattovich G et al. Clinical and virological profiles in patients with multiple hepatitis virus infections. *Gastroenterology* 1993;105:1529–1533.

8. Tsai SL, Liaw YF, Yeh CT, Chu CM, Kuo GC. Cellular immune responses in patients with dual infection of hepatitis B and C viruses: dominant role of hepatitis C virus. *Hepatology* 1995;21:908–912.

9. Jardi R, Rodriguez F, Buti M et al. Role of hepatitis B, C, and D viruses in dual and triple infection: influence of viral genotypes and hepatitis B precore and basal core promoter mutations on viral replicative interference. *Hepatology* 2001;34:404–410.

10. Chen SY, Kao CF, Chen CM et al. Mechanisms for inhibition of hepatitis B virus gene expression and replication by hepatitis C virus core protein. *Journal of Biological Chemistry* 2003;278:591–607.

11. Lin L, Verslype C, van Pelt JF, van Ranst M, Fevery J. Viral interaction and clinical implications of coinfection of hepatitis C virus with other hepatitis viruses. *European Journal of Gastroenterology and Hepatology* 2006;18:1311–1319.

12. Raimondo G, Brunetto MR, Pontisso P et al. Longitudinal evaluation reveals a complex spectrum of virological profiles in hepatitis B virus/hepatitis C virus-coinfected patients. *Hepatology* 2006;43:100–107. **Longitudinal follow-up of co-infected patients demonstrating fluctuating viral dominance.** 🔑

13. Zarski JP, Bohn B, Bastie A *et al*. Characteristics of patients with dual infection by hepatitis B and C viruses. *Journal of Hepatology* 1998;28:27−33.

14. Gaeta GB, Stornaiuolo G, Precone DF *et al*. Epidemiological and clinical burden of chronic hepatitis B virus/hepatitis C virus infection. A multicenter Italian study. *Journal of Hepatology* 2003;39:1036−1041.

15. Shi J, Zhu L, Liu S, Xie WF. A meta-analysis of case-control studies on the combined effect of hepatitis B and C virus infections in causing hepatocellular carcinoma in China. *British Journal of Cancer* 2005;92:607−612.

16. European Association for the Study of the Liver. EASL Clinical Practice Guidelines: management of chronic hepatitis B. *Journal of Hepatology* 2009;50:227−242.

17. Potthoff A, Wedemeyer H, Boecher WO *et al*. The HEP-NET B/C co-infection trial: a prospective multicenter study to investigate the efficacy of pegylated interferon-alpha2b and ribavirin in patients with HBV/HCV co-infection. *Journal of Hepatology* 2008;49:688−694.

18. Liu CJ, Chuang WL, Lee CM *et al*. An open label, comparative, multicenter study of peginterferon alfa-2A plus ribavirin in the treatment of patients with chronic hepatitis C/hepatitis B co-infection versus those with chronic hepatitis C monoinfection. *Gastroenterology* 2009;136:496−504. **Randomized trial evaluating treatment in co-infected patients.** 🔑

19. Chuang WL, Dai CY, Chang WY *et al*. Viral interaction and responses in chronic hepatitis C and B coinfected patients with interferon-alpha plus ribavirin combination therapy. *Antiviral Therapy* 2005;10:125−133.

20. Potthoff A, Deterding K, Trautwein C, Rifai K, Manns MP, Wedemeyer H. Sustained HCV-RNA response and hepatitis Bs seroconversion after individualized antiviral therapy with pegylated interferon alpha plus ribavirin and active vaccination in a hepatitis C virus/hepatitis B virus-coinfected patient. *European Journal of Gastroenterology and Hepatology* 2007;19:906−909.

21. Marrone A, Zampino R, D'Onofrio M, Ricciotti R, Ruggiero G, Utili R. Combined interferon plus lamivudine treatment in young patients with dual HBV (HBeAg positive) and HCV chronic infection. *Journal of Hepatology* 2004;41:1064−1065.

PART III
Clinical Set-up

41 The nurse practitioner and the physician assistant: their role in HCV management

Brenda A. Appolo

Hospital of the University of Pennsylvania, Division of Gastroenterology, Philadelphia, Pennsylvania, USA

LEARNING POINTS

- Nurse practitioners (NPs) and physician assistants (PAs) are non-physician clinicians trained in a variety of medical and surgical disciplines, including viral hepatitis and chronic liver disease management.

- Dedicated gastroenterology/hepatology NPs or PAs are often autonomous hepatology providers skilled in the diagnosis and management of chronic HCV infection and augment the role of their physician colleague.

- The NP or PA model may serve to reduce hepatology physician demands and decompress current hepatology/transplant hepatology physicians as the demands of an ageing population of HCV-infected patients and their treatment grow.

- The NP or PA plays an integral role in the personalized education of the HCV-infected patient, HCV treatment monitoring, and continuity of care.

Introduction

Apart from physicians, designated gastroenterology/hepatology nurse practitioners (NPs) and physician assistants (PAs) can play a vital role in the diagnosis and management of chronic hepatitis C virus (HCV) infection. The specific role of the clinical NP and hepatology PA varies based on individual physician leadership as well as state and institutional regulations with respect to the NP and PA's medical scope of practice. Essentially, certified NPs and

Clinical Dilemmas in Viral Liver Disease, 1st edition. Edited by Graham R. Foster and K. Rajender Reddy. © 2010 Blackwell Publishing.

PAs are utilized as autonomous care-givers in the setting of a wide range of diseases including viral hepatitis B and C. The NP and PA model has been widely implemented in patient care and is a model that exists rather exclusively in the USA, Guam and US military services abroad. Such a model can readily be adopted in others parts of the world as well. Their clinical impact and presence amidst medical care is quite significant and estimates from the American Academy of Physician Assistants indicate that in 2008, 257 million patient visits were made to PAs and 332 million medications were prescribed or recommended by PAs [1].

Nurse practitioner and physician assistant impact

Globally, chronic HBV and HCV infections present an enormous disease burden. According to the Centers for Disease Control, approximately 1.4 million patients in the USA are chronically infected with viral hepatitis B in contrast to the nearly 4 million patients infected chronically with viral hepatitis C. There are 3000 deaths per year related to HBV and 12 000 deaths related to HCV [2]. By 2015, epidemiological projections indicate that although the prevalence of HCV infection may be declining, the number of persons chronically infected for over 20 years could increase substantially, particularly among those individuals born between 1940 and 1965 [3]. This potential swell of chronically infected HCV patients will only increase the demand for well-trained healthcare practitioners in all aspects of patient care and thus will become a major demand on healthcare resources.

That said, the American Association for the Study of Liver Disease (AASLD) commissioned a workforce study in 1999 that examined the need for specialty trained hepatologists and, more aptly, transplant hepatologists. The AASLD thereafter was in the vanguard to also provide formalized postgraduate training for clinical NPs and PAs which, although not necessary for NP or PA practice, has encouraged dedicated NP and PA hepatology careers, some of which primarily focus on chronic HCV management. Thus clinical hepatology/gastroenterology NPs and PAs have in recent years come to the forefront of HCV therapy care coordination, largely due to current and projected demands. In addition to clinical care and education of the HCV-infected patient, NPs and PAs at various academic centres actively participate as sub-investigators in HCV small-molecule treatments poised to influence HCV treatment evolution.

Unfortunately, few studies exist regarding the clinical impact and cost-effectiveness of NPs and PAs in the treatment of liver disease and more particularly viral hepatitis C. However, in 2004, Ahern *et al.* [4] compared the NP with the physician and evaluated their impact on quality of life and treatment outcomes in patients receiving therapy for chronic HCV infection. The treatment outcome data for the NP groups showed a 48% sustained virological response (SVR) rate in genotype 1-infected patients and a 59% SVR rate in genotype 2- or 3-infected patients, compared with 41% and 61% SVR rates respectively in the physician-treated group. While the response rates among the provider groups was not statistically significant, the study highlighted that NPs can provide effective care to chronic HCV-infected individuals.

HCV therapy: getting started

In addition to a routine history and physical, laboratory and radiographic evaluation of the HCV-infected patient considering HCV therapy, assessment of a patient's medical coverage, coping skills, social support network and pre-conceived notions of HCV therapy-induced side effects can be identified and effectively addressed by the NP or PA.

The current standard of care for chronic HCV infection includes once-weekly injections of peginterferon and oral ribavirin twice daily. Medication costs alone average $30 000, depending on which peginterferon is prescribed, the selection of brand versus generic ribavirin, dose and treatment duration. Medication coverage is also dictated by an individual patient's managed care plan and drug formulary and, in some parts of the world, by local policy. A broad knowledge of local and national third-party coverage plans by

the treating specialist is optimal. Prior drug authorizations (pre-approval) are often necessary at baseline and at week 12 on therapy, particularly for Medicaid and Medicare insurance plans in the USA. The NP or PA can effectively spearhead potential approval issues, implement appeals to insurance carriers on behalf of the patient and, more importantly, try to prevent drug interruption related to insurance constraints once therapy commences, which is vital to achieving SVR.

It should also be stressed that in the USA, with our current managed care society, 'approval' does not always denote 'full cost' coverage to the patient, thus leading to the potential for exorbitant out-of-pocket expense to the patient based on individual plans. That said, realistic access to specialty therapy of this nature can be a challenge. Various patient assistance programmes are available to support full cost of HCV therapy or high co-pay cost (also known as 'co-pay compassion' programmes). The NP or PA, through their formal and on the job training, often have first-hand knowledge and practical experience implementing this process with the patient. Certain websites provide specific information on resources available to patients (Table 41.1).

Extensive personalized patient education is also often performed by these health professionals in lieu of their physician counterpart due to the increasing demands on hepatology physicians and transplant hepatology specialists in various regions throughout the USA. As part of the baseline education regarding HCV-induced side effects, 'provider–patient contracts' are often devised and monitored by the NP or PA. This may include the patient's

TABLE 41.1 Patient support websites and recommended provider and practice guideline website resources.

Patient support websites
www.beincharge.com
www.hcvinprison.org/cms
www.hepc-connection.org
www.hepcnetwork.org
www.pegassist.com
www.infergen.com

Recommended websites for patient medication assist programmes and practice guidelines
www.aasld.org
www.amgen.com/patients/assistance
www.beincharge.com
www.cdc.gov/hepatitis/
www.clinicaloptions.com/Hepatitis
www.pegassist.com

signed recognition of common and even rare potential side effects. Personalized materials may also be provided to the patient outlining suggested side-effect management techniques, such as proper pre-emptive paracetamol dosages to palliate or prevent fever and flu-like illness. Moreover, in those of child-bearing age, a patient contract may also include a patient and his/her spouse's recognition that HCV therapy may induce teratogenic side effects and that a commitment to two forms of contraception while on HCV therapy and for 6 months after therapy conclusion are strongly recommended. In addition, it is the NP or PA who conducts the in-office self-injection technique classes at the initiation of therapy.

Treatment initiated: now what?

Invariably patients receiving HCV therapy will have one or more treatment-induced side effects such as, but not limited, to flu-like syndrome, fever, body aches, cough, rash, anaemia and neuropsychiatric problems. The NP or PA is often the first recipient of these complaints via telephone triage or office interface with the patient and therefore can provide emotional support and motivation, and help deduce which side effects necessitate adjunctive therapy or HCV therapy dose modification. Emotional and motivational support is of paramount importance and many practices incorporating an NP or PA develop patient support groups to engender a sense of community.

In addition to on-treatment support of the patient, the NP or PA will triage laboratory studies while on HCV therapy and monitor treatment response rates alongside their physician counterparts. Diligent use of growth factors is widely accepted and coordination of such via the gastroenterology/hepatology NP or PA has replaced previous practice habits of out-sourcing this care coordination to their respective haematology colleagues. Finally, on-treatment response rates and the conscientious monitoring of HCV RNA titres, at set intervals, not only helps predict SVR rates and propel patient motivation but are mandated for continuation of

therapy per the majority of managed care plans in the USA. Therefore, lack of patient follow-up or miscommunication about laboratory assessments on therapy could result in premature discontinuation of therapy at many levels, or compromise patient safety.

Summary

As the clinical knowledge and treatment of chronic viral hepatitis infection evolves, there is a parallel need for trained healthcare professionals. The utilization of physician extenders inclusive of NPs and PAs has helped lead the way to increased access to personalized patient education, chronic viral disease monitoring, treatment and continuity of care. Dedicated gastroenterology/hepatology NPs or PAs are often autonomous hepatology providers skilled in the diagnosis and management of chronic HCV infection and augment the role of their physician colleagues. In particular, the on-treatment monitoring of the HCV-infected patient, as well as side-effect management, is a staple of the NP and PA scope of practice.

References

1. 2008 American Academy of Physician Assistants Census Report. Available from www.aapa.org.
2. http://www.cdc.gov/hepatitis/Statistics
3. Armstrong G, Alter M, McQuillan G, Margolis H. The past incidence of hepatitis C virus infection: implications for the future burden of chronic liver disease in the United States. *Hepatology* 2003:21:777–782. **A significant paper that underscores burden of chronic HCV infection projection, thus enabling the deduction that healthcare resources will need to grow in parallel.** ⚷
4. Ahern M, Imperial J, Lam S. Impact of a designated hepatology nurse on the clinical course and quality of life of patients treated with rebetron therapy for chronic hepatitis C. *Gastroenterology Nursing* 2004:27:149–155. **An important paper that highlights the significant role played by physician extenders.** ⚷

Non-specialist management in general practice of chronic hepatitis C liver disease: cost-effective or foolish cost cutting?

Chris Helen Ford

Lonsdale Medical Centre, London, UK

LEARNING POINTS

- In many developed countries a minority of patients with chronic HCV have received therapy.

- Studies in the UK indicate that a large proportion of patients who are known to have chronic HCV do not access antiviral therapy care pathways.

- In pilot studies with selected patient groups, primary care-led therapy has shown improved uptake of therapy with satisfactory treatment response rates.

Introduction

Hepatitis C virus (HCV) infection is a growing cause of morbidity and mortality around the world. International and national guidelines (e.g. the UK National Institute for Health and Clinical Excellence, which examines both clinical and cost effectiveness of therapies) recommend treatment that is curative in 60–80% of cases [1] and is cost saving in the medium to long term. In many countries diagnosis and treatment rates are poor, for example in the UK around half of estimated cases of HCV infection have been diagnosed, a marked improvement on the high proportion of undiagnosed patients in 2004, but of these a

Clinical Dilemmas in Viral Liver Disease, 1st edition. Edited by Graham R. Foster and K. Rajender Reddy. © 2010 Blackwell Publishing.

mere 2–3% are receiving therapy [2,3]. In other countries, such as France, patients are 6–12 times more likely to gain effective treatment [4]. Interestingly, France treats hepatitis C using a community approach, contrasting with the more traditional 'hospital specialist' model followed by the UK and many other countries. In this chapter I review the question of non-specialist management of hepatitis C with particular reference to the UK model where, it is generally agreed, treatment rates are unacceptably low. The UK model is a good illustration of the problems involved in increasing access to treatment in a system that has relatively few tertiary liver centres but abundant primary care services. As such the system serves as a paradigm for the problems that exist in many countries where access to antiviral therapy is limited by service providers.

Many UK hospitals have insufficient capacity to treat hepatitis C effectively and few can provide a full range of liver services to patients. Less than two-thirds of NHS trusts are confident that they can meet the national target of initiating therapy within 18 weeks of referral [3]. An additional difficulty is discrimination against certain patient groups, notably injecting drug users, who constitute 90% of cases of HCV infection. Many drug users engage poorly with secondary care services, where there is intolerance of missed appointments as well as ongoing prejudice around problems perceived to be self-inflicted.

These problems, together with a national move in England towards a primary care-led NHS with increasing patient choice, have led to the need to look at different, more community-based treatment models for hepatitis C [5]. General practice offers an ideal robust framework, with 98% of the population seen in a year and an average person consulting their general practitioner (GP) as many as five times in that period. General practice offers whole-person care and can deal well with complexity. In other areas primary care has a good track record of managing chronic conditions. Every GP in the UK is likely to have between 8 and 20 HCV-infected individuals (based on an average list size of 1666 and depending on local population demographics) and the position is likely to be similar in many developed countries. Many of these patients will be attending their GP regularly and will be undiagnosed at present, but this situation should improve as knowledge and training about the disease spreads both in the community and among primary care practitioners. There is some evidence of a recent improvement in diagnosis in the UK following government and voluntary sector awareness campaigns: one-quarter of injecting drug users have reported never having had a voluntary confidential test for HCV in 2006 as compared with 51% in 2000, illustrating the value of publicity in improving diagnosis rates. However, in 2006, of those who were infected with HCV, only 54% reported being aware of their disease [6].

UK success in community-based drug treatment

An important factor in the recent increase in diagnosis rates in the UK is the increasing role of GPs in drug treatment. Before 1995 less than 1% of practices treated drug users, but through acquisition of knowledge and skills many more practices have developed an interest in treating drug users and now, overall, more than 30% of practices are treating this patient group, with this figure rising to 50% in some areas [7]. An expanding body of evidence confirms that primary care is an effective setting for delivering treatment for drug dependence. This achievement has required the development of appropriate training, support services and a strong network of primary care practitioners [7]. Traditionally, drug dependency services have been delivered by psychiatric services but the general practice background of primary care physicians ensures that this workforce is not only prescribing substitute medication but also taking on other health needs such as HCV infection. Primary care can also access patients who are excluded from secondary care or who get lost in the transfer from primary to secondary care, making transfer unnecessary for a significant percentage of hepatitis C sufferers.

Primary care: testing and treatment

Testing for HCV in a primary care setting is essential for improving diagnosis and treatment in the UK and elsewhere. Primary care practitioners working with people who inject drugs are uniquely placed to screen this population for blood-borne viruses and surgeries are in an ideal situation to identify those from other high-risk groups such as ethnic groups and past injectors. Studies on care pathways find that many patients with viral hepatitis drop out of care and this often occurs between diagnosis and the specialist clinic. The testing environment is therefore a natural setting for treatment and any system which reduces the relentlessly high non-attendance rate at hospital clinics has an excellent chance of being cost-effective. GP surgeries can provide care in an environment in which the patient's other needs are known and are often already being met, something particularly important for drug users who have a high rate of morbidity. Hospital clinics often struggle to provide this holistic care. Thus the approach in primary care is likely to increase both attendance and compliance rates and thereby improve clinical and cost effectiveness.

Models of community treatment

In the UK, Department of Health Action Plans indicate that all areas should have networks of care for people with hepatitis C. Unfortunately, many of these networks have not worked well, often due to lack of funding and resources rather than good will, and result in high drop-out rates at several points along the patient referral pathway. One study in Nottingham looked at the clinical pathways for newly diagnosed patients with hepatitis C. In the first instance they found that 2.3% were positive but only 49% of these positive results were appropriately referred for specialist treatment, although 64.3% of those from primary care were referred. Of the 49% referred, a mere 27% of those attended and only 10% started treatment, which clearly demonstrates that the existing care pathways are ineffective [8]. In response to this finding, Nottingham set up and evaluated a primary care-based model for the delivery of HCV services, including antiviral therapy, to injecting drug users. The model was simple: a clinical nurse specialist working under the supervision of a secondary care-based hepatitis service was introduced into an inner city general practice in which drug workers and GPs already provided a specialist service to injecting drug users. In this study 353 clients attending opiate substitution clinics in primary care were evaluated and the outcomes evaluated included number of new diagnoses of HCV infection, number of clients assessed as suitable for antiviral treatment, and number of patients treated. Of the sample, 174 HCV antibody-positive clients were identified and 124 were chronically infected with HCV, of whom only six had been previously identified. Of 118 new chronically infected individuals, 86 entered the care pathway and 43 were assessed as suitable for antiviral treatment; more than 30 have so far been treated with outcomes comparable to those obtained in secondary care settings. This study suggests that a primary care-based model is a feasible and effective environment in which to treat hepatitis C in injecting drug users [9] and significantly improves the uptake of antiviral therapy.

Other models have been developed in the UK. There is a pilot primary care delivery scheme in Cornwall, where patients can receive their antiviral therapy in a GP surgery that is geographically isolated from any local hospital. Since it began in 2008 there has been a significant reduction in missed appointment rates (missed appointment rate for the local treatment centre is 30% but in general practice is less than 3%), and excellent patient satisfaction questionnaire results and higher than expected 'completed treatments' have been recorded. The practitioners involved conclude that the key is getting appropriately trained GPs, drug-workers, hepatitis C nurses, and motivated informed patients together in the same local GP surgery building, where a one-stop approach can be adopted. Antiviral therapies, substitute medication, housing, counselling, phlebotomy and immunizations, indeed everything except liver biopsies, can be dealt with at any one time within a primary care setting. In this area, liver biopsies can be performed locally (one in four patients require a liver biopsy to be performed) and thus liver histology can be obtained when required. Continued provision of the service will require further training, monies, secondary support, commissioning and time (Adam Ellery, personal communication, 19 May 2009).

These issues are also found to be key in the variations on these models that are increasingly being developed. The most important elements are a strong clinical network, with flexible support provided by consultants in hepatology or infectious diseases, as well as from specialist nurses, both groups needing a sound understanding of primary care. Within the clinical network a robust assessment process is essential, such that only appropriate cases are treated in the community and all complex cases are referred to secondary care. Naturally, it is important that all clinicians involved work strictly within their own level of competence. However, extensive experience in prescribing opiate replacement therapies to injecting drug users in primary care shows that, as expertise has grown, so too has the level of patient complexity.

Are specialist concerns valid?

Why are some specialists concerned and even opposed to these models? Is it fear of loss of power or clinical concern, or it is that some specialists see that there are many patients who do attend secondary care, so think there is no need to introduce community treatment, even though their own facilities are working to capacity? The perceived risks of treating in a primary care environment are mitigated by patient selection. It is important to clearly identify those patient populations that can be effectively treated in primary care. None of the current models advocate the treatment of complex patients, such as those with cirrhosis or those who have other comorbidities. People who are well, young and with no adverse cofactors and no stigmata or features of advanced liver disease and who, perhaps, have a fear or mistrust of hospitals are the ideal target group for therapy in primary care. This area of work should be compared with progression in other disease areas, such as diabetes, where most care now takes place in general practice [10]. This has occurred over 20 years with increasing complexity being managed in the community. The success of primary care treatment models depends on the 'new' GP who is a highly skilled clinician. Training and ongoing continuing professional development (CPD) for GPs and other primary care practitioners are essential for quality assurance, as well as close partnership between GPs and secondary care.

Is community-based treatment cost-effective?

Currently, there is no robust evidence that primary care-based treatment of hepatitis C is cost-effective, so support for this has to be based on anecdote and opinion. Currently, a large study by the National Treatment Agency in England is trying to assess the unit cost of treatment in different settings and results should be available in late 2009 but early analysis indicates that primary care treatment of chronic HCV is cheaper than therapy in referral centres and evidence to date indicates that it may be equally clinically effective in appropriate treatment groups [11]. When considering costs it is important to remember that treatment in primary care may be cheaper than hospital care because it deals with the less complex cases, and this will have implications on the cost per case at hospital as their caseload becomes more complex and expensive.

Conclusions

The emerging community models of management of chronic HCV infection are valued by patients and GPs alike. Unfortunately, as primary care-based treatment of HCV is a new and rapidly growing area, evidence for the primary care-based treatment of hepatitis C is anecdotal. However, the primary care-based models that do exist evaluate extremely well. With the right patient selection, adequate support, particularly from local secondary care colleagues, and adequate resources, this way forward is in no way foolhardy but is in fact essential if the problem of under-treatment of hepatitis C in the UK is to be in any way addressed and good-quality treatment provided to all those who need it.

References

1. National Institute for Health and Clinical Excellence (NICE). *Peginterferon alfa and ribavirin for the treatment of mild chronic hepatitis C*. NICE Technology Appraisal Guidance 106, August 2006. Available at www.nice.org.uk

2. Health Protection Agency. *Hepatitis C in England: The Health Protection Agency Annual Report 2007*. London: Health Protection Agency.

3. All-Party Parliamentary Group on Hepatology. A Matter of Chance: An Audit of Hepatitis C Healthcare in England 2006. London UK by Hepatitis C Trust. http://www.hepctrust.org.uk/Resources/HepC/Migrated%20Resources/Documents/Other/280_A%20MATTER%20OF%20CHANCE%2023-5-06.pdf

4. European Report Meeting, 31 May 2005. The Hepatitis C Trust and the University of Southampton. The UK vs. Europe: Losing the Fight Against Hepatitis C, 29 September 2005.

5. Creating a patient-led NHS: Delivering the NHS Improvement Plan 17th March 2005 Author and Printer Department of Health http://www.dh.gov.uk/en/publicationsandstatistics/publications/publicationspolicyandguidance/dh_4106506.

6. Health Protection Agency, Health Protection Scotland, National Public Health Service for Wales, CDSC Northern Ireland, CDRHB and the UASSG. *Shooting up: infections among injecting drug users in the UK 2006: An update, October 2007*. London: Health Protection Agency, 2007.

7. Ford C. Supporting GPs in improving substitute prescribing for opiate users in UK general practice. *Heroin Addiction and Related Clinical Problems* 2007;9:31–40. **Data on the advances in opiate prescribing in primary care.** 🔑

8. Irving WL, Smith S, Cater R *et al.* Clinical pathways for patients with newly diagnosed hepatitis C: what actually happens. *Journal of Viral Hepatitis* 2006;13:264–271. **Study of outcomes in patients with chronic HCV referred for therapy showing that relatively few attend.** 🔑

9. Jack K, Willott S, Manners J, Varnam A, Thomson BJ. Clinical trial: a primary-care-based model for the delivery of anti-viral treatment to injecting drug users infected with hepatitis C. *Alimentary Pharmacology and Therapeutics* 2008;29:38–45.

10. Gray A, Clarke P, Farmer A, Holman R on behalf of the United Kingdom Prospective Diabetes Study (UKPDS) Group. Implementing intensive control of blood glucose concentration and blood pressure in type 2 diabetes in England: cost analysis. *British Medical Journal* 2002;325:860.

11. Gossop M, Marsden J, Stewart D, Kidd T. The National Treatment Outcome Research Study (NTORS): 4–5 year follow-up results. *Addiction* 2003;98:291–303.

PART IV
The Future

43 The future of HCV therapy: with or without interferon and ribavirin

Mark Sulkowski

Department of Medicine, Divisions of Infectious Diseases and Gastroenterology/Hepatology, Johns Hopkins University School of Medicine, Baltimore, Maryland, USA

LEARNING POINTS

- Multiple direct-acting antiviral drugs have entered clinical development for the treatment of chronic hepatitis. In general, these drugs have been identified and selected based on their ability to inhibit critical viral steps *in vitro*, including NS3:NS4A protease, polymerase, NS5A.

- The next therapeutic advance in HCV treatment will be protease inhibitors (telaprevir and boceprevir) in combination with peginterferon alfa-2a/2b and ribavirin. Phase II clinical trials clearly demonstrate the essential role of both agents in preventing the emergence of protease inhibitor-resistant virus during therapy and increasing viral eradication.

- Future approaches to HCV treatment are anticipated to include multiple direct-acting antiviral drugs used in combination to suppress viral replication and prevent resistance. The role of interferon and ribavirin in combination with multiple antivirals remains uncertain but trials are underway.

Introduction

Since the discovery of hepatitis C virus (HCV) in 1989 as the major cause of non-A, non-B hepatitis, the identification and screening of HCV-targeted drugs has been hampered by the lack of small animal models and the inability to infect cultured cells. However, over the past 5 years, major advances

Clinical Dilemmas in Viral Liver Disease, 1st edition. Edited by Graham R. Foster and K. Rajender Reddy. © 2010 Blackwell Publishing.

in the understanding of HCV biology and the development of the replicon (autonomous replication of genetically engineered HCV genomes) and infectious virus cell culture systems has led to the identification of candidate antiviral drugs [1,2].

Targeted antiviral drugs are based on the selection of molecules that bind with high affinity to a functional site of HCV target structure, RNA or protein, resulting in interruption of the virus life cycle. The selection of such molecules is based on a detailed understanding of several HCV enzymes critical to viral replication, including NS3 serine protease, a major catalyst in post-translational polyprotein processing, and NS5B RNA-dependent RNA polymerase, a major catalyst in HCV replication. Other potential targets in HCV have been identified, such as NS3 helicase, which serves to unwind viral genomic RNA during replication, and IRES (internal ribosome entry inhibitor), which controls HCV genome translation; however, drugs targeting these processes have not reached clinical development. Nonetheless, multiple specific inhibitors of the HCV protease and polymerase enzymes have advanced to Phase I–III clinical trials in patients chronically infected with HCV. Further, other specific targeted antiviral therapies for hepatitis C (so-called STAT-Cs) such as NS5A inhibitors and novel interferon therapies, such as interferon lambda and recombinant human albumin–interferon alfa fusion protein, are in Phase II and/or III trials (Table 43.1) [3]. While there are many agents in development, the next step forward in the treatment of chronic hepatitis C is likely to be the addition of HCV protease inhibitors (telaprevir and boceprevir) to a backbone of peginterferon alfa and ribavirin. Future research will undoubtedly focus on the replacement of interferon and/or ribavirin in this combination regimen.

TABLE 43.1 Sample of HCV drugs in development.

Protease inhibitors
Telaprevir
Boceprevir
ITMN-191 (R7227)
TMC435350
MK7009
BI 201335

Polymerase inhibitor: nucleoside
R7128
IDX184
PSI-7851

Polymerase inhibitor: non-nucleoside
VCH-759
GS 9190
ANA598
Filibuvir
BI 207127
VCH-916

NS5A inhibitor
BMS-790052
PPI-461
AZD7295

NS4A inhibitor
ACH-806

Cyclophilin inhibitor
DEBIO 025
NIMN 811

Entry inhibitor
PRO 206
ITX5061

Next step forward: protease inhibitors plus interferon alfa plus ribavirin

The NS3 region of the HCV genome represents a multi-functional protein that contains a serine protease inhibitor that, along with a cofactor NS4A, cleaves the viral polyprotein into functional components. The development of NS3 serine protease inhibitors has been problematic because the active site of the enzyme is long, shallow and exposed, making interaction with small inhibitors difficult. Despite these challenges, multiple agents targeting the HCV protease have demonstrated potent antiviral activity in HCV-infected patients. Two drugs have entered the final stage of clinical testing which, if successful, will lead to approval by global regulatory agencies: telaprevir and boceprevir.

Telaprevir

Telapavir (previously known as VX-950) is a peptido-mimetic compound (small protein-like chain designed to mimic a peptide) that binds to and inhibits the HCV NS3-4 serine protease in HCV replicon assays. In early human studies, both the promise and potential Achilles heel of HCV protease inhibitors was revealed. Reesink *et al.* [4] conduced a randomized, dose-escalation, double-blind, placebo-controlled study in persons with chronic HCV genotype 1 infection. Subjects received VX-950, either 450 mg ($N = 10$) or 750 mg ($N = 8$) by mouth every 8 hours or 1250 mg ($N = 10$) by mouth every 12 hours or a matching placebo ($N = 6$). The maximum decrease in HCV RNA level was $-3.46 \log_{10}$ IU/mL in the group taking 450 mg every 8 hours, $-4.77 \log_{10}$ IU/mL in the group taking 750 mg every 8 hours, and $-3.49 \log_{10}$ IU/mL in the group taking 1250 mg every 12 hours. In the groups taking 450 mg every 8 hours and 1250 mg every 12 hours, the maximum decrease in HCV RNA level was observed at day 3 of dosing, followed by an increase in HCV RNA level. Conversely, HCV RNA levels continued to decline to day 14 of dosing in the group taking 750 mg every 8 hours, and two subjects had viral suppression below the limit of detection (10 IU/mL). The initial rapid decline in HCV RNA level was related to the maximal effect of telaprevir (C_{max}), whereas the second phase of the decline was related to the trough concentration (C_{trough}), which was greatest in the group taking 750 mg every 8 hours. To further understand these HCV RNA responses in subjects, particularly those with viral rebound, Kieffer *et al.* [5] investigated viral responses between days 7 and 14, dividing subjects into three groups. In group 1, HCV RNA increased on treatment after an initial decline; in group 2, HCV RNA declined and then reached a plateau; and in group 3, HCV RNA continued to decline to levels below 100 IU/mL. At several time points (dosing on day 14, 7–10 days after dosing, and 3–7 months after dosing), researchers cloned and sequenced the HCV NS3 proteases for an average of 80 clones per subject. As expected, the selection of viral variants with decreased sensitivity to telaprevir during treatment was documented, particularly among those subjects in the groups taking 450 mg every 8 hours and 1250 mg every 8 hours. Low-level resistance to the drug was observed, with several single point mutations in the NS3 protease: position 36, valine→methionine, alanine or leucine (V36M/A/L, roughly fourfold change in IC_{50}); position 155, arginine→lysine, threonine, serine or methionine (R155K/T/S/M, roughly sevenfold change in IC_{50}).

Higher-level resistance to telaprevir was observed with other single or double point mutations in the NS3 protease: position 156, alanine→valine or threonine (A156V/T, roughly 466-fold change in IC_{50}); positions 36 (V36A/M) and 155 (R155K/T, roughly 781-fold change in IC_{50} for the double mutation variant). In long-term follow-up after stopping telaprevir, viral variants with high-level resistance (A156V/T) were rapidly replaced by wild-type virus, suggesting reduced fitness of this variant in the absence of the selection pressure of the drug. Viral variants with low-level resistance with mutations at positions 36 or 155 persisted in some subjects after discontinuation of the drug. Although the long-term clinical significance of this finding remains unknown, this pivotal Phase I study conclusively demonstrated the need for combination therapy to minimize the selection of resistant variants during treatment with protease inhibitors.

Subsequently, telaprevir was studied in combination with peginterferon alfa-2a with or without ribavirin. In the PROVE 1 (Protease Inhibition for Viral Evaluation 1) study, McHutchison et al. [6] randomized treatment-naive HCV genotype 1-infected patients ($N = 263$) to one of three telaprevir groups or to the control group. The control group received peginterferon alfa-2a (180 μg/week), ribavirin (1000 or 1200 mg/day) and placebo for 48 weeks. The telaprevir groups received telaprevir (1250 mg on day 1 and then 750 mg every 8 hours) for 12 weeks in combination with peginterferon alfa-2a and ribavirin for varying durations of therapy: 12 weeks (17 patients), 24 weeks (79 patients) or 48 weeks (79 patients). In this Phase II study, the rate of sustained virological response (SVR) was significantly higher in patients treated with telaprevir in the 24-week (61%, 48 of 79 patients) and 48-week (67%, 53 of 79 patients) treatment groups compared with the 48-week peginterferon/ribavirin control group (41%, 35 of 75 patients). In the exploratory 12-week treatment group, 6 of 17 patients achieved SVR with telaprevir, peginterferon and ribavirin. Viral breakthrough occurred in 7% of patients receiving telaprevir. The rate of discontinuation because of adverse events was higher in the three telaprevir-based groups (21% vs. 11%), with severe rash the most common reason for discontinuation. In the PROVE 2 study, Hézode et al. [7] also tested telaprevir combination therapy in treatment-naive patients ($N = 334$) infected with HCV genotype 1. Similar to the PROVE 1 findings, patients treated with telaprevir (12 weeks) and peginterferon/ribavirin (24 weeks) had an SVR rate of 69%, significantly higher than the SVR rate observed in the peginterferon/ribavirin (48-week)

control group (46%). However, this trial further tested the potential use of treatment regimens of short duration and without ribavirin (peginterferon alfa-2a + telaprevir). In the ribavirin-sparing group, patients treated with peginterferon and telaprevir (12 weeks) were directly compared with those treated with telaprevir and peginterferon/ribavirin (12 weeks). Surprisingly, the SVR rate was substantially lower in the ribavirin-sparing group (36%, 28 of 78 patients) compared with that observed in the ribavirin group treated for the same duration (60%, 49 of 82 patients). More importantly, the incidence of virological failure was markedly higher in the absence of ribavirin. Virological breakthrough due to telaprevir-resistant virus was observed in 24% of patients treated with peginterferon/telaprevir and in only one patient treated with all three drugs. Further, the rate of virological relapse (often with resistant virus) was more common in persons not taking ribavirin. Of note, the triple-therapy regimen of 12 weeks duration had a higher rate of virological relapse (30%) than the same regimen with peginterferon/ribavirin extended to 24 weeks (14%). In the triple-therapy 24-week group, relapse was infrequent (3%) in persons with undetectable HCV RNA at treatment weeks 4 and 12.

Taken together, the Phase I and II clinical trials of telaprevir provide compelling evidence that therapy with three drugs – peginterferon, ribavirin and telaprevir – is more effective than the current standard of care. Further, these studies demonstrate that combination therapy with interferon alfa and ribavirin are critical to the control of pre-existing HCV variants with decreased susceptibility to telaprevir.

Boceprevir

Similar to telaprevir, boceprevir is a mechanism-based inhibitor of the HCV NS3 protease that has potent antiviral activity against HCV genotype 1 in vitro and in vivo [8]. Early in the development of boceprevir, the role of ribavirin was evaluated in a Phase II study of boceprevir plus peginterferon alfa-2b with or without ribavirin in HCV genotype 1-infected patients who had virological non-response to prior treatment with peginterferon and ribavirin ($< 2 \log_{10}$ reduction in HCV RNA at prior treatment week 12). Overall, 357 patients were randomized to multiple treatment groups designed to assess different doses of boceprevir and the need for ribavirin. Early in the course of the trial the independent Data and Safety Monitor Board determined that high rates of viral breakthrough and

TABLE 43.2 Final results of the SPRINT-1 study with boceprevir (B), peginterferon alfa-2b (P) and ribavirin (R).

	P/R	P/R/B Lead-in	P/R/B Lead-in	P/R/B No lead-in	P/R/B No lead-in	P/R/B Low-dose R
Duration of therapy (weeks)	48	48	28	48	28	48
Number of subjects	104	103	103	103	107	59
SVR (%)	38	75	56	67	54	36
Relapse rate (%)	24	3	24	7	3	22
Virological breakthough	0	4	11	5	7	27

treatment failure were occurring in patients randomized to receive low doses of boceprevir and no ribavirin. Accordingly, patients without virological failure ($N = 143$) were switched to receive boceprevir 800 mg (thrice daily) and peginterferon/ribavirin. Patients randomized to the control group (peginterferon/ribavirin) who experienced treatment week 12 virological failure were crossed over to receive boceprevir; in these cross-over patients, the rate of virological response following the addition of boceprevir was lowest in patients with less than 1 $\log_{10}$ reduction at treatment week 12 during the initial therapy (5 of 20 patient achieved undetectable HCV RNA). Virological breakthrough with HCV variants resistant to boceprevir was observed in the majority of patients with treatment failure. Overall, this complex study demonstrated conclusively the role of ribavirin therapy and provided the rationale for 'lead-in' therapy with peginterferon alfa-2b/ribavirin prior to the addition of boceprevir. This rationale includes the reduction of HCV replication and achievement of ribavirin steady-state levels prior to the addition of boceprevir.

In a second Phase II study, Kwo *et al.* [9] evaluated the combination of boceprevir and peginterferon/ribavirin in treatment-naive HCV genotype 1-infected patients. The investigators evaluated the role of lead-in therapy with peginterferon/ribavirin, the effect of treatment duration, and low-dose ribavirin (100–400 mg/day). Overall, higher rates of SVR were observed in subjects randomized to boceprevir, with the highest SVR rate in those treated for 48 weeks and with full-dose ribavirin (Table 43.2). Taken together, this Phase II study indicates that not only is ribavirin a critical part of HCV protease therapy but that the initial dose of ribavirin is also important. In addition, Kwo and colleagues demonstrated that longer duration of therapy (48 weeks) was most important for patients who failed to achieve an undetectable HCV RNA level after

4 weeks of boceprevir (4 and 8 weeks total therapy in the no-lead-in and lead-in groups, respectively). Boceprevir was associated with increased anaemia (necessitating epoetin alfa) compared with placebo, as well as gastrointestinal side effects.

Future steps forward: combination therapy with multiple direct-acting antivirals

Can the role of interferon in the treatment of HCV infection be replaced by the use of other agents? The answer to this question is not known but is critical to the future applicability of HCV therapies. Interferon alfa has several unique advantages in the treatment of HCV, including the absence of viral resistance and infrequent delivery (weekly or biweekly). However, there is considerable variability in responsiveness to interferon alfa among HCV genotype 1-infected patients. Recently, Ge *et al.* found that genetic polymorphism near the *IL28B* gene, encoding interferon-3, is associated with an approximately twofold change in response to treatment with peginterferon/ribavirin. This observation suggests that the selection of interferon in future HCV treatment regimens may be based, in part, on the responsiveness of the patient. Further studies will be needed to evaluate this concept.

At present, no study has demonstrated the eradication of chronic HCV in the absence of interferon therapy. However, Gane *et al.* reported that the combination of an HCV protease, R7227, and HCV nucleoside analogue polymerase inhibitor, R7128, effectively inhibited HCV replication in genotype 1-infected patients treated with combination therapy for 7 or 14 days (Table 43.3). The most important finding was robust viral suppression without evidence of virological breakthrough over the short dosing period.

TABLE 43.3 Preliminary results of the INFORM-1 study of combination HCV protease and polymerase inhibitors.

Cohort	Experimental regimen	HCV RNA change
A	R7128 500 mg orally twice daily/R7227 100 mg orally every 8 hours for 7 days	Mean -3.0 (0.8) $\log_{10}$ IU/mL
B	R7128 500 mg orally twice daily/R7227 100 mg orally every 8 hours for 14 days	Mean -3.9 (0.8) $\log_{10}$ IU/mL
C	R7128 1000 mg orally twice daily/R7227 100 mg orally every 8 hours for 14 days R7128 500 mg orally twice daily/R7227 200 mg orally every 8 hours for 14 days	Range -5.0 to -2.9 One patient < 15 IU/mL at day 14

Nonetheless, these data are preliminary and a substantial amount of research is needed to understand the potential for interferon-sparing regimens.

Summary

The treatment of HCV infection is poised to rapidly evolve over the next 3–7 years, leading to higher SVR rates and, perhaps, shorter duration of treatment. The first advance will be the addition of HCV protease inhibitors to the backbone of peginterferon alfa and ribavirin. Phase II studies of both boceprevir and telaprevir have demonstrated conclusively that interferon and ribavirin are critical components of these regimens. Advances beyond these triple-therapy regimens are less clear but multiple direct-acting antiviral agents are in clinical development and studies of combinations are underway. The key question to be answered is whether interferon is needed to eradicate HCV. This is expected to be answered through carefully designed randomized controlled trials over the next several years.

References

1. Lohmann V, Korner F, Koch J, Herian U, Theilmann L, Bartenschlager R. Replication of subgenomic hepatitis C virus RNAs in a hepatoma cell line. *Science* 1999;285:110–113.

2. Wakita T, Pietschmann T, Kato T *et al.* Production of infectious hepatitis C virus in tissue culture from a cloned viral genome. *Nature Medicine* 2005;11:791–796.

3. McHutchison JG, Bartenschlager R, Patel K, Pawlotsky JM. The face of future hepatitis C antiviral drug development: recent biological and virologic advances and their translation to drug development and clinical practice. *Journal of Hepatology* 2006;44:411–421. **Outstanding overview of the virus and challenges in HCV drug development.** 🔑

4. Reesink HW, Zeuzem S, Weegink CJ *et al.* Rapid decline of viral RNA in hepatitis C patients treated with VX-950: a Phase Ib, placebo-controlled, randomized study. *Gastroenterology* 2006;131:997–1002.

5. Kieffer TL, Sarrazin C, Miller JS *et al.* Telaprevir and pegylated interferon-alpha-2a inhibit wild-type and resistant genotype 1 hepatitis C virus replication in patients. *Hepatology* 2007;46:631–639. **This study provides a snapshot of the issue of pre-existing HCV variants with decreased susceptibility to telaprevir and their potential emergence during treatment as well as the role of interferon in preventing their emergence.** 🔑

6. McHutchison JG, Everson GT, Gordon SC *et al.* Telaprevir with peginterferon and ribavirin for chronic HCV genotype 1 infection. *New England Journal of Medicine* 2009;360:1827–1838.

7. Hézode C, Forestier N, Dusheiko G *et al.* Telaprevir and peginterferon with or without ribavirin for chronic HCV infection. *New England Journal of Medicine* 2009;360:1839–1850. **This study demonstrates the role of ribavirin in combination with peginterferon and telaprevir, resulting in substantially higher SVR rates and lower rate of virological breakthrough and relapse.** 🔑

8. Mederacke I, Wedemeyer H, Manns MP. Boceprevir, an NS3 serine protease inhibitor of hepatitis C virus, for the treatment of HCV infection. *Current Opinion in Investigational Drugs* 2009;10:181–189.

9. Kwo P, Lawitz E, McCone J *et al.* HCV SPRINT-1 final results: SVR 24 from a phase 2 study of boceprevir plus peginterferon alfa-2b/ribavirin in treatment-naive subjects with genotype-1 chronic hepatitis C. *Journal of Hepatology* 2009;50(Suppl 1):S4.

10. Ge D, Fellay J, Thompson AJ, *et al.* Nature. 2009 Sep 17;461(7262):399–401. Epub 2009 Aug 16. PMID: 19684573.

11. Gane EJ, Roberts SK, Steadman CA, *et al.* 'Combination Therapy with a Nucleoside Polymerase (RG7128) and Protease (RG7227/ITMN-191) Inhibitor Combination in HCV: Safety, Pharmacokinetics, and Virologic Results from INFORM-1,' Abstract #193: to be presented at the Meeting of the American Association for the Study of Liver Diseases (AASLD) in Boston, Massachusetts, October 30–November 3, 2009.

44 Protease and polymerase inhibitors for HCV

Christoph Sarrazin

J.W. Goethe-University Hospital, Medizinische Klinik 1, Frankfurt am Main, Germany

LEARNING POINTS

- A large number of direct-acting, highly potent antiviral drugs for HCV infection are in Phase I–III clinical development.

- The new drugs have been shown to inhibit HCV replication within a few days and are associated with effective suppression of viral replication.

- However, the new drugs are associated with the development of antiviral resistance and new additional side effects.

- Combination therapies with HCV NS3 protease inhibitors (telaprevir, boceprevir) with pegylated interferons and ribavirin are currently in Phase III development and it is probable that a new standard of care for treatment-naive genotype 1 patients and probably also genotype 1 relapsers and non-responders will be established shortly and will involve triple therapy consisting of telaprevir/boceprevir in combination with peginterferon and ribavirin. Using this approach, high sustained virological response rates together with significantly shortened treatment durations in many patients are likely to be achieved.

Introduction

Detailed knowledge of the hepatitis C virus (HCV) life cycle and of the structure of HCV proteins, obtained by replicative cell culture systems and crystallographic analysis in recent years, has enabled the development of many promising so-called STAT-C (specifically targeted antiviral therapy for hepatitis C) compounds. Several direct-acting antiviral

Clinical Dilemmas in Viral Liver Disease, 1st edition. Edited by Graham R. Foster and K. Rajender Reddy. © 2010 Blackwell Publishing.

drugs targeting different non-structural HCV proteins (NS3/4A protease, NS5A protein, NS5B RNA-dependent RNA-polymerase) are currently in Phase I–III development (Table 44.1).

Protease inhibitors

Several peptidomimetic inhibitors targeting the active site of the NS3/4A serine protease are currently in clinical trials. Telaprevir and boceprevir are linear tetrapeptide ketoamide derivatives, while ciluprevir, ITMN-191, TMC435350, MK7009 and BI201335 have a macrocyclic structure. Drugs targeting other sites on the surface of the NS3/4A protease have been designed and investigated in preclinical and Phase I studies (i.e. ACH-806, NS4A antagonist) but currently none of these drugs have progressed to Phase II clinical studies.

Monotherapy with protease inhibitors

Phase I studies with protease inhibitors used in isolation showed a sharp initial decline of HCV RNA levels up to approximately 4 $\log_{10}$ within 1–2 weeks [1–3]. In comparison the mean decline of HCV RNA concentration with a peginterferon after 2 weeks is approximately 1 $\log_{10}$ IU/mL [4]. However, because of the high replication rate of HCV and the poor fidelity of its RNA-dependent RNA polymerase, numerous variants (quasi-species) are continuously produced during HCV replication. Among them, variants carrying mutations that alter the conformation of the binding sites of STAT-C compounds can allow development of impaired binding of the specific inhibitor. During treatment with antiviral drugs, these typically occur at low levels and these pre-existing drug-resistant variants have a fitness advantage and can be rapidly selected to become the dominant viral quasi-species. Indeed, during monotherapy

TABLE 44.1 Direct-acting antiviral drugs for HCV in development.

Drug name	Company	Target/active drug	Study phase
NS3/4A protease inhibitors			
Ciluprevir (BILN 2061)	Boehringer Ingelheim	Active site/macrocyclic inhibitor	Stopped
Telaprevir (VX-950)	Vertex	Active site/ketoamide inhibitor	Phase III
Boceprevir (SCH503034)	Schering-Plough	Active site/ketoamide inhibitor	Phase III
TMC435350	Tibotec/Medivir	Active site/macrocyclic inhibitor	Phase II
ITMN-191/R7227	InterMune/Roche	Active site/macrocyclic inhibitor	Phase II
MK-7009	Merck	Active site/macrocyclic inhibitor	Phase II
BI201335	Boehringer Ingelheim	Active site/macrocyclic inhibitor?	Phase II
Nucleoside analogue NS5B polymerase inhibitors			
Valopicitabine (NM283)	Idenix/Novartis	NM107, 3'-val-2'-methylcytidine	Stopped
R7128	Roche/Pharmaset	PSI-6130, 2'-deoxy-2'-fluoro-2'-methylcytidine	Phase II
R1626	Roche	R1479, 4'-azidocytidine	Stopped
Non-nucleoside NS5B polymerase inhibitors			
HCV-796	ViroPharma/Wyeth	Palm 2/benzofuran site inhibitor	Stopped
BILB 1941	Boehringer Ingelheim	Thumb 1/benzimidazole site inhibitor	Stopped
Filibuvir (PF-00868554)	Pfizer	Thumb site inhibitor	Phase II
GS-9190	Gilead	Thumb 1/benzimidazole site inhibitor	Phase I
VCH-759	ViroChem Pharma	Thumb 2/thiophene site inhibitor	Phase II
ANA598	Anadys	Palm site inhibitor	Phase I
NS5A inhibitor			
BMS-790052	Bristol-Myers Squibb	NS5A domain 1 inhibitor	Phase I

with telaprevir and boceprevir, selection of resistant variants with increasing HCV RNA levels despite continued treatment with the inhibitor has been observed within a very few days of therapy [5,6]. Several mutations within the NS3 protease present at different frequencies within the HCV quasi-species and displaying different levels of resistance and replicative fitness have been described by clonal genotypic and replicon-based phenotypic resistance analysis [5–7]. Together with *in vitro* analyses, different but overlapping resistance profiles for the current first-generation NS3 protease inhibitors have been described [5–8] and these include mutations at position R155 within the NS3 protease that seem to be associated with resistance to all protease inhibitors currently in clinical development (Figure 44.1). Detailed clonal sequence analysis for characterization of genotypic resistance in these Phase I monotherapy studies is important but has not yet been presented for all compounds in clinical studies. Interestingly, the R155K resistance mutation has been detected in 0.7% of patients with chronic HCV genotype 1 infection as the dominant variant before initiation of treatment and this was associated with reduced response and breakthrough during subsequent therapy with telaprevir in combination with peginterferon and ribavirin [9].

Combination therapy with peginterferon

To overcome the resistance problems during monotherapy and to investigate a potential additive or even synergistic antiviral activity, combination therapy with protease inhibitors and peginterferon alfa have been initiated. *In vitro* studies have shown that variants harbouring resistant mutations to NS3 protease inhibitors are fully sensitive to interferon alfa [10]. In a clinical Phase I study, a continuous decline in HCV RNA concentrations without viral breakthrough during 14 days of combination therapy with telaprevir and peginterferon alfa-2a was observed. Furthermore, antiviral efficacy seems to be at least additive, with a maximum decline of 5.5 $\log_{10}$ for the combination treatment [4]. A proof of principle study showed the possibility of overcoming previous virological non-response to interferon alfa-based treatment regimens at least in part by combination therapy with boceprevir and peginterferon alfa-2b [3]. However, in a subsequent Phase II trial with longer durations of therapy, up to 24% of patients receiving combination therapy with telaprevir and peginterferon alfa-2a experienced a breakthrough with resistant variants. In addition, high relapse rates (48%) for such a combination treatment schedule was observed [11,12].

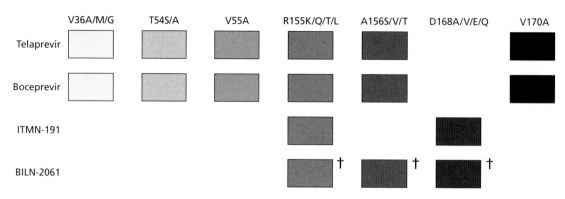

FIG. 44.1 Cross-resistance between different protease inhibitors. † Mutations associated with *in vitro* resistance.

Triple therapy with peginterferon and ribavirin

Because of the problems of monotherapy and combination therapy described above, triple-therapy regimens involving protease inhibitors and peginterferon/ribavirin currently represent the preferred approach for improving treatment outcome in chronic hepatitis C. Telaprevir and boceprevir are currently in Phase III clinical trials and the results of Phase II studies have been presented.

Telaprevir, Phase II, naive patients

Triple therapy of telaprevir with peginterferon alfa-2a and ribavirin for 12 weeks followed by another 12 weeks with combination therapy of peginterferon alfa-2a and ribavirin resulted in a sustained virological response (SVR) rate of 61% and 69% in two studies (PROVE 1 and 2) performed in the USA and Europe in naive genotype 1-infected patients, respectively [11,12]. For the control arms treated with peginterferon alfa-2a and ribavirin for 48 weeks, SVR rates of 41% and 46% were observed. Thus, the triple-therapy approach shortened overall treatment duration from 48 to 24 weeks and achieved an approximately 20% increase in SVR. However, patients without a rapid virological response (HCV RNA undetectable, i.e. < 10 IU/mL at week 4) followed by a complete early virological response (HCV RNA undetectable at week 12) showed relatively high relapse rates after 24 weeks of treatment (42% in the PROVE 2 study), which were reduced by extending treatment to 36 weeks' combination therapy after triple therapy for 12 weeks (PROVE 1 study) [11,12]. Resistance ($\geq 1 \log_{10}$ increase in HCV RNA from nadir or positive HCV RNA ≥ 100 IU/mL in previously negative patients) was observed in 3–7% of patients in the triple-therapy arms. Thus, the addition of ribavirin not only improved treatment response

and relapse rates but also significantly reduced the frequency of development of resistance.

Boceprevir, Phase II, naive patients

An international study in the USA and Europe tested triple therapy with boceprevir, peginterferon alfa-2b and ribavirin in naive patients with genotype 1 chronic HCV for 28 or 48 weeks, with or without an initial lead-in phase for peginterferon alfa-2b and ribavirin alone. In contrast to the studies with telaprevir, treatment with boceprevir was not restricted to 12 weeks' duration but was administered throughout the entire course of therapy. Resistance with breakthrough of HCV RNA levels ($\geq 2 \log_{10}$ increase from nadir and $\geq 50\,000$ IU/mL) was observed in 4–11% of patients. After 28 and 48 weeks, SVR rates of 55–56% and 66–75%, respectively, were reported. Comparable to the trials with telaprevir, patients with rapid virological response benefited most from shortened treatment duration of 28 weeks with SVR rates of 74–82% [14]. Therefore, for both telaprevir and boceprevir, in the ongoing Phase III studies only patients with a rapid virological response will have a shortened overall treatment duration of 24–28 weeks and this approach is likely to dominate future studies.

Telaprevir and boceprevir, Phase II,
non-responders/relapsers

In the first Phase II study with different doses and durations of triple therapy comprising boceprevir, peginterferon alfa-2b and ribavirin in patients who previously did not respond to peginterferon and ribavirin, a maximum SVR of 14% compared with 2% in the control arm was reported [15]. Final analysis of a study of triple therapy comprising telaprevir, peginterferon alfa-2a and ribavirin for 12 or 24 weeks followed by peginterferon and ribavirin for another 12 or 24 weeks revealed promising SVR rates of 38–39% for previous non-responders and 69–76% for previous relapsers. In the control arm receiving combination therapy comprising peginterferon alfa-2a and ribavirin for 48 weeks, SVR rates of 9% for non-responders and 20% for relapsers were achieved [13].

Polymerase inhibitors

Several nucleoside inhibitors targeting the active site of the HCV polymerase as well as non-nucleoside inhibitors binding to different allosteric sites of the RNA-dependent RNA polymerase of HCV have been developed (Table 44.1).

Nucleoside analogues
Valopicitabine

Valopicitabine (NM283), a prodrug of 3′-val-2′-C-methylcytidine (NM107), was the first nucleoside inhibitor of the NS5B polymerase tested in clinical studies. Monotherapy with valopicitabine for 14 days induced HCV RNA decline of up to 1.2 $\log_{10}$ IU/mL in genotype 1-infected patients but nausea and vomiting were observed with the higher doses (400–800 mg daily) [16]. Phase IIb trials in naive and experienced genotype 1-infected patients in combination with peginterferon showed an additive effect, but higher doses (800 mg daily) were not tolerated and dose reductions to 200–400 mg daily were required due to severe gastrointestinal side effects. SVR rates were not superior in comparison with the standard of care [17]. Moreover, *in vitro* studies stated a potential antagonistic effect of ribavirin on the activity of NM107 [18]. Therefore, further development of valopicitabine was stopped.

R1626

The second orally available nucleoside inhibitor to be reported in clinical trials was R1626, the prodrug of R1479 (4′-azidocytidine). A Phase I study in genotype 1-infected patients showed mean viral load reductions of 0.3–3.7 $\log_{10}$ at the end of a 14-day dosing period using medium to high doses of R1626 (500–4500 mg twice daily) [19]. Because of increasing side effects in a subsequent Phase IIa study, treatment-naive genotype 1 patients received lower doses of R1626 (1500 and 3000 mg twice daily) in combination with peginterferon and ribavirin for 4 weeks. Patients treated with triple therapy achieved a significantly higher HCV RNA decline after 4 weeks than those who received the combination of R1626 (1500 mg) and peginterferon alfa-2a only (HCV RNA 5.2 vs. 3.6 $\log_{10}$ IU/mL). However, grade 4 neutropenia ($< 500 \times 10^6$/L) was observed in 39–78% of patients who received peginterferon alfa-2a in combination with R1626 with and without ribavirin [20]. Because of severe infectious disease adverse events in a subsequent Phase IIb study, further development of R1626 was stopped.

R7128

R7128 is the oral prodrug of the nucleoside inhibitor PSI-6130 (2′-doxy-2′-fluoro-2′-C-methylcytidine). Monotherapy with different doses of R7128 for 14 days was well tolerated and showed HCV RNA declines of 0.9–2.7 $\log_{10}$ with no viral rebound during therapy [21]. *In vitro*, different resistant variants for PSI-6130 (S282T) and R1479 (S96T, S96T/N142T) were selected and cross-resistance was excluded [22]. In a subsequent Phase IIa trial, treatment-naive genotype 1-infected patients were treated with R7128 500 or 1500 mg twice daily in combination with peginterferon alfa-2a and ribavirin for 4 weeks. With the higher dose of R7128, after 4 weeks 85% of the patients had undetectable HCV RNA (< 15 IU/mL) [23]. In addition, R7128 was investigated in genotype 2- and 3-infected patients with non-response or relapse to prior peginterferon alfa/ribavirin therapy. Also in this study, 90% of patients achieved a rapid virological response with undetectable HCV RNA after 4 weeks of triple therapy [24]. Further studies with R7128 are ongoing.

Non-nucleoside inhibitors

At least four different allosteric binding sites, named thumb 1/2 and palm 1/2, have been identified as suitable for inhibition of the NS5B polymerase by non-nucleoside inhibitors (Table 44.1).

BILB1941

Increasing oral doses of BILB1941 three times daily for 5 days were given to genotype 1-infected patients with chronic HCV in a Phase Ib study [25]. A significant antiviral response was observed but the trial was discontinued due to gastrointestinal intolerance.

GS9190

Single doses of GS9190 led to a decline in HCV RNA levels by a maximum of 2.5 $\log_{10}$ IU/mL at 24 hours in chronic HCV genotype 1-infected treatment-naive patients. The drug was well tolerated and multiple dosing studies were initiated [26].

VCH-759

Treatment-naive HCV genotype 1-infected patients received different doses of VCH-759 two or three time daily for 10 days. A mean maximum decline of 2.5 $\log_{10}$ at the end of treatment was observed with the highest dose and the drug was well tolerated [27]. Subsequent studies with VCH-759 have not been presented yet.

Filibuvir (PF-00868554)

A Phase I study in treatment-naive HCV genotype 1-infected patients treated with filibuvir for 8 days showed mean maximum viral reductions of 0.97–2.13 $\log_{10}$. Filibuvir was administered two or three time daily at different doses and only mild or moderate adverse events (flatulence, headache and fatigue) were reported [28]. A Phase II study of triple therapy comprising filibuvir, peginterferon alfa-2a and ribavirin has been initiated.

HCV-796

Monotherapy with increasing doses of HCV-796 for 14 days led to a maximum decline in HCV RNA concentrations of 1.5 $\log_{10}$ IU/mL. In a subsequent study HCV-796 was combined with peginterferon alfa-2a/2b. Maximum viral load reductions of 3.2 $\log_{10}$ IU/mL in genotype 1-infected patients and 4.8 $\log_{10}$ IU/mL in genotype 2/3-infected patients were observed after 14 days. The further clinical development of HCV-796 was halted due to liver enzyme elevation in some patients after 8–10 weeks of dosing in the Phase II studies [29].

Resistance

Selection of resistant variants is one of the major problems with the new direct-acting antiviral drugs. For monotherapy with protease inhibitors and non-nucleoside polymerase inhibitors, rapid selection of resistant variants has been demonstrated, whereas nucleoside analogues seem to have a higher genetic barrier to resistance [5–7,19,20,23,26,30]. These resistant variants either occur as normal variants in different subtypes of the virus (0.7% of patients treated with telaprevir have the R155K resistance mutation within the NS3 protease) or occur by chance at low or medium levels because of high viral turnover and error-prone replication of the virus (C316N for example is the predominant variant in the NS5B polymerase of natural genotype 1b isolates and confers resistance to HCV-796) [9,31].

Combination therapy with peginterferon and ribavirin has been shown to reduce the likelihood of resistance developing to protease and non-nucleoside polymerase inhibitors. However, even using triple therapy with protease inhibitors, a significant number of patients experience breakthrough in association with selection of drug-resistant variants (3–11%) [11,13,14]. Furthermore, resistant variants have been detected in patients with relapse after the end of treatment. In these patients, the frequency of resistant variants generally tends to decline during further follow-up after the end of treatment [7]. However, in single patients, even after 3 years, a significant number of different resistant variants have been detected [32].

Another possibility for avoiding the selection of resistant variants followed by viral breakthrough involves combination regimens with direct antiviral drugs only. Studies in the HCV replicon *in vitro* model as well as in chimpanzees have shown the high potential of combination treatment with protease and polymerase inhibitors to eradicate the virus; recently, the first clinical study of the combination of R7128 and ITMN191 has been initiated (INFORM-1 study). In this study patients were treated for up to 14 days with both direct antiviral compounds and no severe adverse events were observed. Moreover, a maximum HCV RNA decline of 5.2 $\log_{10}$ was observed at the end of treatment without any viral breakthrough [33].

References

1. Hinrichsen H, Benhamou Y, Wedemeyer H *et al*. Short-term antiviral efficacy of BILN 2061, a hepatitis C virus serine protease inhibitor, in hepatitis C genotype 1 patients. *Gastroenterology* 2004;127:1347–1355. **Early clinical studies with a first-generation protease inhibitor.** ☞

2. Reesink HW, Zeuzem S, Weegink CJ *et al*. Rapid decline of viral RNA in hepatitis C patients treated with VX-950: a phase Ib, placebo-controlled, randomized study. *Gastroenterology* 2006;131:997–1002.

3. Sarrazin C, Rouzier R, Wagner F *et al*. SCH 503034, a novel hepatitis C virus protease inhibitor, plus pegylated interferon alpha-2b for genotype 1 nonresponders. *Gastroenterology* 2007;132:1270–1278.

4. Forestier N, Reesink HW, Weegink CJ *et al*. Antiviral activity of telaprevir (VX-950) and peginterferon alfa-2a in patients with hepatitis C. *Hepatology* 2007;46:640–648.

5. Sarrazin C, Kieffer TL, Bartels D *et al*. Dynamic hepatitis C virus genotypic and phenotypic changes in patients treated with the protease inhibitor telaprevir. *Gastroenterology* 2007;132:1767–1777. **An important study illustrating the problems associated with resistance.** ☞

6. Susser S, Welsch C, Wang Y *et al.* Characterization of resistance to the protease inhibitor boceprevir in hepatitis C virus infected patients. *Hepatology* 2009;50:1709–1718.

7. Kieffer TL, Sarrazin C, Miller JS *et al.* Telaprevir and pegylated interferon-alpha-2a inhibit wild-type and resistant genotype 1 hepatitis C virus replication in patients. *Hepatology* 2007; 46:631–639.

8. He Y, King MS, Kempf DJ *et al.* Relative replication capacity and selective advantage profiles of protease inhibitor-resistant hepatitis C virus (HCV) NS3 protease mutants in the HCV genotype 1b replicon system. *Antimicrobial Agents and Chemotherapy* 2008;52:1101–1110.

9. Bartels DJ, Zhou Y, Zhang EZ *et al.* Natural prevalence of hepatitis C virus variants with decreased sensitivity to NS3.4A protease inhibitors in treatment-naive subjects. *Journal of Infectious Diseases* 2008;198:800–807.

10. Lin K, Perni RB, Kwong AD, Lin C. VX-950, a novel hepatitis C virus (HCV) NS3-4A protease inhibitor, exhibits potent antiviral activities in HCV replicon cells. *Antimicrobial Agents and Chemotherapy* 2006;50:1813–1822.

11. Hezode C, Forestier N, Dusheiko G *et al.* Telaprevir and peginterferon with or without ribavirin for chronic HCV infection. *New England Journal of Medicine* 2009;360:1839–1850.

12. McHutchison JG, Everson GT, Gordon SC *et al.* Telaprevir with peginterferon and ribavirin for chronic HCV genotype 1 infection. *New England Journal of Medicine* 2009;360:1827–1838.

13. Manns M, Muir A, Adda N *et al.* Telaprevir in hepatitis C genotype-1-infected patients with prior non-response, viral braekthrough or relapse to peginterferon-alfa-2a/b and ribavirin therapy: SVR results of the PROVE3 study. *Journal of Hepatology* 2009;50(Suppl 1):S379.

14. Kwo P, Lawitz E, McCone J *et al.* HCV SPRINT-1 final results: SVR 24 from a phase 2 study of boceprevir plus peginterferon alfa-2b/ribavirin in treatment-naive subjects with genotype-1 chronic hepatitis C. *Journal of Hepatology* 2009;50(Suppl 1):S4.

15. Schiff E, Poordard F, Jacobson I *et al.* Boceprevir combination therapy in null responders: response dependent on interferon responsiveness. *Journal of Hepatology* 2008;48 (Suppl 2):46A.

16. Afdhal N, Godofsky E, Dienstag J *et al.* Final phase I/II trial results for NM283, a new polymerase inhibitor for hepatitis C: antiviral efficacy and tolerance in patients with HCV-1 infection, including previous interferon failures. *Hepatology* 2004;40(Suppl 1):726A.

17. Lawitz E, Nguyen T, Younes Z *et al.* Clearance of HCV RNA with valopicitabine (NM283) plus PEG-inteferon in treatment-naive patients with HCV-1 infection: results at 24 and 48 weeks. *Journal of Hepatology* 2007;46(Suppl 1):9A.

18. Coelmont L, Paeshuyse J, Windisch MP, De Clercq E, Bartenschlager R, Neyts J. Ribavirin antagonizes the in vitro anti-hepatitis C virus activity of 2′-C-methylcytidine, the active component of valopicitabine. *Antimicrobial Agents and Chemotherapy* 2006;50:3444–3446.

19. Roberts SK, Cooksley G, Dore GJ *et al.* Robust antiviral activity of R1626, a novel nucleoside analog: a randomized, placebo-controlled study in patients with chronic hepatitis C. *Hepatology* 2008;48:398–406.

20. Pockros PJ, Nelson D, Godofsky E *et al.* R1626 plus peginterferon alfa-2a provides potent suppression of hepatitis C virus RNA and significant antiviral synergy in combination with ribavirin. *Hepatology* 2008;48:385–397.

21. Reddy R, Rodriguez-Torres M, Gane E *et al.* Antiviral activity, pharmacokinetics, safety and tolerability of R7128, a novel nucleoside HCV RNA polymerase inhibitor, following multiple, ascending, oral doses in patients with HCV genotype 1 infection who have failed prior interferon therapy. *Hepatology* 2007;46(Suppl):862A–863A.

22. Ali S, Leveque V, Le Pogam S *et al.* Selected replicon variants with low level in vitro resistance to the hepatitis C virus NS5B polymerase inhibitor PSI-6130 lack cross-resistance with R1479. *Antimicrobial Agents and Chemotherapy* 2008;52:4356–4369.

23. Lalezari J, Gane E, Rodriguez-Torres M *et al.* Potent antiviral activity of the HCV nucleoside polymerase inhibitor R7128 with PEG-IFN and ribavirin: interim results of R7128 500mg BID for 28 days. *Journal of Hepatology* 2008;48(Suppl 2):29A.

24. Gane EJ, Rodriguez-Torres M, Nelson DR *et al.* Antiviral acitivity of the nucleoside polymerase inhibitor R7128 in HCV genotype 2 and 3 prior non-responders: interim results of R7128 1500 mg BID with peg-IFN and ribavirin for 28 days. *Hepatology* 2008;48(Suppl):1024A.

25. Erhardt A, Wedemeyer H, Benhamou Y *et al.* Safety, phamacokinetics and antiviral effect of BILB1941, a novel HCV RNA polymerase inhibitor, after 5 days oral treatment in patients with chronic hepatitis C. *Journal of Hepatology* 2007;46 (Suppl 1):222A.

26. Bavisotto L, Wang CC, Jacobson IM *et al.* Antiviral, pharmacokinetic and safety data for GS-9190, a non-nucleoside HCV NS5B polymerase inhibitor in a phase-1 trial in HCV genotype 1 infected subjects. *Hepatology* 2007;46(Suppl 1):255A.

27. Cooper C, Lawitz EJ, Ghali P *et al.* Antiviral activity of the non-nucleoside polymerase inhibitor VCH-759 in chronic hepatitis C patients: results from a randomized, double-blind, placebo-controlled, ascending multiple dose study. *Hepatology* 2007;46(Suppl):864A.

28. Hammond JL, Rosario MC, Wagner F *et al.* Antiviral activity of the HCV polymerase inhibitor PF-00868554 administered as monotherapy in HCV genotype 1 infected subjects. *Hepatology* 2008;48(Suppl):1024A–1025A.

29. Villano S, Raible D, Harper D, Chandra P, Bazisotto L, Bichier G. Phase 1 evaluation of antiviral activity of the non-nucleoside polymerase inhibitor HCV-796 in combination with different pegylated interferons in treatment-naive patients with chronic HCV. *Hepatology* 2007;46(Suppl 1):815A.

30. McCown MF, Rajyaguru S, Le Pogam S *et al.* The hepatitis C virus replicon presents a higher barrier to resistance to nucleoside analogs than to nonnucleoside polymerase or protease inhibitors. *Antimicrobial Agents and Chemotherapy* 2008;52:1604–1612.

31. Le Pogam S, Seshaadri A, Kosaka A *et al.* Existence of hepatitis C virus NS5B variants naturally resistant to non-nucleoside, but not to nucleoside, polymerase inhibitors among untreated patients. *Journal of Antimicrobial Chemotherapy* 2008;61: 1205–1216.

32. Forestier N, Susser S, Welker MW, Karey U, Zeuzem S, Sarrazin C. Long term follow-up of patients previously treated with telaprevir. *Hepatology* 2008;48(Suppl):760A.

33. Gane EJ, Roberts SK, Stedman C *et al.* First-in-man demonstration of potent antiviral activity with a nucleoside polymerase (R7128) and protease (R7227/ITMN-191) inhibitor combination in HCV: safety, pharmacokinetics, and virologic results from INFORM-1. *Journal of Hepatology* 2009;50 (Suppl 1):S380.

45 HCV vaccines: coming soon?

David E. Kaplan

Philadelphia Veterans Affairs Medical Center; and Gastroenterology Division, Department of Medicine, University of Pennsylvania School of Medicine, Philadelphia, Pennsylvania, USA

LEARNING POINTS

- HCV viruses are markedly heterogeneous both within and between individuals, a situation that significantly complicates vaccine development.

- HCV entry into hepatocytes requires binding of viral envelope E1/E2 heterodimers to multiple cellular receptors including but not limited to CD81, scavenger receptor B-I and claudin-1. Inhibition of binding of E1/E2 to these receptors could be considered as a vaccine strategy but hypervariability of the virus and virion shielding by lipoproteins may be barriers to development of effective neutralizing antibodies.

- Multiple immunoinhibitory pathways including regulatory T cells, inhibitory costimulation and impaired antigen presentation are induced by HCV in chronic infection, all of which must be considered when designing cellular vaccines.

Introduction

Hepatitis C virus (HCV) infection affects approximately 3% of the world's population including an estimated 2.9 million persons in the USA. While antiviral therapy within the first 2 years of exposure may cure more than 80% of identified acute infections, the impact of early therapy remains limited because the majority of cases are asymptomatic, unrecognized and/or untreated due to lack of medication access or contraindications. Chronic infection and associated chronic hepatitis progress to cirrhosis, often associated with hepatocellular carcinoma, in up to 30% of infected persons

Clinical Dilemmas in Viral Liver Disease, 1st edition. Edited by Graham R. Foster and K. Rajender Reddy. © 2010 Blackwell Publishing.

usually after two to four decades. Antiviral therapy for established chronic infection is associated with suboptimal efficacy, significant morbidity and limited applicability. Thus, preventive or therapeutic vaccine-based therapies hold great promise for significantly ameliorating the burden of HCV disease. However, despite great success with vaccines for other hepatitis and RNA viruses, a vaccine for HCV remains elusive. This chapter reviews the critical factors complicating vaccine development and recent progress.

Factors complicating vaccine development

HCV is an enveloped 9.5-kb ssRNA(+) virus of the *Flaviviridae* family. The most salient virological characteristic of HCV detrimental to vaccine development is the tremendous sequence heterogeneity of viral strains both among (macroheterogeneity, also called genotypes and subtypes) and within (microheterogeneity, also called quasi-species) infected individuals. As a result of an error-prone, non-proofreading viral RNA polymerase that substitutes an estimated 1 in 10^5 nucleotides per replication cycle, coupled with HCV's massive replication rate estimated at 10^{12} virions per day [1], thousands of escape mutations driven by both immune and non-immune selection pressure rapidly generate a swarm of closely related but diverse viral variants (quasi-species) within individual infected subjects. This potential for extreme viral microheterogeneity within individuals is constrained only by viral fitness losses caused by mutations and by the largely genetically determined repertoire of antiviral T-cell responses within each individual. The adaptation of the virus to relatively homogeneous populations within particular regions in the last two centuries has resulted in the evolution of largely geographically defined genotypes, of which six are currently defined. Viral variants within each genotype may vary at up to 10% of nucleotides but variants of different genotypes may differ at up to 34% of positions [2]. Thus, candidate vaccines must cross-protect against the microheterogeneity and macroheterogeneity of possible infecting strains as well as the capacity for the virus to rapidly develop mutations that confer resistance to immunological control.

Combined with the extreme heterogeneity of HCV strains, several technical factors have hampered vaccine development. Until recently, the lack of cell culture-infectious HCV impaired the study of viral pathogenesis and necessitated the development of useful but artificial systems, such as replicons and pseudoparticles, to study HCV entry and replication. The isolation, identification and characterization of the cell culture-infectious HCV JFH1 strain has overcome many obstacles to the study of basic HCV virology but the lack of easily manipulable, immuno-competent small-animal models for HCV continues to limit the study of complex virus–host interactions relevant to vaccine development. The lack of validated correlates of immunological protection that can be measured in vaccine recipients also remains a major obstacle. Despite these significant hurdles, preclinical work in animals and early human clinical trials for several humoral and cell-mediated vaccine approaches remains active.

Concepts in humoral vaccines

Critical to the development of neutralizing antibody-inducing humoral vaccines is an understanding of the mechanisms of HCV entry into permissive cells. Progress in this field has been rapid due to the development of cell culture-infectious HCV clones such as the initial genotype 2 JFH1 clone as well as various HCV pseudoparticles (HCVpp, retroviruses engineered to express HCV envelope proteins). The HCV E1 and E2 envelope glycoproteins, possibly structured as a trimeric association of E1/E2 heterodimers, are both essential for infectivity and hepatotropism [3]. As evidence of the importance of E2–cellular interactions on the viral life cycle, the hypervariable region (HVR1) of $E2_{384-414}$, whose structure is critical for binding to cellular molecules such as CD81, rapidly evolves to escape potentially neutralizing host antibody responses during natural infections [4]. Critical cellular receptors for HCV infectivity include CD81, scavenger-receptor B member I (SR-BI), claudin-1 (CLDN1) and occludin (OCLN). In addition, the low-density lipoprotein (LDL) receptor and glycosaminoglycans

may also play a role [5] (Figure 45.1). In particular, significant progress has been made in understanding the interaction of the HCV E2 protein and the cellular tetraspannin molecule CD81. CD81-deficient hepatoma cell lines normally impermissive to HCV infection can be rendered permissive by CD81 transduction. Soluble forms of the second extra-cellular loop of CD81 and various anti-CD81 antibodies can block HCV infection *in vitro* and critical binding regions within E2 have been identified [3]. In contrast, the details of envelope protein binding to SR-BI, CLDN1 and OCLN are much less well understood. It has been suggested that viral interactions with SR-BI are not HCV sequence specific but that the interaction with SR-BI may be highly dependent on the type of lipoprotein (LDL, very low density lipoprotein) with which HCV associates in the plasma. CLDN1 and OCLN1 appear to be most important for endocytosis of bound virions [5] at a later stage. Thus, at this time, interruption of envelope protein–CD81 interactions appears to be the most favourable strategy for neutralization antibody-inducing vaccines, with the caveat that recent work suggests that associated lipoprotein circulating with HCV could inhibit E2 glycoprotein binding by neutralizing antibodies [6].

Concepts in cell-mediated vaccines

Antiviral T-cell responses, by both CD4 (helper) and CD8 (cytotoxic) T cells, have been demonstrated in both experimental chimpanzee and natural human infection to be critical for spontaneous resolution of HCV infection, which occurs in a sizable minority of patients with acute HCV infection [7]. Vaccines designed to bolster antiviral T cells have been conceived as either preventive or therapeutic approaches. In preventive strategies, the intent of cell-based approaches is to induce the expansion of naive HCV-epitope-specific CD4 and CD8 T cells to expand and establish a stable pool of memory T cells primed to rapidly respond to an early infection by homing to the liver, secreting antiviral cytokines such as interferon-γ and lysing infected hepatocytes. Therapeutic vaccines aim to reinvigorate impaired antiviral T-cell responses in patients with established chronic infection to induce viral clearance, enhance the effect of other antiviral therapies or attenuate fibrosis progression in the absence of viral clearance. Often protein or DNA-based approaches also induce potential neutralizing antibodies in addition to T-cell responses, an effect which could enhance antiviral effects.

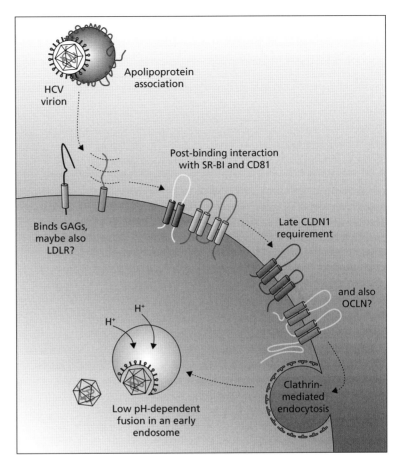

FIG. 45.1 Overview of HCV cell entry. The virion, which circulates in association with lipoprotein complexes, may first bind to hepatocytes via the low-density lipoprotein receptor (LDLR) and glycosaminoglycans (GAGs). Subsequently binding of the E2 protein to cell-surface CD81 and scavenger receptor class B type I (SR-BI), followed later by interaction with the tight junction protein CLDN1 and possibly OCLN, ultimately results in endocytosis of the virion, where it fuses with an endosomal membrane in a pH-dependent process. (From Lanford *et al.* [5] with permission.)

Viral sequence heterogeneity at both the genotype and quasi-species levels is a fundamental obstacle to both preventive and therapeutic vaccine approaches but additional major hurdles in therapeutic vaccination include the myriad of regulatory responses that inhibit antiviral T-cell responses in chronic HCV infection, including but not limited to CD4$^+$CD25$^+$foxp3$^+$ regulatory T cells (Tregs), interleukin (IL)-10-producing T$_R$1 cells, and T-cell exhaustion due to chronic antigen exposure, manifested as expression of the inhibitory costimulatory molecules PD-1 and CTLA-4 [7]. Recent work by several groups has highlighted the importance of PD-1 and CTLA-4 expression on peripheral and intrahepatic HCV-specific T cells, with potential restoration of antiviral effector responses via blockade of one or both of these costimulation pathways [8]. Thus, therapeutic vaccines must not only contend with the variability and mutability of the target sequences but also the capacity of the virus to directly and indirectly inhibit antiviral T-cell effector function.

Vaccine candidates in human trials

In order to address the question of whether an HCV vaccine could be expected soon, the following discussion focuses on the few active immunotherapy programmes that have reached Phase I/II human testing and highlights a few novel approaches. Overall, the experience in human studies has been disappointing but may serve to highlight critical necessary adjustments for future vaccine programmes.

One of the earliest vaccines to enter human clinical trials involved intramuscular administration of alum-adjuvanted recombinant E1 protein (Innogenetics, Gent, Belgium). In early studies, this adjuvanted protein increased anti-E1 antibody levels and modestly boosted anti-E1 T-cell responses in a small cohort of chronic HCV-infected patients [9]. However, development was suspended in 2007 due to unimpressive subsequent clinical trial results.

The next most advanced candidate was IC41 (Intercell AG, Vienna, Austria in collaboration with Novartis, Basel, Switzerland), a vaccine consisting of five synthetic peptides including three HLA-promiscuous CD4 and four HLA-A2-restricted CD8 T-cell epitopes of HCV combined with the synthetic adjuvant poly-L-arginine. In preliminary studies, IC41 induced CD4 and HLA-A2-restricted CD8 T-cell responses in approximately half of uninfected control subjects and in one-third of chronic HCV-infected subjects [10]. However, despite detectable T-cell responses, HCV RNA reductions were infrequent and transient, occurring in fewer than 20% of high-dose vaccine recipients. Furthermore, the vaccine did not appear to significantly improve the phenotype of HCV-specific CD8 T cells [11]. In September 2008, Intercell released preliminary long-term follow-up results of a Phase II study of eight injections of IC41 combined with the Toll-like receptor imiquimod that demonstrated a modest effect on HCV RNA titres, but suggested need to combine future vaccination approaches with other antiviral therapies.

GI-5005 (Globeimmune, Louisville, Colorado), a whole heat-inactivated preparation of *Saccharomyces cerevisiae* engineered to express HCV core and NS3 proteins, also demonstrated modest but sustained reductions in viral titres in a subset of treated patients [12]. However, more recent data suggest that it may be most useful when added to standard interferon-based antiviral therapy in treatment naive patients to improve viral kinetics [13].

Another transgenic viral vaccine, TG4040, a modified vaccinia Ankara expressing genotype 1b core/E1/E2 and NS3 gene sequences, was withdrawn from Phase I/II studies by the its sponsor, Transgene (Lyon, France), apparently after a study in chimpanzees that used the vector for boosting plasmid DNA-primed T-cell responses showed that despite early reductions in HCV RNA titres, three of four chimpanzees progressed to chronic infection when challenged with a related viral strain possessing only 5% sequence difference [14]. Intrahepatic expression of PD-1, CTLA-4 and IDO were shown to correlate closely with failure of the vaccine to improve viral clearance, highlighting the importance of the negative costimulation and T-cell exhaustion in suppression of antiviral T-cell responses.

The first naked DNA-based HCV vaccine to enter Phase I/II clinical trial in humans, ChronVac-C (Tripep, Huddinge, Sweden in collaboration with Inovio, San Diego, California), consists of codon-optimized HCV NS3/4A DNA. Only very early data have been published but show that when 4-monthly injections of 500 µg were injected in three chronic HCV-infected patients, two-thirds mounted HCV-specific T-cell responses that were associated with approximate 1 log viral load reductions [15].

Should an HCV vaccine be developed?

Few studies have addressed the cost-effectiveness of prophylactic or therapeutic vaccines compared with current standard therapy and projected improvements in antiviral therapy anticipated in the near future. One recent study found that a HCV vaccine would only prove cost-effective if it conferred at least 80% efficacy and provided lifelong immunity [16]. No vaccine candidate in development yet approaches this degree of efficacy in any preclinical or clinical study.

TABLE 45.1 Summary of challenges and theoretical approaches to address in future experimental programmes.

Challenge	Theoretical solutions for future study
Microheterogeneity (quasi-species)	Multigenicity, polyvalence, use of consensus sequences
Macroheterogeneity (genotype/subtype variation)	Polyvalence and multigenicity, target E2–CD81 interaction with high affinity/specificity
T-cell exhaustion	Prophylactic rather than therapeutic vaccine, blockade of PD-L1 or CTLA-4, TLR agonism to optimize dendritic cell costimulation
Regulatory T cells	Anti-CD25 monoclonal antibody depletion (e.g. daclizumab, denileukin diftitox), immunostimulatory cytokine therapy (e.g. IL-2, IL-12)
Lack of immunological correlates of immunity in humans	Ongoing human clinical trials

Conclusion: lessons to be learned from early experience

Several lessons can be derived from these early experiences (Table 45.1). First, attempting to boost exhausted or suppressed T cells without concomitantly addressing the mechanisms of exhaustion or suppression is unlikely to yield satisfactory results. Vaccines are more likely to have demonstrable benefit in a prophylactic setting in which antiviral T cells are not yet dysfunctional. Combination of vaccination with blockade of PD-1 and/or CTLA-4 signalling or other strategies to block regulatory T-cell pathways need to be considered. Second, single epitope and/or single genotype vaccines should be expected to be ineffective against heterologous viral challenges. Candidate vaccines should include multiple viral coding regions derived from consensus sequences from several genotypes and/or subtypes to attempt to provide sufficiently broad protection from the myriad of potential strains which vaccinees could harbour or to which they could be exposed. Thirdly, correlates of protective immunity in human subjects need to be more precisely defined and validated. Based on current knowledge, prospects for an HCV vaccine in the near future remain slim. Whether or not HCV vaccines could contribute significantly to clinical care in the era of specifically targeted antiviral therapies for HCV remains unclear.

References

1. Neumann AU, Lam NP, Dahari H *et al.* Hepatitis C viral dynamics in vivo and the antiviral efficacy of interferon-alpha therapy. *Science* 1998;282:103–107.

2. Simmonds P. Variability of hepatitis C virus. *Hepatology* 1995;21:570–583.

3. Stamataki Z, Grove J, Balfe P, McKeating JA. Hepatitis C virus entry and neutralization. *Clinics in Liver Disease* 2008; 12:693–712. **This paper provides a comprehensive up-to-date review of the critical viral entry mechanisms likely to be targeted by prophylactic HCV vaccines.** ⚐

4. Farci P, Shimoda A, Wong D *et al.* Prevention of hepatitis C virus infection in chimpanzees by hyperimmune serum against the hypervariable region 1 of the envelope 2 protein. *Proceedings of the National Academy of Sciences USA* 1996;93: 15394–15399.

5. Lanford RE, Evans MJ, Lohmann V *et al.* The accelerating pace of HCV research: a summary of the 15th International Symposium on Hepatitis C Virus and Related Viruses. *Gastroenterology* 2009;136:9–16.

6. Grove J, Nielsen S, Zhong J *et al.* Identification of a residue in hepatitis C virus E2 glycoprotein that determines scavenger receptor BI and CD81 receptor dependency and sensitivity to neutralizing antibodies. *Journal of Virology* 2008;82:12020–12029.

7. Thimme R, Neumann-Haefelin C, Boettler T, Blum HE. Adaptive immune responses to hepatitis C virus: from viral immunobiology to a vaccine. *Biological Chemistry* 2008;389: 457–467. **Reviews the current understanding of adaptive immune responses against hepatitis C and outlines the myriad suppressive mechanisms that a T-cell-based vaccine must overcome to have potential use in HCV infection.** ⚐

8. Nakamoto N, Kaplan DE, Coleclough J *et al.* Functional restoration of HCV-specific CD8 T cells by PD-1 blockade is defined by PD-1 expression and compartmentalization. *Gastroenterology* 2008;134:1927–1937, 1937e1–e2.

9. Leroux-Roels G, Depla E, Hulstaert F *et al.* A candidate vaccine based on the hepatitis C E1 protein: tolerability and immunogenicity in healthy volunteers. *Vaccine* 2004;22:3080–3086.

10. Klade CS, Wedemeyer H, Berg T *et al.* Therapeutic vaccination of chronic hepatitis C nonresponder patients with the peptide vaccine IC41. *Gastroenterology* 2008;134:1385–1395.

11. Schlaphoff V, Klade CS, Jilma B *et al.* Functional and phenotypic characterization of peptide-vaccine-induced HCV-specific CD8$^+$ T cells in healthy individuals and chronic hepatitis C patients. *Vaccine* 2007;25:6793–6806.

12. Schiff ER, Everson GT, Tsai N *et al.* HCV-specific cellular immunity, RNA reductions, and normalization of ALT in chronic HCV subjects after treatment with GI-5005, a yeast-based immunotherapy targeting NS3 and core: a randomized, double-blind, placebo controlled phase 1b study. *Hepatology* 2007;46(4 Suppl 1):816A.

13. McHutchinson JG, Lawitz EJ, Vierling JM *et al.* GI5005 immunotherapy plus PEG-IFN/ribavirin in genotype 1 chronic hepatitis C patients compared to PEG-IFN/ribavirin alone in naive and non-responder patients: preliminary RVR and viral kinetic analysis from the GI5005-02 Phase 2 study. *Hepatology* 2008;48(4 Suppl 1):1023A–1024A.

14. Rollier CS, Paranhos-Baccala G, Verschoor EJ *et al.* Vaccine-induced early control of hepatitis C virus infection in chimpanzees fails to impact on hepatic PD-1 and chronicity. *Hepatology* 2007;45:602–613.

15. Sallberg M, Diepolder HM, Jung MC *et al.* Antiviral effects of therapeutic vaccination with naked DNA delivered by in vivo electroporation in patients with chronic hepatitis. *Hepatology* 2008;48(4 Suppl 1):1022A–1023A.

16. Massad E, Coutinho FA, Chaib E, Burattini MN. Cost-effectiveness analysis of a hypothetical hepatitis C vaccine compared to antiviral therapy. *Epidemiology and Infection* 2009;137:241–249.

46 New drugs for hepatitis B: what is in the pipeline?

Cihan Yurdaydın, A. Mithat Bozdayı, Ramazan Idilman, Hakan Bozkaya

Department of Gastroenterology, University of Ankara Medical School, Ankara, Turkey

---

LEARNING POINTS

- New drugs currently in development for chronic HBV infection target different aspects of the viral life cycle or the immune response to chronic infection.

- HBV entry inhibitors, viral packaging inhibitors, RNA interference and glucosidase inhibitors are new approaches acting on different molecular targets.

- Several new approaches that aim to augment the immune response have so far produced suboptimal responses, although further efforts in this direction are continuing.

- The concept of liver-targeted drug delivery is a rational approach. Long-term toxicity data of currently available drugs will likely affect future efforts in this direction.

TABLE 46.1 Potential new drugs for the management of chronic HBV infection.

Potential therapies acting at different phases of the HBV life cycle
HBV entry inhibitors
HBV packaging inhibitors
Glucosidase inhibitors
RNA interference
Immunomodulatory approaches
HBV vaccines
Interleukins
Liver-targeted drug delivery
New nucleos(t)ide analogues

Introduction

The arsenal of drugs used to treat chronic infection with hepatitis B virus (HBV) has increased dramatically in the last decade and has favourably affected the natural history of the disease. However, the drawback of the apparent success in the management of hepatitis B is that in many instances treatment needs to be given for an indefinite period and clearance of HBsAg is seldom achieved. Thus, there is still a need for optimization of the management of chronic hepatitis B. A fresh look at the deep involvement of the immune system in the development of chronic infection

and on the life cycle of HBV may provide clues for new drug development (Table 46.1).

Potential therapies acting on different phases of the HBV life cycle

HBV entry inhibitors

The hepatocyte-associated heparin sulphate proteoglycans have been recently identified as attachment receptors for HBV. During cellular attachment, the HBV envelope, consisting of the large (L), middle (M) and small (S) surface proteins, is important. These envelope proteins share the C-terminal S domain and the M and L proteins carry additional N-terminal extensions of 55 and 118 amino acids, designated pre-S2 and pre-S1, respectively. Recent studies have highlighted the importance of the pre-S1 domain within the L HBsAg protein for infectivity of HBV. A myristoyl fatty acid group is bound to glycine at the pre-S1 domain of L protein. The modification of the L surface

Clinical Dilemmas in Viral Liver Disease, 1st edition. Edited by Graham R. Foster and K. Rajender Reddy. © 2010 Blackwell Publishing.

protein by myristoylation and the integrity of the N-terminal 77 amino acids in the pre-S1 domain have been found to be necessary for infectivity of HBV. Eradication of HBV infection with modification of the N-terminal 77 amino acids and the myristoylation step has been shown both *in vitro* and *in vivo* [1]. A Phase I study in humans using HBV entry inhibitors is currently being designed in Germany.

Viral packaging inhibitors

Drugs in development in this category target capsid assembly. The pregenomic RNA (pgRNA) that serves as the template for new virion production has to be first packaged into a nucleocapsid, composed of capsid protein, polymerase and pregenomic RNA. Packaging inhibitors affect the packaging of the pgRNA into nucleocapsids (i.e. they act as allosteric modulators) and exert no effect on viral polymerase. Packaging inhibitors include phenylpropenamide derivatives, such as AT-61 and AT-130, and heteroaryldihydropyrimidines, such as Bay 41-409 and Bay 38-7690 [2,3]. The efficacy of the two latter compounds has been shown both *in vitro* and *in vivo* in a transgenic mouse model and the efficacy of phenylpropenamides has been demonstrated *in vitro*. However, phenylpropenamides are not water soluble and have low bioavailability. Potential toxicity problems need to be overcome for the development of this class of drugs as antiviral agents [3]. On the other hand, heteroaryldihydropyrimidines have been reported to possess a good preclinical pharmacokinetic and toxicology profile [3]. Both classes of drugs have identical antiviral activity against wild-type and drug-resistant HBV.

Glucosidase inhibitors

HBsAg leaves the hepatocyte through the endoplasmic reticulum, where glucosidase enzymes modify the envelope glycoproteins such that these glycoproteins are well suited for appropriate folding and translocation through the endoplasmic reticulum. Glucosidase inhibitors cause misfolding of envelope proteins and thus prevent secretion of virions [4]. Although the use of glucosidase inhibitors seems to be an attractive therapeutic strategy, a serious concern is the possibility that retained HBV envelope proteins may stimulate oncogenic pathways and lead to the development of hepatocellular carcinoma [5].

RNA interference

RNA interference (RNAi), first observed in plants as a natural antiviral defence, is sequence-specific silencing of genes.

Subsequent studies have shown that RNAi is a conserved biological response present in many eukaryotic organisms. It is induced by small molecules of double-stranded RNA (dsRNA). dsRNA-induced gene silencing proceeds via a two-step mechanism. In the first step, the dsRNA is recognized by an RNase III family nuclease called Dicer, which cleaves the dsRNA into small RNA duplexes of 21–23 nucleotides. These small RNA duplexes are called small (or short) interfering RNAs (siRNA). These siRNAs are then incorporated into a multicomponent nuclease complex, the RNA-induced silencing complex (RISC), which identifies substrates through their homology to siRNAs and targets these mRNAs for destruction. Thus, the ability of dsRNA to post-transcriptionally silence gene expression of a gene highly homologues to its own sequence is termed RNAi and Andrew Fire and Craig Mello received the 2006 Nobel Prize for this discovery [6]. The siRNA can target any phase of the life cycle of HBV, although so far efforts have concentrated mostly on inhibition of viral replication.

A disadvantage of siRNAs is that their effects are transient in mammalian cells, persisting no longer than 1 week. Thus ways to circumvent this short-lived effect have been explored. One answer to the problem is short hairpin RNA (shRNA). shRNA is an siRNA production strategy that uses a plasmid or viral vector and involves promoters for continuous shRNA expression. The expressed shRNAs are converted to siRNAs by intracellular processing. Thus, shRNA is processed in the cytoplasm by the cellular machinery into siRNA, which is then bound to RISC. This complex binds and cleaves mRNAs matching the siRNA bound to it.

The antiviral effects of the siRNA and shRNA strategy have been shown in several cell lines *in vitro* and in mice *in vivo*. Several issues such as optimal gene delivery, stability, safety (off-target effects, effect on the innate immune system) and resistance need to be considered for their use in humans. There is anectodal use of shRNA against HBV in humans using a multitargeted RNAi approach to overcome resistance (R. Gish, personal communication).

Immunomodulatory approaches

HBV vaccines

Acute HBV infection is characterized by a vigorous polyclonal and multispecific cytotoxic and helper T-cell response to HBV, whereas these responses are weak or absent in chronic HBV infection. Vaccine therapy aims to eliminate or control HBV infection through induction of a strong

T-cell response. A theoretical concern in vaccine therapy would be that induction of a strong immune response could potentially lead to disease activation which may be deleterious in patients with more advanced liver disease. Several vaccine therapy approaches have been assessed in the recent past, including use of currently available HBV vaccines, a lipopeptide-based T-cell vaccine and DNA vaccines [7]. The latter does not make use of the traditional antigen-based approach but uses plasmid DNA encoding HBV antigens. Thus, antigens are synthesized *in vivo* after introduction of DNA encoding HBV antigens, which apparently prime MHC class I and II T-cell responses with higher potency than conventional vaccine approaches [8].

All these approaches have been tested in humans with limited success. Although a measurable immune response could be obtained in these studies, the overall immune response appears to be still too weak to control HBV infection. The search for optimization of vaccination strategies continues. An example of this is the development of a multiepitope vaccine with selection of a large number of polymerase-derived epitopes, at variance with the use of HBsAg or HBcAg epitopes in previous vaccines. Another potential vaccine development strategy is the use of activated dendritic cells [9]. Although based on a rational theoretical background, vaccine therapy approaches are unlikely to be key players in the management of chronic hepatitis B, at least not in the near future.

Interleukins

Several cytokines that enhance cell-mediated immunity have been tested for the treatment of HBV infection. Among them, interleukin (IL)-12 is a cytokine that promotes cell-mediated immunity by facilitating type 1 helper T-lymphocyte responses, which include secretion of interferon (IFN)-γ from both T and natural killer cells and augmentation of cytolytic T-cell responses. Studies in transgenic mice have shown complete inhibition of HBV replication, mediated most likely through IFN-γ induction. However, the efficacy of IL-12 in human HBV infection, alone or in combination with lamivudine, is limited, despite enhanced T-cell reactivity to HBV and IFN-γ production [10,11]. Similarly, IL-2 and IFN-γ were not efficacious in controlled clinical trials. IL-18, a cytokine promoting cellular immunity in the presence of IL-12, was used in transgenic mice and led to inhibition of HBV replication [12]. In this model, administration of IL-12 and IL-18 in combination had a synergistic antiviral effect. IL-18 has not been tested in humans.

Liver-targeted drug delivery

The concept of site-specific drug delivery aims to increase local drug concentrations and consequently increase efficacy with fewer side effects. In the case of HBV, the aim is to augment liver exposure to the drug. While several approaches can be used, such as site-specific drug carriers like antibodies, peptides and carbohydrate- or peptide-labelled nanoparticles and liposomes capable of recognizing specific proteins expressed on the surface of targeted cells, a strategy tailored to the metabolic pathways of the liver has gained most attention in hepatitis B treatment. Prodrugs metabolized by the cytochrome P450 family of enzymes have been developed for increased liver exposure to drugs such as adefovir and lamivudine. These prodrugs, named HepDirect prodrugs, are cyclic 1,3-propanyl esters containing a ring substrate that renders them sensitive to oxidative cleavage by a cytochrome P450, specifically CYP3A4. The representative prodrug for adefovir is pradefovir. It is metabolically stable and is converted in the liver to adefovir, followed by phosphorylation to the active adefovir diphosphate. This prodrug led to a 12-fold improvement in liver/kidney exposure compared with adefovir dipivoxil, highlighting increased liver and decreased kidney exposure [13]. A Phase II clinical trial with pradefovir treatment for 48 weeks was safe and had significant antiviral activity [14].

Nucleos(t)ide analogues in development

Several nucleos(t)ide analogues are continuing to be developed for possible clinical use in the future; Val-D-cytosine and valtorcitabine, alamifovir and LB80380 are mentioned here briefly.

Valtorcitabine is a prodrug of the nucleos(t)ide analogue Val-D-cytosine. Valtorcitabine was tested in a Phase I/II dose-escalation study which disclosed dose-dependent antiviral activity against HBV in treatment-naive patients. However, Val-D-cytosine has been reported to select for the same mutations as lamivudine [3] and may therefore offer little therapeutic advantage.

Alamifovir is a purine analogue derivative of adefovir, shown to be active against wild-type as well as lamivudine-resistant mutants *in vitro*. In animal species, alamifovir is quickly and extensively metabolized to three metabolites. In a dose-escalation study performed in 66 patients with chronic hepatitis B, 28 days of alamifovir treatment led to viral load reduction ranging from 1.5 to 2.6 log [15]. The drug appears to be safe in humans, although nephrotoxicity had been reported in rats.

LB80380 is an oral nucleotide prodrug and is chemically similar to adefovir dipivoxil and tenofovir disoproxil fumarate. LB80380 is first metabolized to LB80331 and then to LB80317, which is phosphorylated and the triphosphate form of LB80317 inhibits HBV replication following incorporation into viral DNA [16]. Its main excretion route is via the kidneys. *In vitro*, LB80380 has also been shown to be active against HBV strains resistant to lamivudine, adefovir, entecavir and telbivudine. LB80380 has been used in a Phase II clinical study at doses ranging from 30 to 240 mg daily in chronic hepatitis B and was found to be effective in suppressing HBV replication in treatment-naive as well as lamivudine-resistant patients. LB80380 led to mean viral load reductions of $3.0-4.2 \log_{10}$ copies/mL following 4 weeks of treatment in treatment-naive HBeAg-positive chronic HBV infection.

Conclusion

The success of two recently approved drugs in chronic hepatitis B, namely entecavir and tenofovir, with regard to their potent antiviral efficacy and high genetic barrier for resistance, coupled with the very recent report of possible mitochondrial toxicity associated with clevudine, may hamper drug development in hepatitis B in the very near future. However, the management of chronic HBV infection is far from optimal and efforts for further drug development alongside optimization of current treatment strategies, such as combinations of drugs acting at different treatment targets, need to be continued for the sake of our patients.

References

1. Petersen J, Dandri M, Mier W *et al*. Prevention of hepatitis B virus infection in vivo by entry inhibitors derived from the large envelope protein. *Nature Biotechnology* 2008;26:335–341. **Novel entry inhibitors revealed.** 🔑

2. Stray SJ, Bourna CR, Punna S *et al*. A heteroaryldigydropyrimidine activates and can misdirect hepatitis B virus capsid assembly. *Proceedings of the National Academy of Sciences USA* 2005;102:8138–8143.

3. Field J, Lee JY, Locarnini S. New targets and possible new therapeutic approaches in the chemotherapy of chronic hepatitis B. *Hepatology* 2004;38:545–553. **Review of activity in this field.** 🔑

4. Mehta A, Zitzmann N, Rudd PM *et al*. α-Glucosidase inhibitors as potential broad based anti-viral agents. *FEBS Letters* 1998;430:17–22.

5. Wang HC, Huang W, Lai MD, Su IJ. Hepatitis B virus pre-S mutants, endoplasmic reticulum stres and hepatocarcinogenesis. *Cancer Science* 2006;97:683–688.

6. Chen Y, Cheng G, Mahato RI. RNAi for treating hepatitis B viral infection. *Pharmaceutical Research* 2008;25:72–86.

7. Michel ML, Pol S, Brechot C *et al*. Immunotherapy of chronic hepatitis B by anti HBV vaccine: from present to future. *Vaccine* 2001;19:2395–2399.

8. Mancini-Bourgine M, Fontaine H, Brechot C *et al*. Immunogenicity of a hepatitis B DNA vaccine administered to chronic HBV carriers. *Vaccine* 2006;24:4482–4489.

9. Chen W, Zhang Z, Shi M *et al*. Activated plasmacytoid dendritic cells act synergistically with hepatitis B core antigen-pulsed monocyte-derived dendritic cells in the induction of hepatitis B virus-specific CD8-T cell response. *Clinical Immunology* 2008;129:295–303.

10. Carreno V, Zeuzem S, Hopf U *et al*. A phase I/II study of recombinant human interleukin-12 in patients with chronic hepatitis B. *Journal of Hepatology* 2000;32:317–324.

11. Rigopoulou EI, Suri D, Chokshi S *et al*. Lamivudine plus interleukin-12 combination therapy in chronic hepatitis B: antiviral and immunological activity. *Hepatology* 2005;42:1028–1036.

12. Kimura K, Kakimi K, Wieland S *et al*. Interleukin-18 inhibits hepatitis B virus replication in the livers of transgenic mice. *Journal of Virology* 2002;76:10702–10707.

13. Reddy KR, Matelich MC, Ugarkar BG *et al*. Pradefovir: a prodrug that targets adefovir to the liver for the treatment of hepatitis B. *Journal of Medicinal Chemistry* 2008;51:666–676.

14. Lee KS, Lim SG, Chuang WL. Safety, tolerability and antiviral activity of pradefovir mesylate in patients with chronic hepatitis B virus infection: 48-week analysis of a phase 2 study. *Journal of Hepatology* 2006;44(Suppl 2):S274.

15. Soon DKW, Lowe SL, Teng CH *et al*. Safety and efficacy of alamifovir in patients with chronic hepatitis B virus infection. *Journal of Hepatology* 2004;41:852–858.

16. Yuen MF, Lee SH, Kang HM *et al*. Pharmacokinetics of LB80331 and LB80317 following oral administration of LB80380, a new antiviral agent for chronic hepatitis B (CHB), in healthy adult subjects, CHB patients, and mice. *Antimicrobial Agents and Chemotherapy* 2009;53:1779–1785.

47 Hepatitis B – a therapeutic vaccine: hope or hype?

Rosa Di Stefano[1], Antonio Craxi[2]

[1]Department of Hygiene and Microbiology, University of Palermo, Palermo, Italy
[2]Departments of Internal Medicine and Gastroenterology, University of Palermo, Palermo, Italy

LEARNING POINTS

- Therapeutic use of the standard HBV prophylactic vaccine does not sufficiently enhance the immune response in patients with chronic HBV infection. Its effect as a stand-alone agent are inconstant and short-lived.

- Drugs that reduce HBV replication when combined with the immune enhancement and neutralizing response induced by the standard vaccine hold some promise, but the current clinical results are modest at best. The ideal time to immunize (before therapy, at the viral nadir, shortly after) need to be appropriately assessed.

- New vaccines against viral epitopes directly present on the HBV replication complex should be raised. Currently, T-cell-based vaccines have proved disappointing, while DNA vaccines are under development.

Background: why HBV is here to stay

Hepatitis B virus (HBV), a viral agent whose toll in terms of chronic disease and of deaths is among the highest worldwide, is still not curable. Interferon alfas, in standard or pegylated form, and direct inhibitors of the HBV DNA polymerase such as the nucleoside and nucleotide analogues have improved the therapeutic range for chronic hepatitis B [1]. Beside the fact that their efficacy in inducing suppression of HBV DNA remains modest and is frequently limited to the time of administration, their main constraint lies in the persistence of a mini-chromosome carrying a supercoiled form of HBV DNA (cccDNA) within the liver cell nuclei [2]. Persistence of HBV cccDNA is the basis of residual transcription and expression of HBV-encoded proteins, mostly HBsAg, even under the strongest antiviral pressure [3]. Even when transcription has been fully inhibited in the long term, residual HBV DNA may still be present [4] and reactivate under immunosuppression. Thus persistence of episomal HBV DNA and the risk of post-treatment or on-treatment HBV reactivations, if resistance to nucleoside/nucleotide analogues appears, is unavoidable with the current therapeutic regimens. Although in principle it is possible to eliminate residual virus from the hepatocytes without killing the cells [5], up to now it has proven impossible in the majority of patients to clear HBV after reaching a stable plateau of minimal residual viraemia with current potent antiviral agents [6]. These facts emphasize the current need for an effective and afford-able therapy to achieve sustained suppression of HBV replication and remission of liver disease but most importantly of an approach which allows the eradication of infection.

Immune response during HBV infection

Chronic hepatitis B is an immune-mediated disease. Continuing necroinflammatory activity is due to the host immune response rather than to direct viral cytopathic effects [7,8] and HBV persistence, besides the cccDNA reservoir described above, depends on the interaction between the virus and the host, with immune hyporesponsiveness to viral antigens as the dominant factor associated with the chronic carrier state [9,10]. This state of selective immune tolerance to virus-encoded antigens can be broken at the time of HBeAg or even HBsAg seroconversion, which can occur spontaneously during disease exacerbations, following antiviral therapy or through passive transfer of bone marrow from an immune donor [11]. CD4+ and CD8+ T-cell responses have been associated with the phenomenon of seroconversion and with control of infection [12–16]. In addition, the profile and extent of HBV-specific CD8+ T-cell responses are affected by the level of viral replication [17,18]. T-cell reactivity is transiently restored by antiviral therapy in patients with chronic hepatitis B [19] and a combination of antiviral drugs and vaccination had therapeutic long-lasting effects in duck and woodchuck models [20,21].

Several studies have shown that patients able to resolve an acute HBV infection display a strong polyclonal and multispecific CD4+ and CD8+ T-cell response against a range of different epitopes within HBV core, polymerase and envelope proteins that persists long after resolution of acute hepatitis. HBV-specific CD8+ T cells, also known as cytotoxic T cells (CTLs), have been implicated as the principal effector of liver injury by a variety of mechanisms including perforin, Fas-L and tumour necrosis factor (TNF)-α mediated cell lysis and such mechanisms are essential for the elimination of liver cells still harbouring low quantity of virus. However, the lack of massive hepatocyte lysis during recovery from infection suggests that HBV replication is also controlled by intracellular viral inactivation mediated by cytokine production in addition to control by elimination of infected cells. Th1 cytokines such as interferon (IFN)-γ and TNF-α are able to selectively degrade replicating genomes of HBV, thereby eliminating virus without the need to kill the infected cells. HBV clearance is also associated with the production of neutralizing anti-envelope antibodies that can ultimately eliminate the virus. The full development of an efficient antiviral response also requires activation of the components of the innate immune response, including type I interferons, natural killer (NK) cells and NK-T cells, which produce IFN-γ and TNF-α in the liver, and dendritic cells (DCs) that are needed to control and inhibit initial HBV replication and to activate the adaptive immune response.

In contrast, HBV-specific CD4 and CD8 T-cell responses are weak or undetectable in patients who fail to clear the virus and become chronically infected. When a response is present, it only encompasses a restricted number of viral epitopes. During chronic HBV infection, persistently high production of HBsAg and HBeAg can delete or tolerize antigen-specific T cells, thus altering the balance of Th1 and Th2 cytokine responses. Therefore, because viral clearance

may depend largely on non-cytolytic inhibition of viral replication by Th1 cytokines, differences in the cytokine profile of the T-cell responses may be responsible for viral persistence.

The host immune response is paramount in determining the fate of chronic HBV carriers. Some HBV-infected patients never show any features of liver disease during their lifetime, even if they have harboured the virus since birth. However, a considerable number of patients chronically infected with HBV have necroinflammatory liver disease potentially leading to cirrhosis and hepatocellular carcinoma. Direct destruction of hepatocytes by CTLs may not be the only or principal mechanism of damage in patients with chronic liver disease. T cells present in the liver during chronic hepatitis B are not preferentially HBV-specific. Liver injury seems to occur mainly due to the abundant non-antigen-specific mononuclear cells, mostly macrophages, which are the effectors of a delayed-type hypersensitivity reaction.

Hence it would be rational, from a therapeutic standpoint, to manipulate the induction of protective T- and B-cell responses, elicited through vaccination with HBV antigens, to the direct inhibition of virus replication elicited by antiviral therapy [22]. This approach joins a long line of attempts to develop alternative therapeutic approaches for chronic HBV carriers, such as immunostimulation by thymic derivatives or growth factors and adoptive transfer of HBV immunity in experimental models and in humans.

In contrast to passive immunotherapy, which involves administration of drugs as monoclonal antibodies or cytokines that modulate a specific subset of the immune system, therapeutic vaccines act by mobilizing *de novo* the patient's own immune system. In a chronic infectious disease like HBV infection, a therapeutic vaccine should be able to restore deficient immune response in order to control viral replication and prevent complications.

HBV vaccine as a stand-alone therapeutic agent

Since hyporesponsiveness of HBV-specific T cells to antigen stimulation is an important determinant of virus persistence during chronic HBV infection, therapeutic strategies have aimed at correcting or overcoming these deficiencies. The goal of therapeutic vaccination in patient's with chronic HBV infection is to improve the inefficient response of CD4 and CD8 cells as well as to correct the Th1/Th2 cytokine imbalance.

The first pilot study of vaccine therapy was performed by Pol *et al.* [23] who showed that therapeutic vaccination with a pre-S2/S prophylactic vaccine (GenHevac B) decreased viral replication in 50% of treated patients. However, the same authors [24] were later unable to confirm efficacy in a larger multicentre controlled study involving 118 patients randomized to receive five intramuscular injections of a pre-S2/S (GenHevac B) or S vaccine (Recombivax), or no treatment as control group. Although the percentage of patients with undetectable serum HBV DNA, by a low-sensitivity technique, was higher in the vaccine group (16.3%) than in the control group (2.7%) 6 months after the start of vaccination, at 12 months follow-up the number of HBV DNA-negative patients was comparable among vaccinees and non-vaccinees. HBV immunization did not enhance the rate of HBe/anti-HBe seroconversion, and disappearance of serum HBsAg was never seen during the study period.

The characterization of antiviral T-cell responses in 11 chronically infected patients undergoing therapeutic vaccination with a third-generation recombinant vaccine containing HBC pre-S1, pre-S2 and S antigens (Hepacare) revealed significant HBsAg-specific T-cell proliferation with production of a Th2 cytokine profile, i.e. interleukin (IL)-5, but without induction of Th1 cytokines and activation of CD8 T lymphocytes. Vaccination with HBsAg did not influence the HBcAg-specific T-cell proliferation and neither vaccine had significant long-term therapeutic effects compared with the placebo group [25].

One way to enhance the immunogenicity of vaccines consists of combining recombinant HBsAg with anti-HBs immunoglobulin, forming immune complexes to enhance the immunogenicity of HBsAg by increasing its uptake by antigen-presenting cells and thereby the proliferation of HBsAg-specific T cells. In a Phase IIA clinical trial [26], 20 patients with HBeAg-positive chronic HBV infection were immunized with yeast-derived HBsAg/hepatitis B immunoglobulin (HBIG) complexes (YIC) or alum. Half the patients immunized with YIC had a 2 log or greater decrease in HBV DNA with loss or marked reduction of HBeAg and appearance of anti-HBe. In responders a flare of alanine aminotransferase (ALT) occurred, suggesting a cytolytic response to immunization with YIC. HBsAg-stimulated peripheral blood mononuclear cells from responders secreted increased levels of Th1/Th2 cytokines. *In vitro* study of DCs from patients with chronic HBV showed, after stimulation with YIC, increased levels of IL-12, upregulated expression of functional markers on

DCs and effective interactions between DCs and T cells. Thus the therapeutic effect of YIC is associated with both cytolytic and non-cytolytic immune responses. More recently, 242 patients with HBeAg-positive chronic HBV infection were immunized with six injections of YIC 30 μg, YIC 60 μg or alum adjuvant as placebo at 4-week intervals. No significant difference was reached in primary end-points (loss of HBeAg, anti-HBe seroconversion, suppression of HBV DNA) 4 weeks after treatment among the three groups. At the end of follow-up anti-HBe seroconversion rate was 21.8% in the 60-μg YIC group and 9% in the placebo group ($P = 0.03$) [27].

These clinical studies are not strictly comparable because of different protocols in terms of number of inoculations, concentration and composition of doses and criteria of response to vaccine and because of the low sensitivity of some of the tests used to assess HBV replication. Nevertheless, they do suggest that immunotherapy using classical prophylactic vaccines, containing only some of the major antigenic determinants of the viral capsid protein, obtain some degree of reduction in HBV replication in a proportion of chronically infected patients, which is rapidly lost after the end of the immunization schedule. Although no direct data are available, it is tempting to hypothesize that neutralizing anti-HBs antibodies induced by the vaccine could, for a brief period, reduce the number of newly infected hepatocytes. In the long run, subtle changes in HBV nucleocapsid antigenicity in the presence of continuing viral replication would render this partial neutralizing immunity less effective.

It would make sense to downregulate the HBV replication complex at an intracellular level by using a vaccine containing epitopes of the viral core. Unfortunately, immunization with a lipopeptide vaccine containing a single immunodominant HBV core CD8$^+$ T-cell epitope, a T-helper epitope of tetanus toxoid and two palmitic acid molecules (CY-1899) did not show any therapeutic efficacy in terms of changes in liver biochemistry or viral serology [28]. A possible explanation for this failure lies in the inability of this vaccine to access the intracellular compartments where the HBV replication complex is located.

The use of a DNA vaccine could help overcome the issue of low vaccine efficacy seen to date. DNA vaccines activate HBV-specific Th1 T-cell responses in healthy or infected individuals [29,30]. In a recent study [31], 10 HBV carriers with active HBV replication, non-responders to antiviral agents, received a DNA vaccine encoding small and middle HBV envelope proteins, capable of activating both

HBV-specific CTLs and NK cells. Significant modifications in the NK cell repertoire were observed after vaccination, with a specific subset of NK cells (CD56$^+$) secreting increased levels of IFN-γ without cytotoxic activity very early after vaccination and correlating with vaccine-induced HBV-specific T-cell responses. Another study [32] with a DNA vaccine enrolled 12 previously untreated chronic HBV carriers who were injected 12 times with an HBV DNA vaccine in combination with lamivudine. A major feature of this DNA vaccine was that it encoded multiple HBV proteins (i.e. envelope, nucleocapsid and polymerase) and a modified IL-12 gene as adjuvant. Importantly, in this trial, memory T-cell responses were induced and persisted for at least 40 weeks after therapy. These responses correlated with virological responses that were observed in half of the patients. A synergistic effect of the vaccine and the antiviral treatment may be the key to T-cell restoration observed in this study.

Combining HBV vaccine with antivirals: does it work?

Reducing the HBV load by antivirals in order to maximize the efficacy of the neutralizing effect of the vaccine is theoretically appealing. A further boost should be given by the T-cell recovery effect seen at the nadir of viral replication induced by analogues.

HBV vaccine therapy has been assessed in combination with antiviral agents, both interferon alfa and analogues. Only a few studies report the use of combination therapy with interferon alfa and a standard HBV vaccine in adult patients with chronic hepatitis B. These studies have demonstrated that the combination has a weak additional effect against HBV in terms of HBeAg loss and of HBV DNA reduction. In fact, combination therapy with interferon alfa and vaccine may achieve slightly higher response rates in patients who previously did not respond to interferon alfa alone [33] or may increase the durability of HBV DNA suppression after discontinuation as compared with interferon alfa alone [34]. Recently, a Turkish study [35] was performed in children with chronic HBV infection to compare the efficacy of HBV vaccination plus interferon alfa-2b versus interferon alfa-2b monotherapy. Fifty patients were randomized to receive either interferon alfa-2b for 9 months and pre-S2/S vaccine (GenHevac B) at the beginning and 4 and 24 weeks after initiation of interferon therapy or recombinant interferon alfa-2b alone for 9 months. Mean

HBV DNA values were significantly reduced at the end of treatment in the group receiving combination therapy, but no statistically significant difference was found 6 months after the end of treatment. Sustained HBeAg seroconversion was obtained in 13 (52%) treated with combination therapy and in eight (32%) treated with interferon monotherapy. Thus there was only a non-significant trend towards a better sustained response rate in the group receiving combination therapy.

It has been demonstrated that lamivudine treatment of patients with chronic HBV infection, which leads to a reduction in viral load, is associated with an increase in the circulating frequency of HBV-specific CD4 and CD8 cells [36]. However, the recovery of antiviral T-cell responses is only transient, with an early enhancement of T-cell frequency and intensity of responses followed by a persistent decline starting from the fifth to sixth month of treatment. The transitory restoration of virus-specific immunity might provide the perfect platform from which to boost HBV-specific T-cell responses. A clinical trial [37] evaluated the efficacy of a combination of lamivudine and vaccine in 72 patients with chronic HBV infection. All patients received lamivudine 100 mg daily for 12 months. Three months after the start of lamivudine therapy, 15 patients received 12 intradermal injections (once every 2 weeks for 6 months) of a vaccine containing 20 mg of HBsAg. The rate of seroconversion from HBeAg to anti-HBe was significantly higher in patients receiving combination therapy than in those receiving only lamivudine. HBV DNA breakthroughs were never observed on combination therapy.

Another study [32] with a DNA vaccine enrolled 12 previously untreated chronic HBV carriers who were injected 12 times with an HBV DNA vaccine encoding multiple HBV proteins (i.e. envelope, nucleocapsid and polymerase) together with a genetically modified IL-12 gene as adjuvant in combination with lamivudine. Memory T-cell responses were induced and persisted for at least 40 weeks after therapy. These responses correlated with virological responses that were observed for half the patients, thus suggesting a synergistic effect of the vaccine and the antiviral treatment on T-cell restoration.

Recently, a randomized study [38] was performed to evaluate a candidate vaccine composed of HBsAg and a proprietary adjuvant system (AS02) administered simultaneously with lamivudine to patients with HBeAg-positive chronic HBV. The combined administration of vaccine and lamivudine did not improve the HBeAg seroconversion rate compared with the control group. Despite induction of HBsAg-specific lymphoproliferative responses, cytokine production and anti-HBs antibodies, therapeutic vaccination did not demonstrate superior clinical efficacy compared with lamivudine alone.

Conclusions

At present, the use of the standard HBV prophylactic vaccine is unable to sufficiently enhance the immune response in patients with chronic HBV to generate a useful response. However, a combination of drugs that inhibit HBV replication and agents that enhance the immune response against HBV may be of more value, although clinical trials to date are inconsistent and the optimal timing of this approach remains to be determined. New vaccines against viral epitopes present on the HBV replication complex may be required to supplement the effects of vaccines directed against the envelope proteins. Currently, T-cell-based vaccines do not seem to hold much promise, while DNA vaccines are under development.

References

1. Lok AS, McMahon BJ. Chronic hepatitis B. *Hepatology* 2007;45:507–539.
2. Zoulim F. Antiviral therapy of chronic hepatitis B: can we clear the virus and prevent drug resistance? *Antiviral Chemistry and Chemotherapy* 2004;15:299–305.
3. Margeridon S, Carrouée-Durantel S, Chemin I *et al.* Rolling circle amplification, a powerful tool for genetic and functional studies of complete hepatitis B virus genomes from low-level infections and for directly probing covalently closed circular DNA. *Antimicrobial Agents and Chemotherapy* 2008; 52:3068–3073.
4. Raimondo G, Pollicino T, Cacciola I, Squadrito G. Occult hepatitis B virus infection. *Journal of Hepatology* 2007;46: 160–170.
5. Guidotti LG, Chisari FV. Immunobiology and pathogenesis of viral hepatitis. *Annual Review of Pathology* 2006;1:23–61. **Excellent introduction to the complexities of the immune response against hepatitis B.** ●➤
6. Pawlotsky JM, Dusheiko G, Hatzakis A *et al.* Virologic monitoring of hepatitis B virus therapy in clinical trials and practice: recommendations for a standardized approach. *Gastroenterology* 2008;134:405–415.
7. Millich DR. Pathobiology of acute and chronic hepatitis B virus infection: an introduction. *Journal of Viral Hepatitis* 1997;4:25–30.
8. Chisari FV, Ferrari C. Hepatitis B virus immunopathogenesis. *Annual Review of Immunology* 1995;13:29–60.
9. Ferrari C, Penna A, Bertoletti A *et al.* Cellular immune response to hepatitis B virus-encoded antigens in acute and chronic hepatitis B virus infection. *Journal of Immunology* 1990;145:3442–3449.
10. Jung M, Hartmann B, Gerlach J *et al.* Virus-specific lymphokine production differs quantitatively but not qualitatively in acute and chronic hepatitis B infection. *Virology* 1999; 261:165–172.
11. Lau GKK, Liang R, Lee CK *et al.* Clearance of persistent hepatitis B virus infection in Chinese bone marrow transplant recipients whose donors were anti-hepatitis B core and antihepatitis B surface antibody positive. *Journal of Infectious Diseases* 1998;178:1585–1591.
12. Jung MC, Diepolder HM, Spengler U *et al.* Activation of heterogeneous hepatitis B (HB) core and e antigen-specific CD4+ T-cell population during seroconversion to anti-HBe and anti-HBs in hepatitis B virus infection. *Journal of Virology* 1995;69:3358–3368.
13. Jung M, Spengler U, Schraut W *et al.* Hepatitis B virus antigen-specific T-cell activation in patients with acute and chronic hepatitis B. *Journal of Hepatology* 1991;13:310–317.
14. Penna A, Chisari FV, Bertoletti A *et al.* Cytotoxic T lymphocytes recognize an HLA-A2-restricted epitope within the hepatitis B virus nucleocapsid antigen. *Journal of Experimental Medicine* 1991;174:1565–1570.
15. Rehermann B, Fowler P, Sidney J *et al.* The cytotoxic T lymphocyte response to multiple hepatitis B virus polymerase epitopes during and after acute viral hepatitis. *Journal of Experimental Medicine* 1995;181:147–158.
16. Thimme R, Wieland S, Steiger C *et al.* CD8+ T cells mediate viral clearance and disease pathogenesis during acute hepatitis B virus infection. *Journal of Virology* 2003;77: 68–76.
17. Sing GK, Ladhams A, Arnold S *et al.* A longitudinal analysis of cytotoxic T lymphocyte precursor frequencies to the hepatitis B virus in chronically infected patients. *Journal of Viral Hepatitis* 2001;8:19–29.
18. Webster GJM, Reignat S, Brown D *et al.* Longitudinal analysis of CD8+ T cells specific for structural and nonstructural hepatitis B virus proteins in patients with chronic hepatitis B: implications for immunotherapy. *Journal of Virology* 2004; 78:5707–5719.
19. Boni C, Bertoletti A, Penna A *et al.* Lamivudine treatment can restore T-cell responsiveness in chronic hepatitis B. *Journal of Clinical Investigation* 1998;102:1–8.
20. Le Guerhier F, Thermet A, Guerret S *et al.* Antiviral effect of adefovir in combination with a DNA vaccine in the duck hepatitis B virus infection model. *Journal of Hepatology* 2003;38:328–334.

21. Menne S, Roneker CA, Korba BE, Gerin JL, Tennant BC, Cote PJ. Immunization with surface antigens alone and after treatment with 1-(2-fluoro-5-methyl-beta-l-arabinofuranosyl)-uracil (L-FMAU) breaks humoral and cell-mediated immune tolerance in chronic woodchuck hepatitis virus infection. *Journal of Virology* 2002;76:5305–5314.

22. Vandepapeliere P. Therapeutic vaccination for treatment of chronic hepatitis B: rationale, review and prospects for future development. *Viral Hepatitis Review* 2000;6:65–92.

23. Pol S, Driss F, Michel ML, Nalpas B, Berthelot P, Bréchot C. Specific vaccine therapy in chronic hepatitis B infection. *Lancet* 1994;344:342.

24. Pol S, Nalpas B, Driss F *et al.* Efficacy and limitations of a specific immunotherapy in chronic hepatitis B. *Journal of Hepatology* 2001;34:917–921.

25. Jung MC, Gruner N, Zachoval R *et al.* Immunological monitoring during therapeutic vaccination as a prerequisite for the design of a new effective therapies: induction of a vaccine-specific CD4$^+$ T-cell proliferative response in chronic hepatitis B carriers. *Vaccine* 2002;20:3598–3612.

26. Yao X, Zheng B, Zhou J *et al.* Therapeutic effect of hepatitis B surface antigen–antibody complex is associated with cytolytic and non-cytolytic immune responses in hepatitis B patients. *Vaccine* 2007;25:1771–1779.

**27. Xu DZ, Zhao K, Guo LM *et al.* A randomized controlled phase IIb trial of antigen-antibody immunogenic complex therapeutic vaccine in chronic hepatitis B patients. *PLoS ONE* 2008;3:e2565.

28. Heathcote J, McHutchinson J, Lee S *et al.* A pilot study of the CY-1899 T-cell vaccine in subjects chronically infected with hepatitis B virus. *Hepatology* 1999;30:531–536.

29. Roy MJ, Wu MS, Barr LJ *et al.* Induction of antigen-specific CD8$^+$ T cells, T helper cells, and protective levels of antibody in humans by particle-mediated administration of a hepatitis B virus DNA vaccine. *Vaccine* 2001;19:764–778.

30. Rottinghaus ST, Poland GA, Jacobson RM, Barr LJ, Roy MJ. Hepatitis B DNA vaccine induces protective antibody responses in human non-responders to conventional vaccination. *Vaccine* 2003;21:4604–4608.

31. Mancini-Bourgine M, Fontaine H, Scott-Algara D, Pol S, Brechot C, Michel ML. Induction or expansion of T-cell responses by a hepatitis B DNA vaccine administered to chronic HBV carriers. *Hepatology* 2004;40:874–882.

32. Yang SH, Lee CG, Park SH *et al.* Correlation of antiviral T-cell responses with suppression of viral rebound in chronic hepatitis B carriers: a proof-of-concept study. *Gene Therapy* 2006;13:1110–1117.

33. Heintges T, Petry W, Kaldewey M *et al.* Combination therapy of active HBsAg vaccination and interferon-alpha in interferon-alpha nonresponders with chronic hepatitis B. *Digestive Diseases and Sciences* 2001;46:901–906.

34. Senturk H, Tabak F, Akdogan M *et al.* Therapeutic vaccination in chronic hepatitis. *Journal of Gastroenterology and Hepatology* 2002;17:72–76.

35. Helvaci M, Kizilgunesler A, Kasirga E, Ozbal E, Kuzu M, Sozen G. Efficacy of hepatitis B vaccination and interferon-α-2b combination therapy versus interferon-α-2b monotherapy in children with chronic hepatitis B. *Journal of Gastroenterology and Hepatology* 2004;19:785–791.

36. Boni C, Penna A, Bertoletti A *et al.* Transient restoration of anti-viral therapy in chronic hepatitis B. *Journal of Hepatology* 2003;39:595–605.

37. Horiike N, Fazle Akbar SM, Michitaka K *et al.* In *vivo* immunization by vaccine therapy following virus suppression by lamivudine: a novel approach for treating patients with chronic hepatitis B. *Journal of Clinical Virology* 2005; 32:156–161.

38. Vandepapelière P, Lau GKK, Leroux-Roels G *et al.* Therapeutic vaccination of chronic hepatitis B patients with virus suppression by antiviral therapy: a randomized, controlled study of co-administration of HBsAg/AS02 candidate vaccine and lamivudine. *Vaccine* 2007;25:8585–8597. **One of many therapeutic vaccine clinical trials.** ⚷

48 Novel interferons: is there life in the old dog yet?

Graham R. Foster

Queen Mary's University of London, Blizard Institute of Cell and Molecular Science, London, UK

LEARNING POINTS

- Type I interferons are currently administered weekly but alternative delivery systems that allow fortnightly or even monthly administration are in development.

- The type I interferons are a family of cytokines and different members of the family have different properties.

- Attempts to generate novel interferons with superior properties continue.

Introduction

The backbone of antiviral therapy for patients with chronic hepatitis C virus (HCV) infection is the type I interferons, usually administered as a long-acting form of interferon alfa-2a or interferon alfa-2b [1]. In chronic hepatitis B virus (HBV) infection, type I interferon is also still widely used (particularly for HBeAg-positive infection) but their role here is slowly being superseded by the direct-acting oral antiviral agents (see Chapters 29 and 38). In the future it is likely that new oral agents for chronic HCV infection will be developed (see Chapter 44) and it is by no means clear that type I interferon will be required. However, given that prolonged therapy with potent oral antiviral agents does not lead to eradication of HBV, there are many who believe that eradication of HCV will require interferon-based regimens for many years to come. On the other hand, HCV is an RNA virus that can not archive its genetic material in

host DNA (as can the DNA virus HBV) and HCV requires ongoing viral replication to persist. It is therefore reasonable to assume that eradication may be a little easier for HCV than for HBV and therefore an immunostimulant, such as interferon, may not be required. The next few years will see an answer to this controversy as potent antiviral agents for HCV are introduced and their efficacy in the absence of interferon is assessed. I believe that for many patients with chronic HCV infection it will be possible to eliminate type I interferons from the therapeutic regimen but a substantial number of patients will remain who are insensitive to the first- and second-generation oral agents and type I interferons will continue to play a role in patient management for some time to come. Given that type I interferons will continue to be required for some patients, the question arises as to whether current peginterferons will be sufficient or whether new more potent interferons can be developed. There are two approaches to developing a novel interferon: one involves improving the pharmacodynamics of the molecule and engineering a longer-acting interferon, and the other involves modifying the interferon molecule itself to improve its effects. Here I discuss current research in these two areas.

Improving the half-life of type I interferons

Conventional interferon has a very short half-life of only a few hours. However, since its biological effects (chiefly induction of interferon-inducible genes) last for many hours, early clinical trials administered the interferon three times a week. This thrice-weekly dosing was rapidly shown to be effective and although a few studies examined alternative dosing schedules, the thrice-weekly treatment

Clinical Dilemmas in Viral Liver Disease, 1st edition. Edited by Graham R. Foster and K. Rajender Reddy. © 2010 Blackwell Publishing.

regimen became the standard of care, latterly in combination with ribavirin [2]. Developments in chemical pharmacology led to attempts to increase the half-life of interferon by linking the interferon molecule to an inert 'carrier', and studies linking interferon to polyethylene glycol (PEG) soon showed that pegylated interferon was active, well tolerated and led to clinical benefits compared with standard interferon [3]. By design the current peginterferons are used once every week and although there are significant differences in the half-life of the two currently available peginterferons [3], head-to-head comparisons have shown that the differences between the two preparations are modest [4]. The success of the peginterferons has led to studies examining alternative modifications designed to augment the pharmacodynamics of the molecule. The most clinically advanced preparation involves interferon linked to albumin to generate an 'albuminated' interferon [5] that is administered once every 2 weeks. Recently completed Phase III trials show that fortnightly albuminated interferon is not inferior to peginterferon and this product is likely to be licensed in the near future. The change from weekly to fortnightly injections has some obvious benefits to patients, although it will be important to derive user-friendly management plans to ensure that patients administer the doses at the correct time. There is now increasing interest in extending the dosing period still further, perhaps administering the modified interferon every month. Many clinicians are anxious about administering a potent drug such as interferon, with a very long half-life, as there are concerns that prolonged bone marrow suppression may give rise to serious side effects. However, the development of marrow stimulants such as granulocyte/macrophage colony-stimulating factor (GM-CSF), which reverse interferon-induced neutropenia, and the ongoing development of thrombopoietin analogues [6] may persuade clinicians that it is safe to use these very long-acting preparations. Development of monthly interferons is therefore ongoing and there are plans for studies with a number of monthly interferons including albuminated interferons and depot preparations. The results of these trials are awaited with interest.

Modifying the interferon

The type I interferons are a family of different cytokines comprising 12 interferon α subtypes, one interferon β subtype and one interferon Ω subtype. The different subtypes have slightly different properties and their antiviral activity differs considerably [7]. In addition to differences in their antiviral effects, the different type I interferons have marked differences in their immunomodulatory properties, for example interferon α2 is chemotactic, whereas interferon α8 (which has greater antiviral activity) does not induce cellular migration [8]. The differences between the different type I interferons have led to suggestions that it may be possible to select more potent type I interferons that may have enhanced properties. This approach was taken to extremes with the generation of a 'super' type I interferon using gene shuffling and selection techniques that led to the creation of a novel interferon with enhanced antiviral effects, potent Th1 stimulatory effects alongside modest antiproliferative properties [9]. This novel molecule is proof of principle but is unlikely to be further developed for clinical use. However, a number of groups continue to explore the possibility of developing interferons with modified enhanced effects and it will be interesting to see if these studies lead to clinical trials.

The commercial and research interest in developing a new interferon has waned since the success of early clinical trials with oral antiviral agents for HCV. It is probable that studies demonstrating different antiviral effects in the laboratory will not be taken forward into clinical trials in patients unless there is compelling evidence that new interferons will be needed to augment the current small molecules under development.

Conclusion

There is considerable scope for improving both the pharmacology and effectiveness of the type I interferons. However, the current success of small molecules in treating chronic HCV infection suggests that there will be little enthusiasm for expensive clinical trials with drugs that are unlikely to make a substantial contribution to future treatment regimens. The current modified delivery systems for type I interferon are likely to be the last major development in the therapeutic use of these compounds and, perhaps, nearly 50 years after their discovery it is time to consider retiring these valuable drugs. However, it remains conceivable that the new small-molecule regimens for HCV will prove insufficient and, if this is the case, then it is probable that the ongoing laboratory studies with novel interferons will move into clinical trials and it may be premature to write the obituaries for the type I interferons until the new generation of drugs have proved their value in clinical practice.

References

1. D'Souza R, Foster GR. Diagnosis and treatment of hepatitis C. *Journal of the Royal Society of Medicine* 2004;97:223–225.

2. McHutchison JG, Gordon SC, Schiff ER *et al.* Interferon alfa-2b alone or in combination with ribavirin as initial treatment for chronic hepatitis C. *New England Journal of Medicine* 1998;339:1485–1492.

3. Foster GR. Review article: pegylated interferons: chemical and clinical differences. *Alimentary Pharmacology and Therapeutics* 2004;20:825–830.

4. McHutchison J, Sulkowski M. Scientific rationale and study design of the individualized dosing efficacy vs flat dosing to assess optimal pegylated interferon therapy (IDEAL) trial: determining optimal dosing in patients with genotype 1 chronic hepatitis C. *Journal of Viral Hepatitis* 2008;15:475–481.

5. Rustgi VK. Albinterferon alfa-2b, a novel fusion protein of human albumin and human interferon alfa-2b, for chronic hepatitis C. *Current Medical Research and Opinion* 2009;25:991–1002.

6. McHutchison JG, Dusheiko G, Shiffman ML *et al.* Eltrombopag for thrombocytopenia in patients with cirrhosis associated with hepatitis C. *New England Journal of Medicine* 2007;357:2227–2236.

7. Foster GR, Finter NB. Are all type I human interferons equivalent? *Journal of Viral Hepatitis* 1998;5:143–152. **Review of the differences between the different interferons.** ⚷

8. Foster GR, Masri SH, David R *et al.* IFN-alpha subtypes differentially affect human T cell motility. *Journal of Immunology* 2004;173:1663–1670.

9. Brideau-Andersen AD, Huang X, Sun SC *et al.* Directed evolution of gene-shuffled IFN-alpha molecules with activity profiles tailored for treatment of chronic viral diseases. *Proceedings of the National Academy of Sciences USA* 2007;104:8269–8274. **Interesting proof-of-principle study showing that novel interferons with unique properties can be developed.** ⚷

PART V
Ongoing Controversies

49 Is interferon a valuable first-line therapy for HBeAg-positive HBV?

Patrick Marcellin, Rami Moucari, Olivier Lada, Tarik Asselah

Service d'Hépatologie, Hôpital Beaujon, University of Paris, Clichy, France

LEARNING POINTS

- The goal of therapy in chronic HBV (as stated by the EASL guidelines in 2009) is to improve quality of life and survival by preventing progression of disease to cirrhosis, decompensated cirrhosis, end-stage liver disease, hepatocellular carcinoma and death.

- This goal can be achieved if HBV replication can be suppressed in a sustained manner.

- End-points of therapy in HBeAg-positive patients include durable HBe seroconversion (the most satisfactory end-point), or undetectable HBV DNA level for many years with continuous oral therapy, or sustained undetectable HBV DNA level after interferon therapy.

- Therapy with peginterferon, administered for 48 weeks, produces an overall sustained response rate of approximately 30%. Pretreatment factors predictive of treatment response are low viral load (HBV DNA $< 10^7$ IU/mL or 7 $\log_{10}$ IU/mL) and high serum ALT levels (above three times upper limit of normal).

- Peginterferon is an effective therapy for selected patients with HBeAg-positive HBV.

Monotherapy with interferons

Interferon alfa

Six medications are approved for the treatment of chronic hepatitis B virus (HBV) infection: 2 formulations of interferon and 4 oral nucleos(t)ide analogues (lamivudine, adefovir, entecavir, telbivudine and tenofovir) [1–17]. Interferon has been used in the treatment of chronic hepatitis B virus (HBV) infection for many years. Interferon exerts an antiviral effect on HBV infection through two mechanisms [1–3]: (i) it has

a direct antiviral effect by inhibiting synthesis of viral DNA and by activating antiviral enzymes; and (ii) it exaggerates the cellular immune response against hepatocytes infected with HBV by increasing the expression of class I histocompatibility antigens and by stimulating the activity of helper T lymphocytes and natural killer lymphocytes. The immunomodulatory properties of interferon may explain the relatively high HBe and HBs seroconversion rates observed during and after interferon therapy. Thus, interferon induces early diminution of HBV replication (reflected by decrease in HBV DNA in serum) and a late (about 2 months later) increase in serum alanine aminotransferase (ALT) levels. Many controlled studies of interferon in patients with chronic hepatitis B have been reported. In these studies, with various schedules, mean virological response rate was 37% versus 17%, mean HBeAg loss rate was 33% versus 12%, and HBsAg loss rate was 8% versus 2% in interferon-treated groups and the placebo groups, respectively [6] (Figure 49.1). HBsAg loss increases with the time in responders to interferon and is associated with improved outcome [21].

The discrepancies in the results of the different studies could be partly due to the different therapeutic schedules, but are mainly the result of the populations of patients included in these trials. A number of factors are predictive of poor response to interferon [6–9]. Low serum HBV DNA level and high serum ALT levels are predictors of non-response. Also, infection with HBV at birth or early in the patient's life (as is often the case in countries where HBV infection is hyperendemic, such as South-east Asia) is a factor of poor response to interferon.

Pegylated interferons

The efficacy of interferon has improved with the replacement of standard interferon by interferon conjugated with polyethylene glycol (peginterferon). This new form of interferon reduces its elimination by the kidneys, thus significantly increasing its half-life and resulting in more

Clinical Dilemmas in Viral Liver Disease, 1st edition. Edited by Graham R. Foster and K. Rajender Reddy. © 2010 Blackwell Publishing.

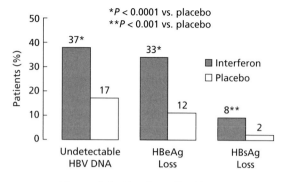

FIG. 49.1 Meta-analysis of interferon alfa trials in patients with HBeAg-positive chronic hepatitis B. The analysis included a total of 837 patients with HBeAg-positive chronic HBV infection from 15 randomized controlled trials (published between 1986 and 1992) that compared interferon with placebo. The superiority of interferon over placebo was shown by the following parameters: undetectable serum HBV DNA (hybridization assays), HBeAg loss and HBsAg loss. (Data from Wong *et al.* [6].)

stable plasma concentrations. Finally, the number of injections has been reduced from thrice to once weekly, thanks to improved pharmacokinetics, which is obviously more comfortable for the patient.

Two peginterferons, which differ in the quality and quantity of polyethylene glycol conjugated to interferon, have been produced: peginterferon alfa-2b, which contains 12-kDa linear polyethylene glycol, and peginterferon alfa-2a, which contains 40-kDa branched polyethylene glycol. The efficacy of peginterferons has been assessed in the treatment of chronic hepatitis B. Large randomized controlled trials have confirmed the efficacy of peginterferons in HBeAg-positive chronic hepatitis B. These studies compared peginterferon monotherapy to the combination of peginterferon and lamivudine and are detailed in the next section.

Combination of peginterferon and lamivudine

In a large randomized controlled study, 307 patients with HBeAg-positive chronic hepatitis B were randomized to receive either the combination of peginterferon alfa-2b 100 μg/week for 32 weeks then 50 μg for 20 weeks and lamivudine 100 mg/day, or peginterferon alfa-2b at the same dose with placebo [9]. At the end of the 26-week post-treatment follow-up, there was no difference in response rates between the group receiving peginterferon monotherapy and the group receiving peginterferon and lamivudine

combination therapy: serum HBV DNA was undetectable by PCR (< 400 copies/mL) in 7% and 9%; HBeAg loss was observed in 36% and 35%; normal ALT was observed in 32% and 35%. Interestingly, a relatively high rate of HBsAg loss was observed (7% in both groups). This study shows that in patients with HBeAg-positive chronic hepatitis B, 26 weeks after therapy, the combination of peginterferon alfa-2b and lamivudine (with the simultaneous regimen used) is not superior to monotherapy with peginterferon alfa-2b with regard to post-treatment response rates. In this study, response was defined by HBeAg loss. Main predictors of response were HBV genotype and pretreatment ALT level. Response was 34% for those with ALT levels under three times the upper limit of normal and 50% for those with ALT levels above five times the upper limit of normal. Response was 60% for genotype A, 42% for genotype B, 32% for genotype C and 28% for genotype D.

In another randomized Phase III trial, a total of 814 patients with HBeAg-positive chronic hepatitis B received either peginterferon alfa-2a (180 μg once weekly) plus oral placebo, peginterferon alfa-2a plus lamivudine (100 mg daily), or lamivudine alone [8] (Figure 49.2). The majority of patients in the study were Asian (87%). Most patients were infected with HBV genotype B or C. Patients were treated for 48 weeks and followed for an additional 24 weeks. After 24 weeks of follow-up, significantly more patients who received peginterferon alfa-2a monotherapy or peginterferon alfa-2a plus lamivudine than those who received lamivudine monotherapy had HBeAg seroconversion (32% vs. 19%, $P < 0.001$; 27% vs. 19%, $P = 0.02$, respectively) or HBV DNA levels below 100 000 copies/mL (32% vs. 22%, $P = 0.01$; 34% vs. 22%, $P = 0.003$, respectively). Rates of suppression of HBV DNA levels to less than 400 copies/mL at week 72 were 14% with both peginterferon alfa-2a monotherapy and peginterferon alfa-2a plus lamivudine, and 5% with lamivudine alone ($P < 0.001$ for both comparisons with lamivudine monotherapy). Sixteen patients receiving peginterferon alfa-2a (alone or in combination) had HBsAg seroconversion compared with none in the group receiving lamivudine alone ($P = 0.001$). The most common adverse events were those known to occur with therapies based on interferon alfa. The safety and tolerability of peginterferon alpha-2a in patients with chronic hepatitis B compares favourably with that observed in patients with chronic hepatitis C, with a lower incidence of common interferon-related adverse events and a significantly lower incidence of depression [22].

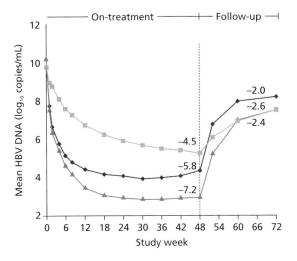
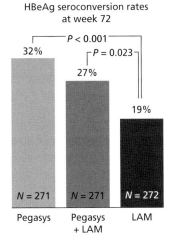

FIG. 49.2 Randomized Phase III trial comprising a total of 814 patients with HBeAg-positive chronic hepatitis B who received either peginterferon alfa-2a (Pegasys) 180 µg once weekly plus oral placebo, peginterferon alfa-2a plus lamivudine (LAM) 100 mg daily, or lamivudine alone. All numbers shown on the graph are log$_{10}$ reduction from baseline. In this randomized controlled trial, 24 weeks after therapy, the rates of response (normal serum ALT, HBeAg seroconversion, serum HBV DNA < 100 000 copies/mL) were higher in the two groups receiving peginterferon alfa-2a (with or without lamivudine) than the group receiving lamivudine (LAM) alone. There was no difference in response rates between the group which received peginterferon alfa-2a alone and the group which received peginterferon alfa-2a plus lamivudine combination. (Data from Lau *et al.* [8].)

In practice: who and how to treat?

The decision to treat or not to treat patients with chronic hepatitis B is mainly based on the severity of the liver disease. Patients should be considered for treatment when HBV DNA levels are above 2000 IU/mL (~ 10 000 copies/mL) and/or serum ALT levels are above the upper limit of normal for the laboratory, and liver biopsy (or non-invasive markers when validated in HBV-infected patients) shows moderate to severe active necroinflammation and/or fibrosis using a standardized scoring system (e.g. at least grade A2 or stage F2 by Metavir scoring). Indications for treatment must also take into account age, health status and availability of antiviral agents in individual countries.

In patients with mild liver disease, treatment is not recommended unless liver fibrosis deteriorates. It should be remembered that the best way to reduce the number of patients with resistance is to select the right patients for treatment, namely those with active liver disease who usually have relatively moderate levels of viral replication and who have a good chance of responding well to therapy and a low risk of developing resistance. For patients with mild disease, the treatment can be delayed with regular follow-up.

Peginterferon monotherapy should be considered in patients without contraindications since this treatment is not associated with resistance and gives the best sustained response rate (HBeAg seroconversion in about one-third) with a definite duration (48 weeks) of therapy. In those patients with HBe seroconversion, the rate of HBsAg loss/seroconversion is high. However, most (about two-thirds) patients with chronic hepatitis B do not develop a sustained response and therefore need prolonged therapy with an analogue.

Conclusion

In the last few years, marked progress has been made in the treatment of chronic hepatitis B. Results after 1 year of treatment with current therapies in HBeAg-positive chronic hepatitis B are presented in Figure 49.3. The efficacy of lamivudine, the first nucleoside analogue, is limited by the high incidence of resistance. Adefovir has better long-term efficacy because of a much lower frequency of resistance. Entecavir and tenofovir have potent antiviral effects, a good safety profile and a low rate of short-term resistance. Telbivudine also has potent antiviral effects, although its long-term efficacy might be hampered by its resistance profile. However, these drugs need to be administered

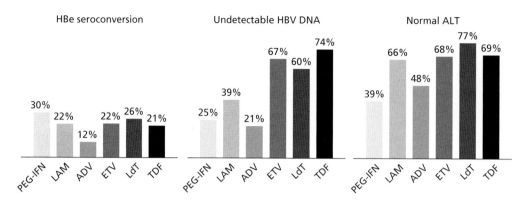

FIG. 49.3 Results after one year of treatment with current therapies.

indefinitely since withdrawal of therapy is generally associated with reactivation and sustained response is uncommon except in HBeAg-positive patients who develop HBeAg seroconversion.

Large randomized controlled trials have demonstrated the efficacy of peginterferon in the treatment of chronic hepatitis B. Peginterferon administered for 48 weeks gives an overall rate of HBe seroconversion of approximately one-third. This sustained response rate is not increased by using the combination of peginterferon and lamivudine. However, it is worth mentioning that combination therapy induced a more rapid and more marked antiviral effect than peginterferon or lamivudine alone. This is the only combination that shows a superior antiviral effect compared with monotherapy. In addition, interestingly, the combination of peginterferon and lamivudine is associated with a much lower resistance rate than lamivudine alone. Therefore, the efficacy of combinations of peginterferon and more potent analogues (such as entecavir or tenofovir) and/or different schedules (e.g. sequential and/or longer duration) need to be evaluated. Quantification of HBsAg has been demonstrated to be a useful marker for predicting sustained virological response and HBs loss in patients with HBeAg-negative chronic hepatitis B treated with peginterferon [23]. The role of this marker in the management of HBeAg-positive patients needs to be evaluated.

The ultimate objective of therapy of chronic hepatitis B is HBsAg loss (with or without HBsAg seroconversion) since this is associated with sustained remission of the disease and improvement in outcome. Therefore future studies should aim to increase the rate of HBsAg loss. HBsAg loss rates obtained with current treatment are around 3–8%,

6 months to 3 years after peginterferon therapy [7–9,24]. The increasing rate of HBsAg loss with time (8% at 3 years, 42% among patients with undetectable HBV DNA) observed in HBe-negative patients needs to be assessed in HBeAg-positive patients [24].

The future of chronic hepatitis B therapy seems to be the combination of different drugs. Ideally, the optimal drugs to combine would meet the following criteria: they should have different sites of action on HBV DNA replication, a potent antiviral effect, an excellent safety profile and should induce a sustained response with HBsAg loss with a limited duration of therapy. Taking into account the drugs available, the combination of peginterferon and entecavir or tenofovir needs to be further investigated. More effective therapy is a major challenge in attempts to decrease the future global burden related to chronic hepatitis B.

References

1. European Association for the Study of the Liver. EASL Clinical Practice Guidelines: management of chronic hepatitis B. *Journal of Hepatology* 2009;50:227–242.
2. Marcellin P, Asselah T, Boyer N. Treatment of chronic hepatitis B. *Journal of Viral Hepatitis* 2005;12:333–345.
3. Hoofnagle JH, Doo E, Liang TJ, Fleischer R, Lok AS. Management of hepatitis B: summary of a clinical research workshop. *Hepatology* 2007;45:1056–1075.
4. Lai CL, Chien RN, Leung NW *et al.* A one-year trial of lamivudine for chronic hepatitis B. Asia Hepatitis Lamivudine Study Group. *New England Journal of Medicine* 1998;339:61–68.
5. Dienstag JL, Perrillo RP, Schiff ER *et al.* A preliminary trial of lamivudine for chronic hepatitis B infection. *New England Journal of Medicine* 1995;333:1657–1661.

6. Wong DKH, Cheung AM, O'Rourke K *et al*. Effect of alpha-interferon treatment in patients with hepatitis B e antigen-positive chronic hepatitis B. *Annals of Internal Medicine* 1993;119:312–323.

7. Marcellin P, Lau GK, Bonino F *et al*. Peginterferon alfa-2a alone, lamivudine alone, and the two in combination in patients with HBeAg-negative chronic hepatitis B. *New England Journal of Medicine* 2004;351:1206–1217.

8. Lau GK, Piratvisuth T, Luo KX *et al*. Peginterferon alfa-2a, lamivudine, and the combination for HBeAg-positive chronic hepatitis B. *New England Journal of Medicine* 2005;352:2682–2695. **First-rate randomized trial evaluating different interferon based regimens.** 🔑⚕

9. Janssen HL, van Zonneveld M, Senturk H *et al*. Pegylated interferon alfa-2b alone or in combination with lamivudine for HBeAg-positive chronic hepatitis B: a randomised trial. *Lancet* 2005;365:123–129.

10. Hadziyannis SJ, Tassopoulos NC, Heathcote EJ *et al*. Adefovir dipivoxil for the treatment of hepatitis B e antigen-negative chronic hepatitis B. *New England Journal of Medicine* 2003;348:800–807.

11. Marcellin P, Chang T, Lim SG *et al*. Adefovir dipivoxil for the treatment of hepatitis B e antigen positive chronic hepatitis B. *New England Journal of Medicine* 2003;348:808–816.

12. Marcellin P, Chang TT, Lim SG *et al*. Long-term efficacy and safety of adefovir dipivoxil for the treatment of hepatitis B e antigen-positive chronic hepatitis B. *Hepatology* 2008;48:750–758.

13. Hadziyannis SJ, Tassopoulos NC, Heathcote EJ *et al*. Longterm therapy with adefovir dipivoxil for HBeAg-negative chronic hepatitis B for up to 5 years. *Gastroenterology* 2006;131:1743–1751.

14. Lai CL, Shouval D, Lok AS *et al*. Entecavir versus lamivudine for patients with HBeAg negative chronic hepatitis B. *New England Journal of Medicine* 2006;354:1011–1020.

15. Chang TT, Gish RG, de Man R *et al*. A comparison of entecavir and lamivudine for HBeAg-positive chronic hepatitis B. *New England Journal of Medicine* 2006;354:1001–1010.

16. Leung N, Peng CY, Hann HW *et al*. Early hepatitis B virus DNA reduction in hepatitis B e antigen-positive patients with chronic hepatitis B: a randomized international study of entecavir versus adefovir. *Hepatology* 2009;49:72–79.

17. Tenney DJ, Rose RE, Baldick CJ *et al*. Long-term monitoring shows hepatitis B virus resistance to entecavir in nucleoside-naive patients is rare through 5 years of therapy. *Hepatology* 2009;49:1503–1514.

18. Lai CL, Gane E, Liaw YF *et al*. Telbivudine versus lamivudine in patients with chronic hepatitis B. *New England Journal of Medicine* 2007;357:2576–2588.

19. Liaw YF, Gane E, Leung N *et al*. 2-Year GLOBE trial results: telbivudine is superior to lamivudine in patients with chronic hepatitis B. *Gastroenterology* 2009;136:486–495.

20. Marcellin P, Heathcote EJ, Buti M *et al*. Tenofovir disoproxil fumarate versus adefovir dipivoxil for chronic hepatitis B. *New England Journal of Medicine* 2008;359:2442–2455.

21. Moucari R, Korevaar A, Lada O *et al*. High rates of HBsAg seroconversion in HBeAg-positive chronic hepatitis B patients responding to interferon: a long-term follow-up study. *Journal of Hepatology* 2009;50:1084–1092. **Long-term follow-up of treated patients demonstrating durability of the response.** 🔑⚕

22. Marcellin P, Lau GK, Zeuzem S *et al*. Comparing the safety, tolerability and quality of life in patients with chronic hepatitis B vs chronic hepatitis C treated with peginterferon alpha-2a. *Liver International* 2008;28:477–485.

23. Moucari R, Mackiewicz V, Lada O *et al*. Early serum HBsAg drop: a strong predictor of sustained virological response to PEG-IFN interferon alfa-2a in HBeAg-negative patients. *Hepatology* 2009;49:1151–1157.

24. Marcellin P, Bonino F, Lau GK *et al*. Sustained response of hepatitis B e antigen-negative patients 3 years after treatment with peginterferon alpha-2a. Peginterferon alfa-2a in HBeAg-negative Chronic Hepatitis B Study Group. *Gastroenterology* 2009;136:2169–2179.e1–4.

50 Most patients with hepatitis C will die from their disease

Graham R. Foster[1], Steven Masson[2]

[1]Queen Mary's University of London, Blizard Institute of Cell and Molecular Science, London, UK
[2]The Royal London Hospital, London, UK

> ## LEARNING POINTS
>
> - The long-term consequences of chronic infection with HCV are unclear.
>
> - Studies over 20–30 years indicate that the majority of patients will not develop significant liver fibrosis.
>
> - Some small-scale selected studies over long periods of time suggest that there may be increasing mortality from hepatitis C with increasing duration of infection. As prospective studies show an increase in the rate of fibrosis with increasing age, many hepatologists believe that in the long term mortality from chronic hepatitis C will increase substantially.

Introduction

Chronic infection with hepatitis C virus (HCV) causes a slowly progressive disease that leads to cirrhosis in a proportion of those who are infected [1]. Once cirrhosis has developed, life-threatening complications (decompensation and/or liver cancer) occur at a rate of 3–6% per year [2]. Although these complications can be treated in a small proportion of patients by liver transplantation, this option is only available to those living in affluent countries with well-developed healthcare systems. Sadly, the majority of patients with chronic HCV infection live in the developing world where access to transplantation is severely limited. Given that the majority of patients with HCV-induced cirrhosis will eventually die from their infection, the debate on the long-term mortality from chronic HCV centres on the proportion of patients who will develop cirrhosis during their lifetime. In this review we focus on this issue and the uncertainties with the current data.

Current data

The proportion of patients with chronic HCV infection who will eventually develop cirrhosis has been estimated by a large number of studies looking at cohorts who have been infected for up to two decades. All these studies have significant methodological flaws and it is therefore not surprising to find that the proportion of patients with cirrhosis differs greatly in the different studies. Superficially the most accurate studies are those in which cohorts of patients infected at a known date by infusion of contaminated blood or blood products are followed for many years. These studies have the enormous advantage of evaluating patients whose date of onset of infection is well established. Such studies normally show that the rate of progression of HCV is relatively slow, with very few patients developing cirrhosis after 20 years [3]. However, such studies involve either patients who have received extensive blood transfusions (and are therefore likely to die as a consequence of their initial, transfusion-requiring, disease) or healthy youngsters (such as women infused with contaminated anti-D) who are likely to progress slowly as they are young and healthy when infected and receive first-rate healthcare. This latter issue is particularly problematic since those infected by contaminated blood often receive preferential healthcare or financial rewards that allow access to high-quality healthcare that may involve interventions (such as alcohol reduction, early

Clinical Dilemmas in Viral Liver Disease, 1st edition. Edited by Graham R. Foster and K. Rajender Reddy. © 2010 Blackwell Publishing.

treatment of diabetes and early treatment of progressive disease) that reduce the rate of hepatic fibrosis progression. It is therefore not surprising to find that these 'ideal' studies usually show that very few infected patients develop significant liver problems. An alternative approach for assessing disease progression in patients with HCV is to look at cohorts (usually hospital-based cohorts) where the date of infection can be ascertained by a careful history [1]. However, such cohorts clearly involve patients attending hospitals with identified disease and it seems likely that such patients will be a group 'self-selected' for progressive disease as asymptomatic patients with normal liver function tests will be less likely to be identified and followed. Studies comparing the outcome of chronic HCV infection have shown that community-based cohorts show much slower rates of disease progression than hospital-based cohorts [4]. Thus the current studies examining the proportion of patients with HCV-related cirrhosis are all flawed to a greater or lesser degree. Nevertheless, valuable data can be obtained from a meta-analysis of these studies and such an analysis has recently been performed and indicates that approximately 16% of patients develop cirrhosis after 20 years [5]. Since these data incorporate studies that have probably overestimated and underestimated disease progression, it is reasonable to assume that this is a reliable estimate.

Disease progression after 20 years

Studies to date allow a reasonable estimate of the prevalence of cirrhosis in patients with chronic HCV infection who have been infected for around 20 years. The lifetime risk of chronic HCV clearly cannot be determined from such studies: in the developed world infection usually occurs in the second decade of life, when drug use is common, and in this context the rate of cirrhosis after 50 years is required to estimate the lifetime risk of cirrhosis. In the developing world it is probable that infection is acquired in early life from contaminated vaccination needles, circumcision and other exposure-prone procedures and in these circumstances the rate of cirrhosis after 70 years needs to be determined to estimate the lifetime risk of HCV-associated mortality. To determine the outcome of chronic HCV infection in the majority of patients it is clearly important to assess the impact over at least five decades and such long-term studies are currently not possible. However, some studies have examined the progression of chronic HCV over time; in one study of patients with histologically proven mild HCV,

a repeat liver biopsy after a short time interval showed an increase in fibrosis in over 30% of patients, suggesting that the progression of chronic HCV is not linear and that the rate of progression of fibrosis increases with time [6]. Other studies have confirmed the view that the rate of fibrosis progression increases with advancing age and these data have led many to conclude that HCV will become more aggressive with advancing age. Given that approaching 20% of patients develop cirrhosis after 20 years and that fibrosis progression will increase with advancing age, it seems reasonable to presume that at least 40% of patients will develop cirrhosis after 40 years of infection. As patients infected in their early twenties with HCV reach their sixth decade, rates of cirrhosis in excess of 50% seem very probable.

Studies in patients infected for many decades

Although the majority of studies looking at the natural history of chronic HCV infection have involved follow-up periods of less than 30 years, a small number of studies have involved patients infected for longer periods of time. A Viennese study examined young men who had been infected iatrogenically some 40 years ago and found a high prevalence of death or liver transplantation 30 years after exposure [7]. In East London we have looked at the prevalence of cirrhosis in people from Pakistan who attended hospital for a liver biopsy and found that approaching 70% of patients over the age of 70 had cirrhosis [8]. Both of these studies may involve some degree of patient selection in that both involved patients attending hospitals and it is therefore possible that the proportion of patients with cirrhosis was unnaturally high. However, in Japan, where the epidemic of HCV probably began a little earlier than in the West, there is growing evidence of increasing mortality and morbidity in the elderly. Thus studies in patients with HCV who have been infected for more than 20 years are sparse and current studies have methodological flaws that may lead to an overestimation of disease progression.

Assessment of the current data

There are currently no hard data to determine the lifetime risk from chronic HCV in individuals infected in early life. However, given that the disease appears to progress more rapidly with increasing age and that at least 16% of patients have cirrhosis after 20 years, it seems reasonable to suppose that more than 50% of patients will develop cirrhosis after 50 years. This estimate of the probability of cirrhosis after 50 years of infection is somewhat less than estimates from the very few studies that have examined patients infected for many decades but, given the concerns that these studies have overestimated the probability of cirrhosis, an estimate of 50% of patients with cirrhosis after 50 years seems reasonable and, arguably, conservative. Since around 5% of patients with cirrhosis will develop life-threatening complications each year, it is likely that at least half of the patients with chronic HCV will develop a significant complication that will lead to their premature demise. In the developed world, one would estimate that the majority of patients will develop complications in their sixth or seventh decade; in the developing world, where infection occurs at a younger age, it seems reasonable to assume that death will occur in the majority of patients in their fifth decade. Given these assumptions the argument that most patients with hepatitis C will die from their infection seems sadly reasonable and accurate.

The assumptions throughout this discussion have focused on the outcome of untreated HCV infection. The growing availability of increasingly effective therapies leads to the realistic hope that most patients with chronic HCV can be cured over the next few decades. However, at present the expensive therapies required to treat patients with HCV are only available in the developed world and therefore it seems likely that the major mortality from HCV will be noted in the developing world. Sadly, the developing world is the reservoir for most of the world's chronic HCV infection and thus it seems probable that over the next few decades most patients with HCV living in the developing world will die from their disease.

References

1. Poynard T, Bedossa P, Opolon P. Natural history of liver fibrosis progression in patients with chronic hepatitis C. *Lancet* 1997;349:825–832. **Major study of fibrosis progression in a large cohort of patients.** ⚷

2. Fattovich G, Giustina G, Degos F *et al.* Morbidity and mortality in compensated cirrhosis type C: a retrospective follow-up study of 384 patients. *Gastroenterology* 1997;112: 463–472.

3. Kenny-Walsh E. Clinical outcomes after hepatitis C infection from contaminated anti-D immune globulin. Irish Hepatology Research Group. *New England Journal of Medicine* 1999;340:1228–1233.

4. Sweeting MJ, De Angelis D, Neal KR *et al.* Estimated progression rates in three United Kingdom hepatitis C cohorts differed according to method of recruitment. *Journal of Clinical Epidemiology* 2006;59:144–152.

5. Thein HH, Yi Q, Dore GJ, Krahn MD. Estimation of stage-specific fibrosis progression rates in chronic hepatitis C virus infection: a meta-analysis and meta-regression. *Hepatology* 2008;48:418–431. **Important meta-analysis of fibrosis progression studies.** ⚷

6. Ryder SD, Irving WL, Jones DA, Neal KR, Underwood JC. Progression of hepatic fibrosis in patients with hepatitis C: a prospective repeat liver biopsy study. *Gut* 2004;53:451–455.

7. Ferenci P, Ferenci S, Datz C, Rezman I, Oberaigner W, Strauss R. Morbidity and mortality in paid Austrian plasma donors infected with hepatitis C at plasma donation in the 1970s. *Journal of Hepatology* 2007;47:31–36.

8. D'Souza R, Glynn MJ, Ushiro-Lumb I *et al.* Prevalence of hepatitis C-related cirrhosis in elderly Asian patients infected in childhood. *Clinical Gastroenterology and Hepatology* 2005;3: 910–917.

51 Most patients with hepatitis C will die with their disease

Ronald L. Koretz

David Geffen-UCLA School of Medicine, Los Angeles; and Division of Gastroenterology, Olive View-UCLA Medical Center, Sylmar, California, USA

LEARNING POINTS

- In order to avoid selection bias, the natural history of hepatitis C is best established by following entire cohorts of patients who are identified at the time of disease onset.

- Natural history studies of cohorts of patients identified at the time of infection with HCV have found that the vast majority (at least 80–90%) will never develop end-stage liver disease and/or hepatocellular carcinoma.

- Considerations of epidemiological data of hepatitis C prevalence and the annual incidence of hepatitis C-related deaths also demonstrate that most HCV-infected patients will never develop symptoms of decompensated cirrhosis or hepatocellular carcinoma.

Abraham Lincoln reportedly said 'We cannot escape history'. With regard to chronic hepatitis C virus (HCV) infection, this sage observation is an important piece of advice. Patients with HCV infections have two fundamental concerns, namely how likely are they to develop problems with end-stage liver disease (from cirrhosis) and, if they are going to develop any, what can be done to reduce the likelihood of that happening. In order to frame any treatment decision about hepatitis C, it is necessary to understand what would happen if we did not treat (in other words, appreciate its natural history). The following discussion develops a perspective about the untreated outcome in chronic hepatitis C.

Clinical Dilemmas in Viral Liver Disease, 1st edition. Edited by Graham R. Foster and K. Rajender Reddy. © 2010 Blackwell Publishing.

The large majority of individuals infected with HCV fail to clear the virus and become chronically infected [1]. Once the chronic viral infection is established, only a few individuals spontaneously clear it. However, from a patient's perspective, the issue is not the presence of abnormal biochemical, histological or serological findings but rather the presence of symptoms. This is not an unimportant consideration. If the only long-term consequence for a patient is that tests (signs) remain abnormal but he or she remains free of liver symptoms and ultimately dies of some unrelated cause, is there any reason to worry?

With regard to symptoms of 'hepatitis', almost all individuals with chronic viral hepatitis have none or, at worst, only some mild fatigue that does not interfere very much with their daily activities [2]. Occasionally, individuals do complain of substantial fatigue. Of course, fatigue is common in uninfected patients as well, so not every infected patient who complains of fatigue will have that symptom because of the HCV infection. The threat that chronic hepatitis C presents to infected patients is the development of decompensated cirrhosis and/or hepatocellular carcinoma. Thus, the issue of interest is how often patients with chronic hepatitis C actually progress to end-stage liver disease. There are data available in this regard.

Published 'natural history' studies from tertiary liver centres have suggested that it takes, on average, about 20 years to develop cirrhosis and 30 years to develop hepatocellular carcinoma in patients infected with HCV [3,4]. While the observation is technically true, it is limited to the subgroup of patients who (i) were referred to that centre and (ii) developed cirrhosis or cancer. It is incorrect to assume from this observation that *all* patients who are infected with HCV will progress to these end-points in two or three decades. In fact, in order to calculate the probability that end-stage liver disease will occur, one needs to look at the outcomes in complete cohorts of people identified at the time of infection.

Let us consider the problem of selection bias. Virtually every patient with hepatitis C at a liver transplant centre has developed end-stage liver disease. On the other hand, none of the infected patients identified at the time of donation at a blood bank are having any problems. These observations show that somewhere between 0 and 100% of infected patients will have hepatic morbidity and mortality. This is an intuitively obvious, but unhelpful, conclusion. (It should be appreciated that while hepatitis C is the leading cause of liver transplantation, this is a consequence of the high prevalence of the infection in the population; even if only a small percentage develop end-stage liver disease, the absolute number is large.)

Several studies have followed entire cohorts of patients who were identified shortly after infection. A 'recall' study was done for patients who had been identified as having developed non-A, non-B (almost all due to HCV) post-transfusion hepatitis in the 1970s [5]. For each such patient, a control patient was identified who had been transfused but had not developed this disease. Over the 20-year follow-up, those who had hepatitis had overall survival curves that were superimposable on those who did not have hepatitis, although there were more hepatic deaths in the hepatitis group. When these data were updated after 25 years of follow-up [6], the all-cause mortality continued to be comparable in both groups (69%). The liver-disease related mortality was slightly higher in the group that developed hepatitis than in the one that did not (4% vs. 1.7%; $P < 0.01$).

Between 1972 and 1980, our group at UCLA identified 90 individuals with non-A, non-B (again, mostly HCV) post-transfusion hepatitis; 26 of them were in the above noted study. Employing life-table analysis, we calculated the probabilities of developing liver failure over time, assuming that no patient would die of any other cause in the interim, and of dying of some non-hepatic cause [7]. Over the first 15–20 years after becoming infected, the probability of having clinical evidence of liver failure was 15–20%. On the other hand, the probability of dying of something else during that same time was about 50%. A subsequent analysis, looking at the first 20–25 years, found that the risk of end-stage liver disease over that more extended period of time continued to be less than 20% [8], as no further episodes of liver failure had occurred. (By absolute numbers, only 8 of 90, or 9%, patients have developed liver failure.) In fact, to

date (30–35 years after the transfusions), we are not aware of any further instances of liver failure in this cohort (R. Koretz, unpublished data).

In the late 1970s, large numbers of young women in Ireland and Germany were treated with an HCV-contaminated immunoglobulin (used for prophylaxis against Rh incompatibility). Twenty years later, clinical evidence of end-stage liver disease was present in less than 1% [9–11]. Similar experiences were described for 67 children infected by contaminated blood within the first few years of their lives [12] and 31 others who were transfused and infected at birth [13]. The durations of follow-up were almost 20 [12] and 35 [13] years. At that time, no subject had any overt end-stage liver disease and only a few even had histological evidence of progressive liver disease.

In the 1990s, a large bank of frozen sera was uncovered. The specimens came from military recruits who were participating in an epidemiological study of a streptococcal outbreak between 1948 and 1954. Seventeen of these sera were found to be positive for antibody to HCV [14]. The fates of these men were sought 45–50 years later and only two (13%) of them had developed clinical evidence of liver failure.

The question of the rate of progression to end-stage liver disease can be addressed with latent phase calculations. A latent phase represents the time between the initial appearance of a disease (in this case, the initial infection) and the subsequent development of a recognizable clinical end-point. According to classical epidemiological principles, the average latent phase is the prevalence of the disease (the number of HCV carriers in the population) divided by the incidence of the end-point (in this case, the annual number of deaths due to chronic hepatitis C). There are at least 3 million hepatitis C carriers in the USA [1,15]. There were slightly fewer than 7500 deaths attributable to hepatitis C in 2004 (and the numbers were actually slightly lower than in 2002 and 2003) [16]. Thus, on average, it would take approximately 400 years for hepatitis C to progress to liver death. Since the symptomatic manifestations preceding the death only arise a few years earlier, we have corroboration of the fact that the large majority of infected patients (at least 80–90%) will not be troubled during their lifetimes.

Latent phase calculations do assume that the population is in a steady state. However, because most of these carriers were infected in the 1960s, more end-stage liver disease may emerge in future years (assuming that the patients do not die of some coexistent morbidity first). Furthermore, some patients receive liver transplants and, while their livers 'die', they do not (and are not included in the annual mortality data). However, if the annual mortality rate (the denominator) is doubled, tripled or even quadrupled, the average latent phase would still be 100–200 years.

Some of the hepatitis C deaths may actually be due to concomitant factors such as alcohol or non-alcoholic steatohepatitis. If this is the case, the number of deaths used in the denominator (deaths attributed to hepatitis C) would be smaller (and the latent phase of hepatitis C not associated with these other treatable conditions would be longer).

Given the data from the cohort studies and the epidemiological observations, it must be that the large majority of patients will never develop liver failure, even in the absence of any treatment. Individuals with chronic HCV infections may not clear the virus and thus will die with HCV in their bloodstreams. However, at least 80–90% of them will not die of any HCV-associated liver disease.

References

1. National Institutes of Health. NIH consensus statement on management of hepatitis C: 2002. *NIH Consensus and State-of-the-Science Statements* 2002;19(3):1–46.

2. Di Bisceglie AM, Goodman ZD, Ishak KG, Hoofnagle JH, Melpolder JJ, Alter HJ. Long-term clinical and histopathological follow-up of chronic post-transfusion hepatitis. *Hepatology* 1991;14:969–974.

3. Tong MJ, El-Farra NS, Reikes AR, Co RL. Clinical outcomes after transfusion-associated hepatitis C. *New England Journal of Medicine* 1995;332:1463–1466.

4. Kiyosawa K, Sodeyama T, Tanaka E *et al.* Interrelationship of blood transfusion, non-A, non-B hepatitis and hepatocellular carcinoma: analysis by detection of antibody to hepatitis C. *Hepatology* 1990;12:671–675.

5. Seeff LB, Buskell-Bales Z, Wright EC *et al.* Long-term mortality after transfusion-associated non-A, non-B hepatitis. *New England Journal of Medicine* 1993;327:1906–1911.

6. Seeff LB, Hollinger FB, Alter HJ *et al.* Long-term mortality and morbidity of transfusion-associated non-A, non-B and type C hepatitis: a National Heart, Lung, and Blood Institute Collaborative Study. *Hepatology* 2001;33:455–463. **This is the largest prospective cohort study of post-transfusion hepatitis C and found that less than 5% of the originally infected patients had developed liver failure 25 years later.** 🔑📖

7. Koretz RL, Coleman E, Abbey H, Gitnick G. Non-A, non-B post-transfusion hepatitis. *Annals of Internal Medicine* 1993;119:110–115.

8. Koretz RL, Abbey H, Gitnick G. Non-A, non-B posttransfusion hepatitis at the quarter century. *Hepatology* 1998;28:673A.

9. Kenny-Walsh E for the Irish Hepatology Research Group. Clinical outcomes after hepatitis C infection from contaminated anti-D immune globulin. *New England Journal of Medicine* 1999;340:1228–1233.

10. Barrett S, Goh J, Coughlan B *et al.* The natural course of hepatitis C virus infection after 22 years in a unique homogenous cohort: spontaneous viral clearance and chronic HCV infection. *Gut* 2001;49:423–430.

11. Wiese M, Berr F, Lafrenz M, Porst H, Oesen U. Low frequency of cirrhosis in a hepatitis C (genotype 1b) single-source outbreak in Germany: a 20-year multicenter study. *Hepatology* 2000;32:91–96.

12. Vogt M, Lang T, Frosner G *et al.* Prevalence and clinical outcome of hepatitis C infection in children who underwent cardiac surgery before the implementation of blood-donor screening. *New England Journal of Medicine* 1999;341(22):866–70.

13. Casiraghi MA, de Paschale M, Romano L *et al.* Long-term outcome (35 years) of hepatitis C after acquisition of infection through mini transfusions of blood given at birth. *Hepatology* 2004 Jan;39(1):90–6.

14. Seeff LB, Miller RN, Rabkin CS *et al.* 45-year follow-up of hepatitis C virus infection in healthy young adults. *Ann of Intern Med* 2000 Jan 18;132(2):105–11. **This is the cohort study with the longest follow-up, namely four to five decades and, while the numbers are small, only 13% (2 of 17) developed manifestations of end-stage liver disease.** 🔑📖

15. Edlin BR. Five million Americans infected with the hepatitis C virus: a corrected estimate. *Hepatology* 2005 Nov;42(5 Pt 2):213A.

16. Wise M, Bialek S, Finelli L, Bell BP, Sorvillo F. Changing trends in hepatitis C-related mortality in the United States, 1995–2004. *Hepatology* 2008 Apr;47(4):1128–35.

Index